AGE-PROOF YOUR BODY

Your Complete Guide to Lifelong Vitality

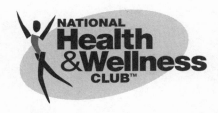

Health & Wellness Reference Library™

ALSO BY ELIZABETH SOMER

AGE-PROOF YOUR BODY

Your Complete Guide to Lifelong Vitality

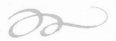

ELIZABETH SOMER, M.A., R.D.

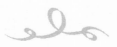

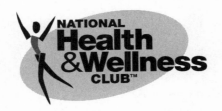

Health & Wellness Reference Library™

BOOK DESIGN by *Susan Hood*

COVER DESIGN

Tom Carpenter
Director of Book Development

Jenya Prosmitsky
Cover Designer

Gina Germ
Photo Editor

Heather Koshiol
Book Development Coordinator

PHOTOGRAPHY CREDITS
Front Cover: Stone/Lori Adamski Peek; ©Melanie Carr/Image State; Stone/Les Weis; ©Bob Daeminrich; Stone/Charles Thatcher; ©Frank Siteman/Stock Boston. Back Cover: Stone/Ian O'Leary; ©Melanie Carr/Image State; CCOA Archive; ©Tim Mantoani/Image State.

The Library of Congress has cataloged a previous edition of this title.

National Health & Wellness Club
12301 Whitewater Drive
Minnetonka, MN 55343
www.healthandwellnessclub.com

To my papa, Rolly Somer

One of the most soul-stirring blessings of my life has been to grow up in the current of my father's passion for life. I may no longer have his hand to hold, but his vitality shines more brightly now than ever before, illuminating every day of my life and helping to guide my children as they grow into their versions of vitality.

Foreword

The best cooks use the finest ingredients in their recipes; they wouldn't dream of using wilted lettuce in their salads or rancid oil in their dressings. Each one of us is like a chef, blending the ingredients from our daily habits, which contribute to or detract from our recipes for healthy, long lives. We don't often think of our lives as we age as being a result of the ingredients we put into them, but what we eat, how we move, and the way we think contribute importantly to how and when we grow old and to what degree we enjoy living in the meantime.

We live in an age of medical miracles where bone marrow transplants and coronary bypass surgery have become routine procedures. These technological breakthroughs of modern medicine still reflect the old paradigm of "rescue and repair," which emphasizes treating rather than preventing disease. Abundant evidence now indicates that a health-care approach—with a goal of promoting health and preventing illness—costs less than the disease-care approach with its expensive diagnostic and therapeutic interventions. More importantly, focusing on prevention will help us achieve the ultimate goals—a high-quality life and sustained good health. The best news is that the individual has considerable control in making those goals happen. We can improve our diets. We can become more active—both physically and mentally. We can choose to stop the insult from cigarette smoke and more.

Most people are willing and eager to make changes that will improve their chances of living well; however, there is a bewildering, and often contradictory, array of information available to the general public on ways to achieve optimal health and reduce the risk for age-related declines in health and function. Some of that information is accurate, but much of it is not. Some popular information is even harmful.

Elizabeth Somer has worked to summarize much of the vast and still-growing scientific literature about ways to age-proof our bodies, from basic advice to eat more vegetables and exercise more to the latest research on supplements, hormones, and phytochemicals. Employing her esteemed professional judgment and drawing on the help of many experts, she has separated the facts from the hype and provided the essential "take-home" messages about what really works, what doesn't, why, and at what cost.

She recognizes that as we age, health is more than the absence of disease: What we ultimately want is to live vital and passionate lives filled with purpose, joy, and fulfillment. The skills, tools, and guidelines for transforming our lives to achieve and maintain health and vitality for a lifetime are in this book. Elizabeth Somer makes it easy to understand that when you age-proof your body, you begin to engage in an ongoing, dynamic process that brings rewards far greater than just longevity. She even shows you how to make it fun!

Here is a fact-based, comprehensive, easy-to-read book on how to empower yourself to die young—as late as possible.

—JEFFREY BLUMBERG, Ph.D., F.A.C.N.
USDA Human Nutrition Research Center on Aging
Tufts University

Acknowledgments

Many friends and colleagues donated their valuable time and thoughts to this book. A special thank you to Nancy Clark, Gayle Cromwell, Lovey DelSarto, Victoria Dolby, Norm Eburne, Sandra Gleason, Janet Haley, Betsy Horton, Ralph LaForge, Bill McAuliffe, Barbara Mullard, David Ralstin, Brooke Richert, Melinda Riley, Jill Saletta, Daryl Seidentop, Mary Starrett, Joy Taylor, Jeanette Williams, Christina Young, my agent, David Smith, Miriam at the library, and especially my family—Patrick, Lauren, and William.

I also want to thank the researchers who have pioneered the theories and ideas on vitality and aging, and who were so gracious in explaining these concepts and their research with me, including George Armelagos, Ph.D., Holly Atkinson, M.D., Jeffrey B. Blumberg, Ph.D., F.A.C.N., Robert N. Butler, M.D., C. Wayne Callaway, M.D., Larry Christensen, Ph.D., Leonard Cohen, Ph.D., William Connor, M.D., Douglas Darr, Ph.D., Sharon Edelstein, Sc.M., Bess Dawson-Hughes, M.D., Johanna Dwyer, D.Sc., R.D., Mary Enig, Ph.D., Helen Gensler, Ph.D., Michael Green, Ph.D., Robert Heaney, M.D., David Jenkins, M.D., Robin Kanarek, Ph.D., Darshan Kelley, Ph.D., Susan Krebs-Smith, Ph.D., R.D., Sarah Leibowitz, Ph.D., David Levitsky, Ph.D., Paul Mills, Ph.D., Byron Murray, Ph.D., Daniel Nixon, M.D., Ed Pierce, Ph.D., Herbert Pierson, Ph.D., Judy Putnam, Ph.D., William Pryor, Ph.D., George Roth, M.D., Robert Russell, M.D., Robert Sack, Ph.D., Adria Sherman, Ph.D., Varro Tyler, Ph.D., Sc.D., Thomas Wadden, Ph.D., Walter Willett, M.D., Ph.D., Margo Woods, D.Sc, Margo Wootan, D.Sc, and Gary Zammit, Ph.D.

Contents

Before You Begin This Book

When I was twenty-one
I had just begun.
When I was forty-two
I was nearly new.
When I was fifty-three
I was hardly me.
When I was sixty-four
I was not much more.
When I was seventy-five
I was just alive.
But now I have eighty-six, I'm as clever as clever.
So I think I'll be eighty-six for ever and ever.

> adapted from *The End*
> by A. A. Milne

Most of us are eager to push back the hands of time. In fact, three out of every five of us want to live to be 100, according to a survey by the Alliance for Aging Research; 67 percent of those polled believe it's within their control, and nine out of every 10 people say they'd adopt a more positive outlook on life, eat more nutritious foods, and exercise regularly to reach this goal.

Their hopes are not far off the mark. The evidence shows that up to 70 percent of cancers result from lifestyle, including what we eat and how we live. More than half of all heart disease cases are preventable and osteoporosis, a disease of thinning bones, is almost entirely preventable with a change in lifestyle. The list of avoidable age-related diseases is seemingly endless. That's particularly good news, since most of us are more concerned with illness, disability, and loss of independence in our later years than we are with dying. Few people want a longer life if it means years spent in a nursing home or lost to Alzheimer's disease.

But the powerful benefits of a few simple changes in lifestyle go beyond just being a healthy grandparent. New research from respected institutions, such as the National Institute on Aging and Tufts University in Boston, show that we easily can stretch our life expectancies from the current 76 years to as much as 100 years by making some simple changes in what we eat and how we move. We might even push beyond life's ultimate finish line of 120 years by making additional dietary changes. The sooner you take the longevity plunge the better; however, it's never too late to jump on the anti-aging bandwagon and reap the benefits of all that good food and activity have to offer.

Improving on a Good Thing

"EFFORT IS THE MEASURE OF A MAN."

William James

Improving the odds of living as long and fully as you can imagine is not as monumental a task as you might think. Most of us have at least some joy, laughter, and playfulness in our daily routines. We are fortunate to have at least a few, if not many, nurturing relationships. We even do a bit of exercise every day, even if it's only walking from the parking lot to the grocery store.

All that most people need to do is improve on a good thing. That's what this book is all about. *Age-Proof Your Body* provides a wealth of suggestions on how to tweak a pretty healthy life into a very healthy one to boost your chances for living longer, happier, and better.

What Can You Expect from This Book?

"BEGIN AT ONCE TO LIVE."

Seneca

Perhaps you picked up this book because you're noticing the beginnings of aging, such as a stiff joint here or a gray hair there. Or maybe you like the hand you've been dealt and don't want to lose your edge as you age. Whatever the longevity recipe you've been handed by inheritance or have chosen, you can make use of those ingredients to the fullest, starting today.

In this book you'll gain the tools to begin a quest for well-being and passion that will last a lifetime. If you follow the simple guidelines outlined in *Age-Proof Your Body,* you can expect to:

- decrease your risk for numerous diseases
- improve your immunity and resistance to colds, infections, and disease
- reduce your body fat
- increase both muscle strength and flexibility
- improve your chances of living a long life without having to rely on others or a nursing home for your daily care
- experience enhanced sexuality in the second 50 years
- have a more youthful appearance
- enjoy life more
- have more energy for what you want to do and waste less energy on needless worries, tensions, and negative thoughts
- heal more quickly and recover faster from illnesses
- increase your aerobic capacity (i.e., endurance)
- feel more fully alive

Not bad for starters! And, it's only the beginning.

Living Vitally

"LET EACH OF YOU DISCOVER WHERE YOUR CHANCE FOR GREATNESS LIES.
SEIZE THAT CHANCE, AND LET NO POWER ON EARTH DETER YOU."
from the movie Chariots of Fire

I reviewed literally thousands of scientific studies while researching this book. All of the anti-aging guidelines in this book reflect this thorough review of the literature. While more pieces of the anti-aging puzzle will continue to unfold, we already have in our grasp reliable, sound, and necessary habits that will slow aging and prevent age-related diseases.

But the goals of this book extend far beyond just living longer, or even living more healthfully. My wish is that all who read this book will incorporate into their vision of their future selves the quality of vitality. I hope that you will strive every day not only to live well, but to live passionately—to incorporate into your daily routine some small glimmer of your higher self, so that by the time you reach your one hundredth birthday, vitality and the joy of life will have settled on you like an elegant cloak. The focus of this book is to provide the tools to fashion a life that will let you live both long and joyfully. Your vitality quest starts today, and everything you need for the journey is in the following pages.

—ELIZABETH SOMER, M.A., R.D.

RECLAIMING YOUR VITALITY

Chapter 1

WHAT IS THIS THING CALLED AGING?

"I always wanted to be somebody, but I should have been more specific."

Lily Tomlin

What does it mean to age? Technically speaking, Dr. Denham Harman from the University of Nebraska College of Medicine defines biological aging as ". . . the accumulation of changes in the cells and tissues that increase the risk of death." If this is the only "biomarker" of aging, then from birth on and escalating after age 30, we all are in the process of dying.

Luckily, that's not the case. When each component of aging is analyzed, from loss of cell function to the onset of most degenerative diseases from heart disease to cancer, repeatedly we find that it is not age but years of abuse that wear down the body's ability to regenerate itself. Stop the abuse and encourage the repair processes, and all physiological functions should retain much of their youthful vitality.

Even the superficial signs of the passage of time—from wrinkles and stooped posture to a feeble or frail appearance—can vanish when a person's approach to life is vital and enthusiastic. An 80-year-old who mountain climbs, takes ballet classes, is working on her college degree, or tackles life with a passion not seen in most 20-year-olds is hardly "old" by anyone's standards, and she radiates the beauty unique to healthy, happy people.

Researchers are finding that the oldest old are much healthier than traditional views of aging would predict. Often they are more vital than people 20 years younger. When the oldest old in the world are compared, from the Okinawans to the Hunzas living in the Himalayas (both peoples typically live past 100 years), they all exhibit the same qualities. They have *stretched their middle years*, not prolonged their old years, and they are remarkably healthy and robust. Even in the general population, people with healthful lifestyles live longer and are more likely to live disease-free compared to their unhealthy neighbors.

The message is loud and clear. Aging has much more to do with how you live and who you are than with chronology. Having a clear mental picture of who you want to be when you're 100 years old can help shape your life each day to reach that goal.

What Are Your Vitality and Longevity Goals?

In your journal or on a piece of paper, answer the following questions:

1. What does aging mean to you?
2. What is your image of the perfect older person?
3. What aspects of aging do you want to avoid?
4. What aspects of aging do you want to nurture and encourage?
5. Reflect on your subtle beliefs about aging. Do you assume people's minds deteriorate with age? Do you expect people to become more debilitated or more serene as they age? Do you expect to become weakened or empowered in later years? What negative and positive images do you have of aging, and where did they come from? What body shape do you assume old people should have? Make a list of your assumptions on the left-hand side of the page, and then argue against these assumptions in the right-hand column.
6. List your most precious memories and then review your list. What has given your life the most meaning up to this point? How can you add more meaning to your life every day to extend your years and boost your enjoyment of life?

How Long Can We Expect to Live?

"No life that breathes with human breath
Has ever truly longed for death."

Lord Tennyson, 1830

We've more than tripled the average life expectancy since the 1700s, from 25 years to 76 years today. But that still is a far cry from what scientists estimate is our maximum lifespan of 120 years.

THE SPAN OF A LIFETIME

1 life =
120 years
480 seasons
1440 months
6240 weeks
43,800 days
1,051,200 hours
63,072,000 minutes
3,784,320,000 seconds

Before we begin our longevity journey, there are a few terms that should be clarified, such as *life span, life expectancy,* and *active life expectancy.* These terms might sound as though they mean the same thing, but they are very different. While the second has changed exponentially in the past century, the third has made only modest improvements, and the first hasn't given an inch in the entire history of humankind.

Life span refers to the maximum number of years any human has ever lived. With everything on your side—from the best longevity genes nature has to offer to a perfect lifestyle and a lot of good luck—the longest a person can hope to live is approximately 120 years. (There are no hard facts to back up isolated reports of extreme longevity.) Anything short of this 120-year mark essentially is premature aging.

With the research accumulating on why we age and the advancements in genetic engineering (see Chapter 2), there is the possibility that future generations will tamper with this cutoff point. But for now, 100 to 120 years is the best you can hope for, and reaching this maximum life span eludes most of us.

WHAT DO YOU EXPECT OUT OF LIFE?

That brings us to the most important issue of longevity: life expectancy. Life expectancy is how long a person can expect to live. It is based on a number of factors, most of which are within our control.

Longevity is a modern luxury. Life expectancy for the human race in general has seen dramatic changes in the past 100 years. The human species survived for hundreds of thousands of years—more than 99 percent of our time on earth—with a life expectancy of only about 18 years. Chinese archeological finds dating back 10,000 years show that most people died young and violently. In one dig, only three of the 173 total skeletons uncovered (or 1 percent of the population) showed signs of having lived more than 50 years. Early Iron Age and Bronze Age cave dwellers had the same maximum life span as modern humans, about 120 years, but life was so violent for most men and childbirth was so risky for women that most would not reach drinking age. Up until the Roman Empire, only 2 to 3 percent of the population survived past the age of 65. Even by the late 1700s, half the population of the world was under the age of 16.

In short, in the old days, the elderly were honored because they were more rare than gold. In those days, most of our current health and aging concerns, from eating well and exercising to routine dental checkups and deciding whether or not to take hormone replacement therapy at menopause, would have been moot.

As recent as the turn of the century, life expectancy was still only 49 years. Since then, more than 25 years have been added to the average person's life expectancy at birth, primarily because of improved diagnosis, treatment, and prevention of infectious disease, along with lifestyle habits that include better diet, more exercise, and improved work conditions.

In this century alone, women have increased their average life expectancy by 71 percent, while men's life expectancy has improved by 66 percent. This steady improvement is expected to continue, although at a slower rate and always with the cutoff point at 120 years.

The good news about life expectancy statistics is that they improve with age. That is, the longer you live, the farther ahead you are of the population average. So, while your life expectancy at birth is 76 years, if you can make it to 45 in good health and are not a smoker, you have a good chance of living to age 80. If you live to 80 in good health, your chances of living even longer increase compared to the average person. Longevity is the one race in life where the farther you get, the longer you've got.

In essence, you have time on your side when it comes to life expectancy . . . *if* you use that time well. The amazing variation in the signs of aging from one person to the next is evidence that the underlying causes of these changes are modifiable. One person wrinkles heavily by age 45; another appears virtually wrinkle-free at 70. One 80-year-old is stooped and shuffles; another walks upright and briskly. Many 75-year-olds are world travelers, taking college classes, playing tennis daily, or starting new careers, while some 50-year-olds complain of stiff joints and low energy.

These vast differences are constant reminders that besides the genes you were given, much of what we consider as "getting older" is a reflection of what we think and how we live. Studies on twins repeatedly show that only about 15 to 20 percent of aging is due to genetics; the other 80 to 85 percent is linked to lifestyle and attitude. The better care you take of yourself today and the more vitality you welcome into your life, the more healthy tomorrows you are likely to have.

ACTIVELY PURSUING LIFE

Which leads us to the most important longevity term: active life expectancy, which is what this book is all about. Active life expectancy is the maximum number of healthy, disease-free years a person can expect to have. This is where a person has the most control, since the majority of chronic and crippling diseases that undermine health in the later years can be avoided with a few changes in what you eat, how you live, what you think and believe, with whom you spend your time, and how much you move. The choice is yours.

What Are the Biomarkers of Age?

"IF A MAN HASN'T DISCOVERED SOMETHING THAT HE WILL DIE FOR, HE ISN'T FIT TO LIVE."

Martin Luther King, Jr.

Wouldn't it be wonderful if there were simple tests you could take at your annual physical that would chart your biological age—that is how fast your body is aging? That way, you could tell if taking the latest anti-aging hormone or making a change in your diet was turning back the clock.

Unfortunately, identifying predictable biomarkers—accurate and specific measurements of how fast the body is aging—is easier said than done. As yet, scientists have not found a measurable sign of aging that arrives predictably during a limited time span and that is inevitable and irreversible. What makes the hunt even harder is that the aging process begins much earlier than is commonly assumed. At the very core of your trillions of cells, aging already has set in by the time you are 20 or 30 years old. It's just that the signs don't show up on the surface for another 30 to 40 years. For example, by the time people are 35 years old, they have attained their maximum bone density. From this point on, they are losing bone. How quickly they lose it depends on what they eat and how they exercise. Muscle mass and strength also start to wane in the thirties, while heart disease is percolating as early as the teen years.

Another confounding factor is that individual uniqueness increases as we age, so two 60-year-olds are biologically and psychologically less akin than two 18-year-olds. Consequently, the older you get, the more difficult it is to determine how old your body really is.

That doesn't mean no one is trying. Researchers at the National Institute of Aging are exploring reliable biomarkers, from loss of short-term memory to changes in pain sensitivity. In the future, we probably will take a series of longevity tests that produce a score. A score of 95 might mean you would live to 110, while a score of 60 might mean you have only until age 72, give or take a few years. A low score at an early age could be the incentive to make changes while there's still time.

One rough estimate of aging can be obtained from monitoring athletes over time. Even a fine-tuned athletic body loses about one-half percent of performance for every year of life after about age 30. If this is a true benchmark for decline, then any greater loss of function is not aging, but an indicator of abuse or disuse. If you maintain optimal function through diet, exercise, attitude, and lifestyle so that you lose only one-half percent of mental or physical function each year after age 30, then by age 65 years you will have lost only 15 percent of your original vigor and you should have a wealth of vitality left by the time you reach 120 years.

On the other hand, a sedentary life with little attention to how you fuel your body through diet and thoughts can speed the aging process to 2 percent or more each year. By the time you reach age 65, you've lost up to 70 percent or more of the vigor you had in your youth. The numbers add up and are all in your favor if you choose to play your cards well.

Do Women Live Longer Than Men?

"HONOR WOMEN! THEY ENTWINE AND WEAVE HEAVENLY ROSES IN OUR EARTHLY LIFE."

Johann von Schiller

Until recently, more women died during childbirth than did men in battle, making the life expectancy for women even worse than men's. It wasn't until the 1600s that rich women could expect to live as long as their husbands (into their twenties). Surviving childbirth for the average woman did not improve until the mid-1800s to early 1900s.

That all changed in the twentieth century. Today, men may sit in the Oval Office, have walked on the moon, and hold the record for running a marathon, but it is women who will live to talk about it. In only a few decades, women not only closed the gap but raced ahead of men in life expectancy.

Worldwide, women are winning the longevity race. Compared to men, Greek women enjoy the Mediterranean sun five years longer, Japanese women have six more years to spoil their grandchildren, U.S. women have seven more years of retirement, and Russian women have 10 more years of smelling the roses and

AVERAGE LIFE EXPECTANCY

Time/Year	Men	Women
1900	48.3 years	51.5 years
1950	66.0	71.7
1990	72.1	79.0

gathering memories. In fact, only the men in Nepal outlive their women, and only by one year.

Modern women also are hardier than men when it comes to surviving disease. For example, 170 boys are conceived for every 100 girls, but girls have closed the gap by adolescence, primarily because more male fetuses are miscarried and those boys who are born are more likely to die from infections, disease, and accidents. In later years, men are up to seven times more likely than women to die from heart attack, stroke, cancer, respiratory diseases, accidents, and AIDS. "Approximately one-third of the difference in life expectancy between men and women is attributed to biological or genetic factors," says Robert N. Butler, M.D., Director of the International Longevity Center at Mt. Sinai Medical Center in New York. According to Dr. Butler, women have stronger immune systems, possibly as nature's way of ensuring that they survive pregnancy and childbearing.

WHY CAN'T A MAN BE MORE LIKE A WOMAN (OR VICE VERSA)?

Women have time on their side for a number of reasons. First, there is the hormone factor. A high ratio of the female hormone estrogen to the male hormone testosterone protects a woman from heart disease and stroke—at least until menopause, when estrogen levels drop and a woman's heart disease risk escalates to that of men's.

Second, the secret might be in the genes. One theory states that the male sex chromosome Y might contain the stumbling block for reduced life span. Some disorders such as muscular dystrophy affect only men and can be traced to that missing segment of DNA that makes a Y chromosome a Y instead of a female X. Dr. Denham Harman at the University of Nebraska College of Medicine in

Omaha speculates that the female X chromosome is protected from damage during the early stages of development in the womb and that this allows girl babies a better chance at long-term survival.

A third possibility is that men's greater muscle mass and increased metabolic rate undermine longevity by speeding cell death, much in the way the remote control on a television fast-forwards a movie. On the other hand, men's battle with longevity could be traced to their feistier, more aggressive and competitive natures, or to the fact that they work in higher-risk jobs. Whether it's in their cells or in their attitude, men in general tend to live faster and harder and die younger than women.

While women live longer than men, they don't always live better. Women, once they get sick, are less likely than men to regain their health, and the extra years are likely to be spent depending on others' care. Women are more likely to struggle with rheumatoid arthritis, depression, osteoporosis, and other "age-related" diseases, while men who live longer than average also live stronger and more independently.

For example, after age 65, 71 percent of men live independently, while only 54 percent of women can boast the same. By the time he reaches 85, a man has about a 50 percent chance of still maintaining his independence; a woman has only a one-in-three chance. The main reasons why older women fare worse than older men are economics and lifestyle. One in every five women over the age of 75 is below the poverty line; lack of resources has as much if not more to do with health status and longevity as gender. Women also start out with less muscle and are less likely than men to maintain what muscle they do have. Consequently, their weakened physical condition leads to disability, frailty, osteoporosis, and other debilitating conditions.

Women don't have to take the decree of frailty as gospel, just as men don't have to take this longevity news lying down! "Up to two-thirds of the difference in longevity between men and women can be traced to choices, such as drinking and smoking, diet, and exercise," says Dr. Butler. By making a few healthy changes, a woman can prepare for a robust and independent life in later years, while a man can significantly shrink the longevity gap.

Most men aren't willing to trade in their testosterone for more estrogen, but they would do well to live (and act?) a little more like a woman. For example, they could eat more like a woman. Women, on average, consume more fruits, vegetables, and whole grains, while men consume more red meat, beer, and liquor. Trading in the 8-ounce steak and alcohol for more dark green leafy vegetables, whole-wheat rolls, and fruit salads would help men lower blood fat levels and manage their weight, which in turn lowers the risk for heart disease, hypertension, and diabetes.

Women also are more apt to attend to routine medical tests that increase the chance of early diagnosis and treatment of disease. In addition, they seek medical attention more readily when things go wrong.

Then there's the communication issue. "While men may have their old boy networks and camaraderie in the locker room, they generally aren't willing to go so far as to admit they have emotional issues, let alone share them with friends," says Dr. Butler. Women are much freer in venting grief, worries, and intimate issues with friends and family.

All of these behaviors are associated with improved health, speedy recovery from illness, and longer life. Something as simple as taking a few moments to relax each day or seeking advice can help protect men from a variety of ills, from depression and alcoholism to arrhythmias and cancer.

In short, women can avoid frailty and men can close the longevity gap by taking charge of their health today. "Adding life to your years requires *physical fitness* that includes a healthful diet, regular exercise, and not smoking; *purposeful fitness*, which means developing a purpose beyond yourself; and *social fitness* by developing a network of friends you can turn to during a crisis," recommends Dr. Butler.

How Diet and Exercise Can Maximize Longevity: Promising New Findings

"IT IS MUCH CHEAPER AND MORE EFFECTIVE TO MAINTAIN GOOD HEALTH THAN IT IS TO REGAIN IT ONCE IT IS LOST."

Kenneth H. Cooper, M.D., M.P.H., chairman and founder of the Cooper Aerobics Center in Dallas

Of all life's gifts, none is as important as health. You can have boundless money, fame, possessions, experiences, and opportunities, but all of these pale without health. With health, almost anything is possible. A fit, healthy body and mind provide the stamina and energy to achieve most goals.

No one can avoid getting older, but there's no reason to look or feel old. Change how you eat, think, exercise, and live and you'll not only add years to your life but can count on those extra years as some of your finest. In fact, the traditional enfeebled and ailing elderly person will someday be a distant and vague memory of an unenlightened era.

However, while more than 70 percent of people believe they can stretch their years, only one in every 10 people meets even minimum standards for a healthful diet or engages in even modest daily activity. It takes determination to live long and vitally, and it requires a daily commitment to take care of yourself.

Remember, the purpose of anti-aging is not to extend life in order to live more years as an "old" person, but to delay the onset of the aging process and lengthen the healthy middle years. That means taking charge of your health today. The sooner you grab onto your health and vitality, the longer you can stretch those healthy middle years and the slower you will glide into old age. The good news is that it is never too late to slow the ticking of the aging clock.

Looking Back to the Future

Developing a lifelong plan for vitality means knowing where you are going. Who do you want to be when you're 100 years young? What do you need to do today to get there?

Grab a pencil and a piece of paper and find a comfortable spot where you won't be disturbed. Imagine that it is your one-hundredth birthday. You are healthy, fit, happy, and full of life. What do you look like? How do you feel? Who surrounds you? Where are you? How do you spend your time?

Now, as a 100-year-old, take a moment to look back over your life. What did you do all those years to help yourself stay healthy, fit, and vital? What did you eat? How did you exercise? With whom did you spend time? What relationships did you nurture, and which ones did you discontinue? What were your hobbies? At what fulfilling jobs did you work? What challenges did you assume?

Are you creating a life *today* that will help you reach your vitality and longevity goals? What are you doing that supports these goals? What will you change?

Chapter 2

HOW DOES AGING HAPPEN?

"Youth, large, lusty, loving—
Youth full of grace, force,
    fascination.
Do you know that Old Age
    may come after you with
    equal grace, force,
    fascination?"

Walt Whitman

W e can't avoid getting old, but we don't have to age. By following the recommendations in this book, you can avoid most of what once were considered inevitable consequences of aging. By taking good care of yourself, you can sidestep some of the "metabolism meltdown" listed below and can expect to look, act, and feel at least 20 years younger. Not bad for a start!

Metabolism Meltdown: What Happens to Our Bodies As They Age?

"NOTHING IS MORE DISHONORABLE THAN AN OLD MAN, HEAVY WITH YEARS, WHO HAS NO OTHER EVIDENCE OF HIS HAVING LIVED LONG EXCEPT HIS AGE."

Seneca

Left to its own devices, starting somewhere between the ages of 20 and 30, the body starts a gradual decline in many major systems, including the immune and muscular systems. The metabolic rate slows, the digestive tract becomes sluggish, and the endocrine system slips. A decrease in glucose tolerance increases the risk of diabetes, and an increase in blood pressure contributes to heart disease. Hair cells stop producing pigment, so most of us develop at least a few gray hairs, sometimes as early as our thirties. Some people turn totally gray or white, while others lose their hair entirely. Oil glands in the scalp dry out, so the hair might become more brittle or break more easily. The skin wrinkles, although the extent depends in large part on sun exposure, history of smoking, nutrition, and genetics. The skin also loses some of its elasticity, again more as a result of sun exposure than of age. The skin is less moist and might even feel chalky. The upper layers produce fewer cells, so the skin is thinner and prone to bruises. Reduced blood supply to the skin causes paleness, but this is easily remedied by increased exercise.

Sight, sound, and smell also are affected. By age 40, most people notice they can't read the print on a food label no matter how far away they hold the package. The lens of the eyes thickens and becomes less smooth and elastic, while the pupil gets smaller and the muscles that help it widen and narrow are less responsive. Hearing peaked during puberty and has been on the decline ever since. By the forties and fifties, hearing loss is noticeable and a person may find it difficult to block out background noise. High-frequency noises are the first to go, especially in men, which might explain why husbands don't hear their wives as well.

The gradual loss of smell affects appetite by diminishing a person's ability to taste. This partially explains why some older people heavily salt or sweeten their foods. (Zinc deficiency also can lower taste in older persons and can be remedied by taking a multiple vitamin and mineral supplement that contains 15 to 20 milligrams of zinc.)

A person's figure changes over the course of decades. Cartilage is one of the few tissues that continues to grow throughout life. Consequently, the ears and nose grow longer, starting around age 30. Waistlines broaden, while shoulders might narrow. Unless a person continues to exercise, a loss of muscle and a gain in fat weight are inevitable as the decades pass.

Hormone levels change with age, resulting in cessation of menstruation at menopause for a woman and perhaps loss of libido in a man. The drop in estrogen for women can affect skin tone, vaginal lubrication, emotions, mental function and memory, and sex drive. Men's testosterone levels drop by as much as 40 percent between the ages of 30 and 80. Other hormones, such as growth hormone and DHEA, also drop with age, possibly reducing muscle strength, vigor, and immune function. (See Chapter 5 for more on these hormones.)

MATTER OVER MIND

- At the age of 75, the film producer-director Cecil B. DeMille premiered his seventieth film, *The 10 Commandments*.
- At age 71, Michelangelo was appointed chief architect of one of the world's greatest architectural undertakings—St. Peter's in Rome. He worked on the project for 18 years until his death at age 89.
- At age 69, America's most famous architect, Frank Lloyd Wright, began what is often considered his best work—the house at Falling Water.
- After age 80, the Italian composer Giuseppe Verdi wrote two of his greatest operas.
- Until his death at age 86 and despite failing eyesight, Claude Monet, the father of French Impressionist painting, was still painting his famous *Water Lilies.*

It is obvious from these and many other examples that talent and intellectual ability can bloom in the later years. Yet no other aspect of aging causes more distress and confusion than the thought of losing mental acuity and with it our personalities, talents, and memories. Many people incorrectly assume that mental function deteriorates with age; consequently, serious mental problems such as Alzheimer's disease often progress undetected because they are misdiagnosed as natural memory loss. But senility is not inevitable with age.

Almost all deterioration of mental function comes from disease, not from the aging process. Granted, people lose a few brain cells as they age, but they don't lose brain function. In fact, most brain cells are lost prior to puberty. After that, the rate slows considerably, at least until about age 60.

Any normal reduction in mental capacity, such as slowed reaction time or trouble with short-term memory, might result from changes in blood pressure, reduced blood supply to the brain, changes in sleep patterns that affect brain activity, stress, or changes in hormones or brain chemicals called neurotransmitters. Of course, some changes in the brain could result from self-fulfilling prophecies: the more a person complains of memory loss, the more likely he or she will experience more of the same. Many of these changes in body and mind are modifiable by making a few simple alterations in diet, exercise, and thinking.

Theories of Aging

"PEOPLE GROW OLD ONLY BY DISCARDING THEIR HOPES AND DREAMS. YEARS MAY WRINKLE THE SKIN, FADE VISION, OR STOOP POSTURE, BUT ONLY LOSS OF PASSION WRINKLES THE SPIRIT!"

Anonymous

Why does the body change with time and age? In essence, aging is the result of accumulating loss of functioning cells. These effects are most noticeable in muscles and nerves, since their capacity to regenerate is limited.

Numerous theories attempt to explain this gradual decline in cell function, but no one really knows why we age. In centuries past, the ravages of old age were attributed to demonic forces. In the machine age it was postulated that aging was a sign the body's machinery had worn out. Today, scientists theorize that aging might result from a number of factors, acting alone or together in the body.

THE ABUSE THEORY

The most practical of all the current theories on aging is the Abuse Theory, which states that longevity depends on how well we treat our bodies. An abundance of evidence shows that people live longest when they:

1. eat a low-fat, fiber-rich diet;
2. exercise regularly;
3. limit alcohol and avoid tobacco and drugs;
4. maintain a healthful weight;
5. have a positive attitude toward life;
6. wear seat belts.

How Fast Are You Aging?

Here's a quick test of how your lifestyle is affecting your aging process. All the questions below pertain to lifestyle habits that you can change or modify. Of course, family history of disease, your age, the age at death of your ancestors, and luck also are key influences of life expectancy and would modify the final score.

Women, on average, live about seven years longer than men. Your average life expectancy is your starting point. Respond to the statements below and add and subtract years as directed to obtain your approximate life potential.

	Women (Average life expectancy: 79)	**Men** (Average life expectancy: 72)
1. Add two years for every "yes" answer to the statements below.		
a) I am in excellent health.		
b) I maintain a trim weight.		
c) I exercise daily.		
d) I consume a low-fat, high-fiber diet.		
e) I avoid consuming excess calories.		
f) I eat seven to nine servings of fruits and vegetables every day.		
g) I maintain a cholesterol level under 200mg/dl.		
h) I get at least seven hours of quality sleep each night.		
2. Add an additional one year for every "yes" answer to the following statements.		

	Women (Average life expectancy: 79)	Men (Average life expectancy: 72)

a) I am in good health
   (ignore if you already answered
   "yes" to 1(a) above).

b) I limit meat intake to
   three weekly servings (3 ounces each).

c) I take a moderate-dose
   multiple vitamin and mineral
   supplement with extra vitamin E.

d) I am generally happy and
   satisfied with my life.

e) I cope with stress and avoid
   unnecessary stress when possible.

f) I eat five to six servings of fruits
   and vegetables every day (ignore
   if you already answered
   "yes" to 1(f) above).

g) I am in a long-term,
   satisfying relationship.

3. Subtract five years for
   every "yes" answer to the
   statements below.

a) I am very overweight.

b) My blood cholesterol is
   over 200mg/dl.

c) I eat too much fat and not
   enough fruits and vegetables.

d) I use tobacco.

e) I don't have an annual
   physical examination by an
   M.D.

	Women (Average life expectancy: 79)	**Men** (Average life expectancy: 72)

4. Subtract two years for every "yes" answer to the statements below.

a) I am in poor health.

b) My blood pressure is high.

c) My blood sugar is high.

d) My blood cholesterol is greater than 200mg/dl or my HDL cholesterol is under 60mg/dl.

e) I drink more than five alcoholic beverages each week.

f) I am overweight (ignore if you already answered "yes" to 3(a) above).

5. Subtract one year for every "yes" answer to the statements below.

a) I don't use sunscreen.

b) I don't use seat belts.

c) I am not in a long-term relationship.

d) I have no close friends.

Total the numbers to obtain a rough estimate of what your life expectancy is, given your current habits. Keep in mind that you can improve these odds by making changes today in what you eat, how often you exercise, and how you live.

7. effectively handle stress;

8. seek medical care when needed;

9. have ample money, education, support, and self-confidence; and

10. live in middle- to upper-income communities.

THE WEAR-AND-TEAR THEORY

Life can kill you. Or so say proponents of the Wear-and-Tear Theory of aging, who assert that daily life simply wears out the body's tissues. Consuming too much fat over time raises blood cholesterol levels, which leads to heart disease. Sunbathing makes skin susceptible to wrinkling and cancer. Alcohol consumption wears down the liver and leads to premature disease and death. Almost anyone over 65 has some joint damage from years of walking, lifting, bending, jogging, squatting, or dancing.

Unlike machines produced on an assembly line, however, every human body is different. Some people are more prone to osteoarthritis, possibly because their cartilage is less resilient. Others increase their chances of developing osteoarthritis by being overweight, which places additional stress on the joints. Atherosclerosis, wrinkling, loss of muscle tone, and numerous other wear-and-tear disorders can be greatly modified by diet, exercise, and how you live. In short, genetics and lifestyle are as much to blame for how the body "wears" as aging.

The Wear-and-Tear Theory also doesn't explain why the body stops repairing itself. Machines can't fix themselves or build new parts, but our bodies have a complex repair system that quickly remedies engine problems every day, usually putting us back in action without a sign of malfunction. What causes the body to stop repairing broken parts? Other theories, discussed below, address this question.

THE CROSS-LINKAGE THEORY

Repair processes cease when cell communication breaks down, according to the Cross-Linkage Theory of aging. This theory states that cells generate defective cell "messengers" that then tell the cell to produce defective or cross-linked proteins including enzymes. These useless proteins accumulate and eventually reduce cell function, interfere with cell repair, or cause cell death. What causes the defective messengers is unknown, but many researchers suspect that highly reactive compounds called free radicals are to blame.

THE FREE RADICAL THEORY

Like David and Goliath, the body may be brought down by infinitesimal oxygen fragments called free radicals found in air pollution, fried foods, tobacco smoke, and normal metabolic processes. A free radical attacks and damages the genetic code and the protective coatings, called membranes, of cells. Free radicals also halt energy production by damaging the cells' powerhouse centers (the mitochondria). Some researchers speculate that the rate of mitochondrial damage might determine life span.

After thousands of free-radical attacks on each cell every day, over decades the cells become damaged or abnormal. Due to immune cell damage, the body gradually loses its resistance to colds, infections, and disease. Eventually the cell dies and only a "clinker" remains. In fact, the cell age of tissues is determined by the number of clinkers present.

Luckily the body's antioxidant system, comprised of vitamins, minerals, enzymes, and other compounds, sweeps up and deactivates free radicals. This is why it is essential to stockpile a strong antioxidant defense and minimize any lifestyle habit that generates free radicals.

The body is exposed to free radicals throughout life, yet the damage seems to escalate in the later years. This suggests that the aging human body needs greater amounts of antioxidants to compensate for other lagging systems. (See Chapters 4 and 9 for more information on free radicals and antioxidants.)

THE IMMUNE THEORY

The main job of the body's immune system is to separate friend from foe, letting normal cells flourish while destroying everything damaging, from germs to renegade cancer cells. Sometimes immune processes malfunction as a result of aging and attack body tissues, rather than foreign substances, leading to tissue destruction. Studies on animals support this theory of aging. Animals with vigorous immune systems live approximately 77 percent longer than those with poorly functioning immune systems.

While there's a big difference between humans and mice, the link between immunity and aging might cross species. Poor diet and medication use in later years can interfere with nutrient absorption and compromise immunity. In addition, intestinal absorption and the availability of some immune-enhancing nutrients, such as vitamin B_{12}, decrease as a person ages, thus increasing dietary requirements to maintain health. Several studies report improved immunity when a person follows the guidelines of the Anti-Aging Diet (see Chapter 7) and consumes a low-fat, high-fiber diet, takes a moderate-dose multiple supplement, and exercises in moderation.

THE WASTE PRODUCTS THEORY

Like your car, your refrigerator, and the earth itself, the body depends on an efficient means of removing waste. Anything that interferes with this system could contribute to aging. When one or more of the body's waste-removal systems malfunctions, byproducts accumulate in cells, clogging normal metabolic processes and potentially damaging or killing the cell.

No one knows why the aging body becomes less efficient at handling wastes. However, accumulation of damage caused by free radicals, including the buildup of yellow-brown pigments called lipofuscin, is likely a primary contributor. Low intake of vitamin E results in greater accumulation of lipofuscin, and marginal deficiencies of several nutrients, such as the B vitamins and iron, are associated with accumulation of abnormal byproducts of metabolism and reduced mental functioning.

TELOMERES: THE TICKING CLOCK THEORY

In the 1960s, a scientist named Leonard Hayflick noticed an interesting characteristic of cell growth. Placed in a flask and fed well, cells continued to thrive by reproducing themselves, but only up to a point. Then, after a set number of replications, the cells grew old and died. No cell tested lived forever.

This "Hayflick limit" is specific to each type of cell. For example, cells from chickens divide 15 to 35 times, while cells from mice achieve only 14 to 28 replications. Human cells fare better at about 50 to 60 generations. Hayflick theorized that some kind of cellular clock counts the generations and triggers cell death. According to the Ticking Clock Theory, life span and aging might be arranged and enforced somewhere within the cell.

That somewhere might be at the ends of the DNA strands within each cell. These end segments, called telomeres, are like the handles on a jumprope. They protect the DNA cord from unraveling and allow complete replication of the entire DNA strand during cell division. However, each time the DNA splits during cell replication, one notch on the telomere handle is lost. After a set number of cell divisions, the telomere is used up and the cell can no longer replicate. These dead or damaged cells interfere with neighboring cells, creating a haphazard cascade effect that could result in aging. In essence, the telomere is like a ticking clock that determines life span. If scientists could measure telomere length, it might serve as the most accurate biomarker of aging. In the future, there may be ways to directly affect telomere length by tampering with the enzymes responsible for its shortening. According to this theory, stop that internal clock and you can stop the aging process.

In the meantime, even if you can't stop the clock, you can slow it a bit. Several things speed up cell division, which amplifies telomere demise. Sun exposure, infections and injury, radiation exposure, stress, and tobacco use increase cell turnover. On the other hand, restricting calories slows cell turnover and extends life span.

Protecting the DNA from free-radical attacks also might extend the life of the telomere. Preliminary evidence shows that building antioxidant defense systems does, in fact, lengthen the life of some species. Granted, extrapolating results from roundworms to humans is a big leap, but the possibilities are exciting. Extending the life span from three to an unheard-of six weeks in a worm is equivalent to giving the average human life span a boost to 150 to 240 years!

You Can Reverse the Aging Process

"TO KNOW HOW TO GROW OLD IS THE MASTER WORK OF WISDOM,
AND ONE OF THE MOST DIFFICULT CHAPTERS IN THE GREAT WAR OF
LIVING."

Henri Frédéric Amiel

Aging doesn't happen overnight. The slow loss of youth begins in your twenties, when you still think you're indestructible. The sooner you jump on the anti-aging bandwagon and start supplying your body with all the nutrients it needs for optimal functioning, the more likely you will hold onto that youthful health, sidestep the slow demise of aging, enjoy life to its fullest, and dramatically reduce medical costs later in life. For this reason, it's important to be aware of the subtle first signs of poor health. For example, did you know that mood swings might be caused by a vitamin deficiency rather than a glitch in your personality? That dry skin might be easily remedied with a little more oil in your diet? Or that fatigue might be a sign you need more iron, not more coffee?

Most of us know that what we eat is important to how we feel, and we've made some changes. We've cut fat intake from 42 percent to 34 percent of total calories and are trying to eat the recommended servings of fruits and vegetables. We've switched from potato chips to baby carrots, from chocolate ice cream to fat-free frozen yogurt, and we put low-fat milk in our caffè lattes. Hey, many of us even know our cholesterol levels!

While all of those changes are commendable, many of us think we're doing better than we really are. According to a recent survey by the American Dietetic Association, 90 percent of adults think they eat a healthful diet, when in fact only 1 percent meet the dietary guidelines outlined in the USDA's Food Guide Pyramid.

Seeking medical help and having an annual physical exam to monitor blood cholesterol, blood sugar, weight, blood pressure, and other parameters of health status are important. But being healthy is about taking charge of your health every day.

One place to start is your diet. Do you really know how well you're doing diet-wise? You might be surprised at how what you eat might be affecting how

Assessing the Tests

Recording your food intake in a daily journal is one way to assess your eating habits. Another helpful test includes anthropometric measurements of the body. Anthropometric measurements include height, weight, upper arm circumference, fat-fold thickness, and head circumference. Measurements and interpretation of results should be conducted by a trained health professional such as a physician, a registered nurse, or a registered dietitian.

Laboratory tests of blood, urine, or tissues can detect vitamin or mineral deficiencies at an earlier stage than can a physical examination. For example, measurements of red blood cell volume, serum ferritin, or total iron-binding capacity provide feedback on iron status. Blood albumin levels are a clear indicator of protein status. Blood levels of various enzymes also are indicators of nutritional status. Low blood alkaline phosphatase indicates zinc deficiency; low levels of glutathione peroxidase in red blood cells suggest a selenium deficiency; and red blood cell transketolase activity reflects vitamin B_1 status. Most laboratory tests other than hematocrit and hemoglobin for iron-deficiency anemia, however, are often too cumbersome and expensive to conduct as part of a typical physical exam, so you must request them.

Most unorthodox tests for nutritional status are inaccurate and unreliable. Hair analysis can detect toxic metal concentrations in the body, such as mercury, lead, arsenic, aluminum, or cadmium, but numerous environmental factors, such as tobacco, smoke, water, sweat, shampoos, and hair sprays, alter the mineral composition of hair and disqualify hair analysis as a reliable method of nutritional analysis.

Cytotoxic testing promises to identify and treat disorders by testing the blood for food allergies. However, the information obtained from cytotoxic testing (and from any test that promises a simple and complete analysis of a person's nutritional status and that is conducted without the supervision of a physician) is unreliable and misleading.

A thorough evaluation of nutritional status assesses a person's physical condition, his or her growth and development patterns, the level of nutrients in the blood and urine, the quality and quantity of nutrient intake, and the body's ability to absorb and utilize ingested nutrients. Information on the use of medications, level of stress, history of disease, living conditions, availability of food and food preparation equipment, knowledge of nutrition and proper eating habits, and cultural patterns also should be included in a complete nutritional assessment.

you look, feel, and age. Marginal nutrient intakes can have profound yet subtle effects on well-being, vitality, and aging. The symptoms of poor nutrition are vague, so they progress unnoticed or we explain them away as being "all in our heads" or with the observation "I'm just getting older" or "I was born this way." In fact, all it might take is a few simple dietary changes to look and feel good, if not great.

The effects also can be immediate. While heart disease or osteoporosis may require a lifetime of poor eating habits, the sparkle in your eye or a healthy smile is a sign of what you've eaten in the last few months. The warning signs of a bad diet listed in the table on page 29 will help you assess your dietary intake and decide what, if anything, needs improvement. Use this information to work with your physician to prevent age-related diseases and to help slow the aging process. Chapter 10 includes information on how to improve your diet to prevent specific conditions.

SIGNS OF A BAD DIET

Hair and Scalp

THE SIGNS: Dry, thin, lackluster hair

Hair that splits or breaks, or is dry and tangles easily

Hair loss and/or dandruff

Premature graying or changes in hair color

Nails

THE SIGNS: Poor growth

Nails that chip or are weak

Brittle, fragile nails, or nails with ridges

Skin

THE SIGNS: Dull, dry skin

Sun-damaged skin, sagging skin, easy bruising

Flaky, itchy, or rough skin

Mouth, Teeth, and Gums

THE SIGNS: Cracks at the corners of the mouth, soreness, or burning of the tongue

Bleeding gums

Periodontal disease

Cavities

Eyes

THE SIGNS: Vision loss caused by cataracts or macular degeneration

Sensitivity to bright light, burning, itching

Bloodshot eyes, poor vision

Mood and Energy

THE SIGNS: Tiredness, lethargy

Mild depression, irritability, mood fluctuations

Chapter 3

EXPLORING VITALITY

"Sow a thought, reap an act;

Sow an act, reap a habit;

Sow a habit, reap a character;

Sow a character, reap a destiny."

Anonymous

e are surrounded by living examples of vitality:

- Christopher Reeve, the actor who played Superman in the movie and now is a daily inspiration to everyone as he faces and beats one of life's hardest lessons, rising above a neck injury that has left his body paralyzed.
- Katharine Hepburn, the actress whose vigor and spirit continues to inspire us. She was in her fifties with three more Oscars to win. She was 60-plus when she played the 40-something Eleanor of Aquitaine in *The Lion in Winter;* in her seventies in *On Golden Pond;* and in her eighties in *Love Affair.*
- Huston Smith, the author, student, and teacher of world religions who exudes an aura of peace and joy so strong it is felt even when watching him on television.

These are just a few of our mentors of vitality. Each of us has people much closer to us—in our homes, offices, schools, or neighborhoods, or sitting next to us at church—who possess that same passion for living. Most of us have ourselves experienced the joy and aliveness of vitality, though perhaps not as often as we'd like. Most vital people, in fact, live what they would call ordinary lives, yet they're filled with extraordinary experience.

Vitality is the spark of life itself and is the fuel for a happy life. Choosing to live longer is not the goal—the true goal is to live those extra years vitally.

What Is Vitality?

"... THEY WANT SOMEBODY TO TELL 'EM THEY HAVE A CHANCE AT THE I-N-G OF LIFE AND NOT JUST THE E-D."

Tom Robbins, from Jitterbug Perfume

There is more to longevity than a low cholesterol level and more to vibrant living than an exercise program. Vitality provides the passion that makes getting older worth it.

Vital people exude a spirit, gusto, or *joie de vivre* (joy of life) so radiant that it forms our first impressions of them. We're attracted to them like moths to a light. Vital people make us smile. They wake us up. We feel better, happier, and more hopeful just being around them. We describe them as positive, energetic, comfortable with themselves, centered, curious, uplifting, optimistic, or resilient; they describe themselves simply as normal or happy, but wonder why other people aren't having as much fun. Vital people appreciate all of life. They enjoy life in general and in almost all of its aspects, while other people glimpse only isolated moments of the same enthusiasm.

But vitality goes even deeper than just taking joy in life. According to the *Oxford Dictionary,* the word *vitality* means "the principle of life" or "the ability to sustain life." Vitality *is* life or aliveness expressed to its fullest. The quest for longevity, therefore, is an empty goal unless it encompasses the striving for vitality or life's source.

Vital Dreaming

One way to nurture vitality is to visualize it, or picture it in your mind. Visualizations give you the chance to see life as it could be if vitality and health were in full bloom. There are no right or wrong ways to visualize; just accept and enjoy whatever comes to mind.

Find a comfortable, quiet place where you won't be disturbed, preferably just before you go to bed at night or just after awakening in the morning. Close your eyes and for a few moments pay attention to your breathing—the drawing in and the going out of your breath. When you feel calm, consider the following questions and try to picture in your mind and even feel in your body the answers:

1. What does vitality mean to you?
2. How does it feel to be energized with vitality? What does it feel like to be emotionally at peace, feeling no anger, fear, or depression? How does it feel to have a heart filled with love, trust, and compassion?
3. What would you look like as a vital person?
4. What would you do in your life to nurture your vitality?
5. What brings you joy? What helps you feel and give love, delight, and wonder?
6. At what moments in your life have you felt vital? Describe how you felt.
7. What people, events, traits, experiences, or other things tie your life together and give it meaning? Look to these as a starting point to vitality.

Now, take a long look at yourself in a mirror. What do you see that you like? What resembles the looks and feelings of vitality you just identified in the visualization? What do you see that you want to change? How will you go about bringing your daily life into a focus on health and vitality?

A Roadmap to Vitality: Advice from Vital People

I interviewed many vital people for this book. Here are a few of their recommendations for getting the most out of life:

Live in the present, and enjoy it.

Think positive.

Don't take your health for granted.

Be grateful for every single thing life has to offer.

When you're feeling down in the dumps, do something for someone else; it will help you forget your woes.

No matter what comes along, know that you can handle it.

Be good to people; it always pays off.

Don't take yourself too seriously.

Accept that no one goes through life scot-free.

Do what you love and love what you do.

Keep moving.

Where Does Vitality Come From?

"SEIZE THE MOMENT OF EXCITED CURIOSITY ON ANY SUBJECT TO SOLVE YOUR DOUBTS; FOR IF YOU LET IT PASS, THE DESIRE MAY NEVER RETURN, AND YOU MAY REMAIN IN IGNORANCE."

William Wirt

Everyone has the potential for and the right to vitality. Granted, growing up in a household of encouragement, joy, silliness, and vitality certainly boosts the odds of developing it yourself, but many vital people came from less-than-happy child-hoods. Still more have suffered serious illness or tragedy, yet continued to appreciate life despite the odds.

With as yet no research on the topic we can only speculate that there might be a genetic predisposition to vitality. Even if some aspects of vitality are inherited, in large measure it is how you nurture your genetic potential that makes all the difference in life. In essence, each of us comes into this life as a canvas with only the rough outline of a picture. Life hands us the paints, the brush, and the palette; it's up to us whether we create a Monet or a fiasco.

More Advice from Vital People

When things seem overwhelming, remind yourself that "It's only life."

Be necessary.

Practice random acts of kindness (put a dime in someone else's parking meter, cook a hot meal for a housebound senior, hold the door for a stranger, let someone with fewer purchases go ahead of you in line, buy someone flowers when it isn't his or her birthday).

Don't fret about the future; it's a waste of time.

Never retire.

Learn something new every day.

Don't be afraid to make mistakes; they're only signs you're stretching your wings and growing a little.

Be resourceful. If you can't get where you want to go one way, try a different route.

Do things because you love them, not because you expect fame or fortune.

Throw out the television and get involved in life.

Be outrageous.

Hang out with happy people.

THE VITALITY CONTINUUM

Like most aspects of our physical and mental makeup, each of us probably has a unique continuum for vitality that ranges from merely existing to sheer joy—say, on a scale of 1 to 10 where 1 equals existing and 10 equals maximum vitality. Where you are on that continuum depends on the choices you make each day. The ultimate goal is to live at the upper end of the scale most of the time.

Every baby is born overflowing with vitality and wonder at life. As an adult, it takes practice to hold onto or rekindle that natural-born vitality by adding a depth that comes only from experience and maturity. Vital people are exposed to the same world as everyone else; their adversities might be no different than their neighbors'. The difference is that they focus on positive times and try to view even hard times in a positive light. As a result, uplifting experiences, feelings, thoughts, and beliefs come far more frequently and intensely to them than to other people. Everyone can push their natural-born right to vitality by taking charge of their life and their physical, emotional, mental, and spiritual well-being.

The Link Between Health, Attitude, and Vitality

"WHEN FATE HANDS US A LEMON, LET'S TRY TO MAKE A LEMONADE."
Dale Carnegie

Taking care of the body by eating well and exercising, not smoking, drinking in moderation, and sleeping well clears the way for vitality to shine. But vitality has an emotional component as well. It is difficult to feel vital when you're depressed, fatigued, or stressed. People who develop a positive, trusting attitude toward life are less likely to suffer from disease, from cancer and heart disease to migraines and urinary problems. When they are ill, they're more likely to recover and recover quickly. Vitality can even master terminal illness and shine through amidst some of life's biggest challenges. In fact, often it is during a crisis that a person realizes that life is too short and too precious to be spent any other way but vitally.

Even when faced with a terminal condition, vital people look for meaning, purpose, and even humor in their experience, discovering ways to appreciate life even when they're dealt a bad hand. They also are less likely to be dependent on others for their daily care in the later years than people who clutch onto negative, angry, or hopeless thoughts.

The link between vitality and health is a win-win relationship. Embracing vitality boosts energy, helps maintain health, and reduces the risk of disease and premature aging. In turn, a healthier body encourages positive thinking and fuels vitality. Nurturing both works in your favor for health, happiness, and longevity.

Conversely, not taking care of your health, eating poorly, not exercising, living a stressful lifestyle, allowing negative thoughts, or surrounding yourself with depressing people dampens or even snuffs out vitality, which leads to more damaging behaviors, disease, and premature death.

Vitality is a choice, but it takes courage and determination to pursue it. Researchers at the University of California at San Francisco found that people who allowed themselves to be overcome by stress, fatigue, or depression were much more likely to lose sight of vitality and health. Negative life events or poor work environment had little effect on happiness or well-being. The old saying "Don't let life get you down" is worth heeding!

Even More Advice from Vital People

Take responsibility for yourself; don't blame anyone else for what happens in your life.

Be the kind of person you would want to have as a friend.

Love others because you want to, not because you expect anything from them.

Take risks.

Don't let pain get you down. If something hurts, it's going to hurt whether you're lying in bed or climbing a mountain. You might as well enjoy the view!

Don't bear grudges.

Be curious about everything.

You're old when you feel sorry for yourself.

You may not be perfect, but you're good enough.

What makes people young or old is how they think.

Never give up!

Put all the vital people in the world into one room and you wouldn't find a curmudgeon in the batch. Vitality begins and ends with attitude. Vital people are grateful for life. They don't avoid life's problems, but they do minimize the things they can't change and view unpleasant experiences as temporary. Vitality is the opposite of the "victim mentality," whereby people blame anyone and anything but themselves for their problems. Vital people instead ask, "How can I change, fix, or improve this situation?"

You can reach that upper end of your vitality continuum by filling your mind and life with vital thoughts and actions, layer upon layer. Listen to your thoughts. Do they reaffirm vitality or bury it? Thoughts that negate vitality sound like this:

"You can't do this."
"You can't handle this."
"You're likely to fail."
"This is going to be awful."
"This will never work."

Thoughts that nurture and reinforce vitality sound like this:

"I can handle this."
"I'm enjoying this adventure no matter what the outcome."
"I'll learn and grow from this experience."
"I love what I'm doing."
"This is fun!"

Remember, attitude is everything, and attitudes spring from thoughts. You choose your thoughts. If you want to be old, think "can't," "won't," or "shouldn't." The sooner you start, the quicker you'll age.

If you want to live vitally and long, choose to think youthfully and be playful. Focus on all you have to be grateful for and take good care of it. Try new experiences, surround yourself with nurturing relationships, and keep your sense of humor. If you plan to live a long life, be prepared to work on your attitude.

KEEP LAUGHING

"Keep your sense of humor." That is the most common advice given by vital people. "Don't take yourself too seriously" is another.

Vital people are playful. They're not afraid to be silly, spontaneous, or vulnerable. Vital people get a "kick" out of things and find humor even when life tries to bring them down. If you don't feel this way, hang around someone who does. The humor is contagious!

Vital people also are likely to be a bit outrageous and adventuresome, willing to take risks and inclined to make their own rules. Vital people define themselves; they don't let others or society decide who they are.

One way to nurture this playfulness is to never "act your age." If you act your age when you're 40 years by slowing down, not taking up Rollerblading, mountain climbing, ballet, the clarinet, or any other hobby (because "people your age don't do those sorts of crazy things"), image how feeble, dependent, and inactive you'll be by the time you're 90! And how can you live to be 120 if you stop living at 40?

Some of the healthiest and oldest people in the world live in Okinawa, where it is common for people to celebrate their one-hundredth birthday. When asked, these oldest old attribute their longevity to diet and to "yuimaru," which comes from the Japanese words for "circle" and "connection." Feeling necessary and sharing gives meaning and fun to everyday living.

Another way to kindle joy is to challenge set patterns. Routine and habit, though comfortable, can dampen an inventive, light-hearted approach to life. Try living from a new angle, even if it's by taking a small step, such as reading the paper at a different time of day or ordering something new at a favorite restaurant. Keep each day fresh and open to joy.

CURIOSITY VERSUS FEAR

Vital people are curious, open, and willing to learn. They ask questions, want details, and have an insatiable appetite for knowledge. That's what makes a vital person so interesting, someone you want to know. Curiosity and playfulness keep vital people young.

Anxiety, stress, and fear kill curiosity and, thus, vitality. As Dr. Gerald G. Jampolsky says, "Love is the absence of fear." Being curious and willing to try new things requires that a person push past fear, self-doubt, or negative beliefs and take the risk. It means viewing problems, troubles, barriers, and fears as opportunities for growth, rather than as reasons to retreat from life. It takes courage to live a long and vital life, but when you think of the alternative, it's worth it!

HAVE A PURPOSE

Bertrand Russell, the British philosopher, resigned at age 88 from the Campaign for Nuclear Disarmament to establish a more militant group called the Committee of 100. The year before he died at age 98, he stated that his purpose in life was sparked by three passions: "the longing to love, the search for knowledge, and the unbearable pity for the suffering of mankind."

What is your life's purpose? How do you want to answer the question "What good came from my life?" Your answer tells a lot about how you should live each day and also gives you insight into the source of your vitality. As the German philosopher Friedrich Nietzsche said, "He who has a *why* to live can bear with almost any *how*."

When life loses its meaning, the desire to live fades. "The highest suicide rates are in white men over the age of 80 who have lost a purpose in life and are absorbed in meaninglessness," says Robert N. Butler, M.D., Director of the International Longevity Center at Mt. Sinai Medical Center in New York. The search for meaning in life can take on a new depth as we age, given dimension by our experience, pain, struggle, triumphs, loss, and discovery.

Vitality is closely woven into the meaning and purpose we give to every moment of our lives. It has nothing to do with possessions, fortune, fame, or status, but much to do with how open we are to love and happiness. Vital people have a clear sense of what gives their lives meaning. This personal philosophy underlies their daily decisions and actions. Usually the purpose involves giving; that is, being of service to others, helping to make the world a slightly better place, or bringing joy to others' lives.

Sometimes we actively define what gives our lives significance; other times it lands in our laps unexpectedly. My life's purpose was revealed years ago while participating in a guided imagery in a college class. The teacher had asked us to close our eyes, relax, and let our imaginations carry us. She asked us to imagine we were climbing a mountain. The path was winding and it took some time to reach the summit, where someone was waiting. The person was to hand us a present, and then we were to walk back down the mountain. After the guided imagery, the class discussed what each one of us had visualized.

Like many of the students in the class, I had been met by a sage, sort of a

Gandolf or Merlin-like character. My sage was sitting at a fire overlooking the surrounding mountain peaks. It was that magic time when daylight meets darkness. I sat down by the fire next to my imaginary sage, who pulled from his robes a simple brown suede pouch tied with twine, much like those little bags that hold marbles. I peeked into the bag to find a fistful of pea-sized crystals that caught the firelight and twinkled. I put the bag into my back pocket, stood up, and started back down the mountain. As I walked, the crystals fell out of the pouch and sprinkled on the ground, covering my trail with jewels.

From that brief journey into my imagination I realized that my purpose in life was to leave sparkles wherever life took me and that I could always find my way back up the mountain by following the joy I left behind.

If you plan to live a long life, you'd better know why you're here. Each person's life purpose and source of vitality is as unique as his or her fingerprints. No two people can follow the same path to vitality. Thus you must take time to ask yourself some very important questions, such as

- What do I choose as the meaning and purpose of my life?
- What do I want to accomplish during this lifetime?
- What do I want to be remembered for?
- If it were the last day of my life and I was reviewing my time here on earth, what would I want to look back on with pride? What regrets do I want to avoid?
- Why do I want to live a long and healthy life? How will I use those extra years constructively?

RESILIENCE: IT'S ALL IN YOUR HEAD

Vital people bounce back. They have their ups and downs, sadness and grief, failures and losses. But they meet the challenge, experience the pain, then return to vitality. In fact, vital people may seek experiences that have the potential for discomfort. They are willing to live and love fully, even if that love brings potential pain or loss. They are willing to move to a new city, start a new career, and speak out against the crowd, because they know the long-term benefits are worth it, even if the short-term process is uncomfortable.

Go for It

"IF YOU WANT TO LIVE TO BE 100 OR OLDER, YOU CAN'T JUST SIT AROUND WAITING FOR IT TO HAPPEN. YOU HAVE TO GET UP EACH DAY AND GO AFTER IT!"

George Burns

Developing a vital personality and approach to life isn't achieved overnight; it takes a lifetime of practice to grow into and strengthen your vitality, just as it takes daily exercise to keep your muscles strong. It isn't easy to change, but it *is* possible, and it's the desire to better ourselves that makes us human and makes life valuable.

First, you must build a healthful life that fulfills basic needs for feeling safe, feeling connected to other people through family and friendships, nurturing love in every act of life, building respect both for yourself and for others, and taking care of your body with healthful habits. According to the psychologist Abraham Maslow, only when these basic needs are fulfilled can a person focus on more profound issues of vitality and spirituality. Sometimes you have to start gradually, finding small ways to work joy and health into daily experiences, starting with any aspect of your health, from the physical, mental, and emotional to the social or spiritual.

ACTING AS IF . . .

If you don't feel vital, start by changing how you think or act. The feelings may catch up. Anything becomes a habit if repeated often enough. Research shows that when people adopt a healthful lifestyle, eat well, exercise regularly, and keep stress at bay they start feeling better about themselves. They also enjoy life more and have a more positive attitude. Vitality is like a snowball rolling downhill. The more you incorporate vital qualities into your life, the more vital and enthusiastic you will feel and the easier it becomes to connect with that wellspring of life within you.

Identify one aspect of your life that you want to change. Even if you don't feel that way yet, start by "acting as if" you already have mastered that change. For example,

- if you are struggling to start an exercise program, tell yourself several times daily that you are an exerciser, then "act as if" you feel comfortable with your new exercise routine. Rehearse success by visualizing yourself exercising effortlessly and enjoying the experience. To support this attitude, surround yourself with people who are enthusiastic about their exercise, read books that will motivate you to stick with it, and/or put stars on the calendar for every day you successfully meet your exercise goals.
- To feel more energetic, start with something as simple as how you walk. Start walking as if you were self-confident and energetic. Walk with long, powerful strides, with your head high, your shoulders back, your chin up, and your arms swinging freely at your side. Do it every day until it becomes habit.
- If you want to bring more laughter into your life, surround yourself with people who make you laugh, watch comedy shows on television, rent silly movies, put up a bird feeder in the backyard, volunteer at a daycare center, and/or read funny books. Avoid people, activities, thoughts, and behaviors that rob you of humor, and slowly replace them with more positive people and experiences.

Include something every day in your life that excites you and brings you joy (if possible make it your job, your family, and your friends or community). Stop reading the paper or listening to the news, and start spending the extra time with positive-thinking people and listening to music or motivational tapes. Replace negative thoughts with positive ones and repeat positive affirmations throughout the day. And slowly, without your even noticing it, vitality will come to you.

Just Do It

When it comes to changing attitudes, the basic advice to "just do it" is about as useful as a crash course in walking on water. However, there is a pearl of wisdom in this advice. Attitudes—from optimism to hopelessness—are learned responses, not cut-in-stone personality traits. Basically, negative thinking is just a bad habit, and habits can be changed. Here are a few tips for adjusting your attitude:

1. Start replacing negative thoughts with positive ones. Interpret setbacks as temporary and specific learning experiences. Attribute favorable situations to enduring causes.
2. Surround yourself with positive people; attitudes often rub off.
3. Don't let one setback contaminate your whole life; keep it contained and in perspective.
4. Believe in your ability to stretch your limits. (Studies of college students found that their level of hope more accurately predicted college performance than did SAT scores or high-school grades.)
5. Improve your diet and exercise regularly to alleviate depression, hostility, and negative thinking.
6. Push the limits of your comfort zone. Research from the University of Chicago shows that peak experiences come from matching challenges to abilities. People are most likely to feel invigorated when their skills are pushed to the limit by a hefty challenge. On the other hand, anxiety is likely when the task is more than their skills can handle, while apathy is a product of never taking risks or stretching boundaries.

The secret is to keep learning, experimenting, adventuring, and challenging yourself. Cultivating a positive approach to life takes time and effort, but it's well worth it. Besides, think of the alternatives!

Ageless, Timeless

"GO OUTSIDE, TO THE FIELDS, ENJOY NATURE AND THE SUNSHINE, GO OUT AND TRY TO RECAPTURE HAPPINESS IN YOURSELF AND IN GOD. THINK OF ALL THE BEAUTY THAT'S STILL LEFT IN AND AROUND YOU AND BE HAPPY!"

Anne Frank

Vitality is the fuel that makes the journey of life fun, and possibly longer. It is a process, not an endpoint. Even 100-year-young vital people say they are still learning more about how to appreciate life. Each of us must pass through many of life's doors and experience many failures, successes, losses, and gains before vitality reaches its full expression. We are like roses slowly unfolding. Only age can bring us into full bloom.

Chapter 4

STACKING THE DECK
AGAINST AGING

"Should you fail to pilot your own ship, don't be surprised
at what inappropriate port you find yourself docked."

Tom Robbins, from Jitterbug Perfume

Staying young depends on a healthful diet, daily exercise, a positive attitude, and a supportive lifestyle, with a hefty dose of heredity thrown in. Basically, nature deals us the cards, but we play our own hand. And we're allowed to stack the deck.

While specific guidelines for each of these facets in the longevity game will be outlined in future chapters, there are a few anti-aging cards that are so potent they deserve a chapter all to themselves. Read on!

Antioxidants Against Age

"TODAY, YOU DON'T HAVE TO WORRY ABOUT GROWING OLD, YOU
HAVE TO WORRY ABOUT RUSTING."

George Burns

As was discussed in previous chapters, disease is not a matter of age, but is a result of accumulating damage over time. Antioxidants are key players in damage control.

A wealth of evidence has accumulated showing that the antioxidant nutrients, including vitamins C and E, the carotenoids, selenium, and zinc

- play a leading role in the prevention of age-related diseases.
- stimulate the immune system, thus protecting the body from disease and infection that can lead to premature death.
- protect the nervous system and brain from oxidative damage associated with age-related memory loss and nerve function.
- function at the very foundation of the body's biological clock, preventing or at least slowing the damage that underlies aging itself.

Free-radical damage to our cells' genetic code escalates as we age; consequently, anything that reduces free-radical production or counteracts free radicals, including the antioxidants, becomes important in staying young as we grow older. (See chapters 2 and 9 for more on free radicals.)

WHAT YOU CAN EXPECT FROM ANTIOXIDANTS

More than 200 published studies consistently show that a diet rich in antioxidants prevents disease and possibly premature aging. More than 130 studies show a protective effect of fruits, vegetables, and their antioxidants in preventing numerous types of cancers, including cancers of the bladder, breast, pancreas, esophagus, lungs, larynx, oral cavity, cervix, stomach, ovary, endometrium, colon, and rectum. "Although every study done to date, and probably every future trial, can be critiqued over one issue or another, the accumulating evidence is such that this approach [increasing intake of antioxidants] may turn out to be one of the most important disease prevention strategies of the 90s," states Harinder S. Garewal, M.D., Ph.D., Assistant Director, Cancer Prevention and Control, Arizona Cancer Center and Tucson VA Medical Center.

For example,

- Men and women who maintain high blood levels of beta carotene are at low risk of dying from cardiovascular disease and other causes, state researchers at the Dartmouth Medical School in New Hampshire. A total of 1,188 men and 532 women with an average age of 63 years supplemented their diets daily with 50 milligrams beta carotene. More than eight years later, those with the highest initial beta carotene levels showed almost half the risk of dying from cardiovascular disease or from any cause compared to those who entered the study with low beta carotene levels.

• Nutrition intervention studies on more than 29,000 people between the ages of 40 and 69 in Linxian, China, show that taking a multiple vitamin and mineral supplement containing antioxidants, especially vitamin E, beta carotene, and selenium, reduces the risk of premature death by 9 percent, the risk for esophageal cancer by 17 percent, and death from heart disease by almost 40 percent. A second study conducted by the same group found that antioxidant supplements also significantly lowered total mortality (by 13 percent), gastric cancer mortality (by 20 percent), and mortality from other cancers (by 19 percent).

• A U.S. study of health professionals age 40 to 75 years concluded that taking at least 100IU of vitamin E daily reduced heart disease risk by up to 40 percent.

• Seniors who supplement with vitamin E are less likely to die prematurely from any cause, report researchers at the National Institute of Aging in Bethesda, Maryland. Of the 11,178 subjects ages 67 to 109 years who were studied, those who took vitamin E supplements had a 27 percent lower risk of all-cause mortality, a 41 percent reduction in heart disease risk, and a 22 percent reduction in death from cancer. Combining vitamin C with vitamin E lowered all-cause mortality even further.

HOW ANTIOXIDANTS COMBAT THE RADICALS

On a cellular level, antioxidants are the advocates of vitality because they are uniquely effective in combating the oxygen fragments called free radicals (also called oxidants). Free radicals have an extra electrical charge called an electron. Since electrons usually come in pairs, having an unpaired electron makes free radicals highly unstable. In an effort to neutralize their extra charge, free radicals attack cell membranes, proteins, and even the genetic code within cells, stealing an electrical charge. This reaction neutralizes the free radical but generates a new one, since the attacked membrane or protein is now short one electrical charge.

Left unchecked, this chain reaction of destruction is much like the process called oxidation that rusts metal or turns butter rancid, but in your body it means cell membranes are weakened, the powerhouse centers of the cell called the mitochondria break down, proteins are scrambled, and the genetic code is altered. The end result is damaged, devitalized, or dead cells. As discussed in Chapter 2, the accumulation of free-radical damage in tissues is a major contributor both to the aging process and the diseases associated with aging.

Unless you're willing to give up breathing, which is a main source of these oxygen fragments, there is no avoiding free radicals. We also ingest them in food, especially fried or fatty foods. The body generates these renegades as natural by-products of metabolism. Even damaged tissue spews out free radicals, which interferes with the repair and healing of new tissue. In fact, the DNA in each cell of your body alone receives about 100,000 free radical "hits" every day. If you smoke or breathe cigarette smoke, drink alcohol, eat a high-fat diet, live in an area with air pollution, or are exposed to ultraviolet light from the sun, your hits per day are likely to be much greater.

You can't avoid the free radicals that gradually undermine youth and vitality, but you can combat them with antioxidants. In fact, the body has an elaborate antioxidant defense system comprised of enzymes (such as superoxide dismutase, catalases, or glutathione peroxidase), molecules (including numerous phytochemicals, the carotenes, and coenzyme Q10, to name only a few), vitamins (vitamin C and vitamin E), and minerals (selenium and zinc) whose job is to block the action of free radicals.

So if our antioxidant system is so efficient, why do we age? The body's antioxidant system can be overwhelmed when exposed to excessive amounts of free radicals. Even if 99.9 percent of all free radicals were erased by an active antioxidant system, the remaining 1,000 free radical "tears" each day to your cells' genetic code, proteins, and membranes would result in millions of wounds over the course of a lifetime. It is this backlog of cellular debris that contributes to the aging process and its associated diseases. Although you cannot entirely prevent this buildup, you can slow it down by boosting your antioxidant system.

HOW DO YOU KNOW YOU'RE GETTING ENOUGH ANTIOXIDANTS?

While you can't peek into your cells to judge the war's outcome, you can get a frontline report by how you feel and look. A well-stocked antioxidant system will help maintain a youthful appearance, healthy body, and clear mind. Numerous studies report that people who consume ample amounts of antioxidants from either food or supplements and maintain high blood levels of these nutrients also are the least likely to develop heart disease, cancer, cataracts, arthritis, and other diseases. They additionally are more likely to be physically strong and active and least likely to require assistance in caring for themselves as they age.

Boosting the body's antioxidant system takes effort. Most people don't eat enough fruits, vegetables, and other antioxidant-rich foods when they're young, and the deficit worsens with age as intake drops even further and the body's needs rise to an all-time high, in some cases to levels higher than can be supplied realistically from diet alone. That's why you must stockpile your antioxidant defense system so it is well armed every day.

This means combining diet with supplements. William Pryor, Ph.D, Boyd Professor of Chemistry and Biochemistry and Director of the Biodynamics Institute at Louisiana State University, suspects that the level of many antioxidants needed to stimulate immunity and prevent disease can be met only by combining food and supplements. Supplements provide the extra levels of many antioxidant nutrients, but fruits and vegetables are goldmines for the thousands of health-enhancing phytochemicals.

How do you know if your antioxidant system is well armed and winning the anti-aging war? More than 50 measurements can test free-radical damage (also called oxidative stress status, or OSS) in the body. Tests measuring compounds in blood and urine called isoprostanes are the most promising, but measurements of a gas called pentane in exhaled breath or compounds called TBARS (thiobarbituric acid-reactive substances) in blood also directly reflect a person's OSS. Dr. Pryor speculates that high levels of these free radical red flags are "... an early marker for the development of cancer." Ask your physician about the availability of any of these tests in your area, and make sure you're getting enough antioxidants, by:

1. following the Anti-Aging Diet outlined in Chapter 7;
2. avoiding foods that generate free radicals, such as fried foods, processed foods made with oils, and fatty foods in general; and
3. taking antioxidant supplements, such vitamin C, vitamin E, the carotenoids, selenium, coenzyme Q10, and others.

CHOOSING AN ANTIOXIDANT SUPPLEMENT

There are no "magic bullets" or one-pill approaches when it comes to turning back the hands of time. No nutrient works in a vacuum, so it's no surprise that the antioxidants also work as a team, one facilitating the effects of another. Researchers at the University of Tokyo concluded that vitamin C is very efficient at recycling vitamin E, thus prolonging and strengthening the antioxidant defense system. In turn, the antioxidant glutathione helps recycle vitamin C. Although beta carotene is less potent than vitamin E, it functions at the interior of membranes or lipoprotein compartments more effectively. On the other hand, many of the antioxidant phytochemicals, such as the flavonoids or polyphenols in fruits and vegetables or coenzyme Q10 (see below), inhibit the formation of free radicals, thereby increasing concentrations of antioxidant vitamins in tissues. So, when considering an antioxidant supplement, choose one that supplies a wide variety of antioxidants, not just a single nutrient. (See Chapter 6 for specific dietary guidelines and supplement dosages to ensure optimal antioxidant intake.)

The Phytochemicals

"YOU CAN'T TURN BACK THE CLOCK. BUT YOU CAN WIND IT UP AGAIN."

Bonnie Prudden

Phytochemicals are not vitamins or minerals, nor are they fiber or complex carbohydrates. Yet they could explain why fruits and vegetables, soybeans, and green tea help prevent cancer. While they have no specific nutritional value, they are the nutrients of the future.

Phytochemicals are naturally occurring compounds found in fruits, vegetables, seeds, legumes, and grains. *Phyto* is derived from the Greek word for plant. Every vegetable and fruit contains thousands of these chemicals that protect plants from harmful effects of the environment. In essence, phytochemicals are a plant's elixir of life. By the benevolent hand of Mother Nature, phytochemicals also help cells stay normal in human tissue by blocking one or more stages of cancer development. Phytochemicals inactivate cancer-causing substances, stimulate the immune system, protect the heart against disease, and help prevent cataracts.

While scientists have long known that vitamins, minerals, and fiber in fruits and vegetables are beneficial, more recent evidence shows that beyond nutrients, certain phytochemicals in these foods are particularly health-enhancing and disease-preventing.

Take cancer, which is a multi-stage disease. At almost every step along the pathway leading to cancer are one or more phytochemicals in fruits and vegetables that will slow or even reverse the process. People who eat the most fruits and vegetables, or at least eight servings daily, are about half as likely to have cancer as those who eat the typical two to three servings daily.

The research on phytochemicals is in its infancy, but it appears that some fruits and vegetables have an added phytochemical punch. Carrots and green leafy vegetables are particularly effective in lowering lung cancer risk. For colon cancer, the cruciferous vegetables, such as broccoli and cabbage, and possibly carrots, are very effective. For cancers of the larynx, throat, mouth, and esophagus, fruit seems to be consistently important. But a lower cancer risk is really related more to high intake of a wide variety of fruits and vegetables than to overconsumption of any one plant.

Does cooking destroy phytochemicals? Yes and no. Some phytochemicals, such as beta carotene, are lost to a certain extent during cooking. Others, such as the indoles in cabbage and broccoli, increase as a result of cooking, either because heat softens undigestible plant tissue, making the compound more accessible for digestion, or because cooking converts inactive compounds into health-enhancing substances. The bottom line is to eat a wide variety of cooked and raw vegetables and fruits to maximize your intake of all phytochemicals.

MOTHER NATURE'S BEST INVENTIONS

Food	Phytochemical	Function
Fruit	Ferulic acid Caffeic acid	Decrease cancer-causing nitrosamines. Solubilize carcinogens.
Dark green/orange fruit/vegetables	Carotenoids: *lutein*, lycopene, alpha or beta carotene, canthaxathin	Antioxidants. Help prevent blindness in seniors by replacing lost pigment in the retina. Lower the rate of cancers of the lung, breast, and other sites. Protect the immune system.
Berries/nuts/grapes	Ellagic acid	Antioxidant. Stops DNA mutations.
Green tea	Flavonoids	Antioxidant.
Cruciferous vegetables	Indoles	Help regulate estrogen. Decrease cancer risk.
	PIETC Phenols:Flavonoids	Inhibits lung cancer. Antioxidants.
	Sulforaphane	Inhibits cancer growth.
Citrus fruits	Monoterpenes (including limonene)	Inhibit breast cancer.
Tomatoes/green peppers/strawberries	P-Coumaric acid Chlorogenic acid Lycopene	Inhibit carcinogens, decrease nitrosamines. Protect DNA (antioxidant) cell proteins and fats.
Beans	Saponins Phytosterols Phytoestrogens	Decrease cholesterol. Slow colon cancer growth. Help regulate estrogen. Decrease breast cancer.
Garlic/onions	Sulfur compounds	Inhibit cancer. Decrease heart disease.

THE FLAVONOIDS

How many apples, onions, and other fruits and vegetables did you eat yesterday? If you're like most people, you could double the amount and still fall short of optimal. Besides being the most nutrient-packed, fiber-rich, fat-free items on the supermarket shelves, these foods also tote a whopping dose of flavonoids that lower heart-disease risk, according to researchers at the National Public Health Institute in Helsinki. In their study, those who ate the most flavonoid-rich foods had only 69 percent the heart-disease risk of other people. While taking extra antioxidants helped improve the heart-disease risk for other people, these vitamins did not make up the difference obtained from flavonoids. Although tables listing flavonoid concentrations are not readily available, in general, the best sources of flavonoids include onions, apples, kale, broccoli, endive, celery, cranberries, grapes, green tea, and citrus fruits.

But what are flavonoids? These phytochemicals are found in an abundance of fruits and vegetables, spices such as curcumin (curry powder), and green tea. Almost all of these compounds scavenge free radicals, inhibit the formation of certain cancer-causing substances, stimulate the immune system, and modulate certain cellular defense systems. Most reduce cancer formation or progression.

GREEN TEA

Replacing coffee with green tea once or twice during the day might be good for your health. Green tea contains at least 10 compounds that reduce cancer risk, many of which are flavonoids, according to a study from the University of California at Berkeley. Two human cancer cell types were exposed to each of these 10 compounds. Four of these compounds, beta-ionone, nerolidol, cadinene, and beta-caryophyllene, significantly inhibited breast cancer cells. While these compounds also curtailed cervical cancer cell growth, beta-ionone showed the most potent anticancer effects.

THOSE OTHER CAROTENES

Beta carotene makes the headlines, but it is actually only one of more than 500 carotene-like compounds, called carotenoids, found in dark orange or green fruits and vegetables. These relatives to beta carotene include alpha carotene, lycopene, lutein, zeaxanthin, cryptoxanthin, and canthaxanthin. While beta carotene can be converted to vitamin A, many of the other carotenoids can't. However, in some cases their antioxidant capabilities are even more potent than beta carotene's.

Lycopene, the carotenoid that made tomatoes famous, has come into its own. A recent study from the University of the Negev in Israel reports that lycopene is a more potent antioxidant than either alpha or beta carotene, especially in the prevention of endometrial, breast, prostate, and lung cancers. It might take up to four times more alpha carotene and 10 times more beta carotene to match the anticancer effects of lycopene.

BEANS: PHYTOCHEMICAL GOLD MINES

Navy, black, kidney, or soy—any bean you name is a powerhouse of phytochemicals. Phytosterols in beans might slow or even prevent colon cancer. Phytoestrogens, such as daidzein and genistein, in soy products keep tiny tumors from connecting to capillaries, so the tumors literally suffocate and die. Phytoestrogens also alter estrogen production, which might reduce the risk for developing breast cancer and lessen the symptoms of menopause. Saponins prevent cancer cells from multiplying and also might lower blood cholesterol, thus lowering heart-disease risk.

Garlic and Longevity

"EAT LEEKS IN MARCH AND WILD GARLIC IN MAY,
AND ALL THE YEAR AFTER PHYSICIANS MAY PLAY."
Old Welsh rhyme

It was placed in King Tutankhamen's tomb, possibly to ensure eternal life. It was a remedy for the Great Plague in Europe. It was put on pillows during childbirth to ensure an easy delivery. And today, it is suspected to be a frontline defense against infections, heart disease, and cancer. Garlic is the common thread that links your 20th-century kitchen to the gardens of Babylon, ancient Egypt, and prerecorded history.

In the days before cutting-edge science, there was folk medicine and garlic was at the helm. While many herbal remedies fell by the wayside with the advent of modern medicine, this black sheep of the lily family (cousin to chives, daffodils, onions, and tulips) not only held its own, but exchanged its folksy demeanor for a scientific lab coat.

Since the mid-1980s alone there have been hundreds of studies conducted on garlic and its 200-plus constituents. An overwhelming number support what the ancients knew: garlic is effective in the prevention and treatment of numerous conditions, including infections, heart disease, and cancer, as well as in stimulating the immune system.

A POOR MAN'S PENICILLIN

As legend has it, in Marseilles during the Great Plague, four thieves were released from prison to cart away the dead. Rather than succumb to the deadly disease, they remained healthy. Their good fortune was attributed to their daily drink of wine laced with garlic.

Modern scientists have isolated numerous sulfur-containing compounds in garlic that have potent antibacterial effects, destroying germs' ability to grow and reproduce, in much the same way that penicillin fights infections. Fresh garlic also is helpful in the treatment of fungal infections, including urethritis, athlete's foot, vaginitis, and candida albicans (yeast infections). Garlic even may help combat viruses, something no man-made drug is able to do.

While most researchers agree that garlic is an age-old standby in germ warfare, controversy rages over what exactly it is in garlic that has the effect. Byron Murray, Ph.D., Professor of Microbiology at Brigham Young University in Provo, Utah, believes the active ingredient is allicin, a sulfur compound produced when garlic is crushed or sliced. "The more allicin there is in a product, whether it is fresh garlic or commercial garlic powder, pills, or oils, the better is its anti-viral ability," says Dr. Murray.

"Allicin is too unstable to be of much use," counters Herbert Pierson, Ph.D., Vice President of Preventive Nutrition Consultants, Inc., in Woodinville, Washington, and former toxicologist for the National Cancer Institute in Bethesda, Maryland. "Allicin also is indiscriminate; it probably kills both the harmful and beneficial bacteria and irritates the stomach lining, possibly contributing to [stomach] ulcers." In reality, allicin is quickly converted to other sulfur compounds within minutes of cooking or hours of storage, so a person must chow down on the raw clove to get any allicin at all.

The Garlic Lover's Tool Kit: Part 1

For the garlic connoisseur, here are a few tips for selecting top-grade garlic.

1. Pick large, plump, and firm bulbs.
2. Color is not important between January and May, but from June on, choose the whitest garlic you can find.
3. The sheath should be tight and unbroken.
4. Avoid soft, spongy, or shriveled garlic.
5. Store fresh garlic in a cool, well-ventilated place.
6. For long-term storage, place peeled cloves in a jar with olive oil and refrigerate.
7. For a few tasty garlic recipes, see the Recipe section of this book (try Three-Bean Market Soup, Linguini with Clams, Vegetable Lasagna Rolls, and Garlic Spinach).

A HEARTWARMING TALE

Researchers worldwide report that compounds in garlic decrease blood cholesterol levels by as much as 12 percent. Fresh garlic or odor-modified garlic capsules also raise HDL cholesterol (the "good" cholesterol) and reduce cholesterol manufacture in the liver.

Garlic additionally reduces the stickiness of blood cell fragments called platelets, which in turn reduces blood clotting and artery clogging. Garlic counteracts a hormone-like substance called thromboxane that causes the arteries to spasm. Consequently, the blood is more fluid and passes more easily through the blood vessels, reducing the risk for heart attack, stroke, and high blood pressure.

Compounds in garlic also might help mobilize fats already deposited into the arteries, thus helping to reverse the disease process. The more garlic consumed, the greater the benefit to the heart. Again, researchers disagree on what in garlic protects the heart. Many admit they have no idea. "Garlic is a chemical nightmare," says Dr. Pierson. "Allicin converts to 40 to 50 different sulfur compounds, depending on whether it is aged, boiled, fried in oil or dried. Some of these compounds lower blood cholesterol, others reduce platelet [clumping], still others eventually might be recognized as pain relievers." Dr. Pierson also points out that other, as yet untested, compounds in garlic, including saponins and phenolic compounds, also could have health-enhancing capabilities. "It is likely that in the future we will recognize a synergistic effect of many of these substances," he theorizes.

In contrast to the highly unstable allicin, most of the compounds in garlic suspected to lower cholesterol or reduce blood clotting are resistant to heat, storage, or processing. In some cases, lightly cooking garlic creates new sulfur compounds, like ajoene, that also help protect the heart.

GARLIC AGAINST THE BIG "C"

The Codex Ebers, an Egyptian medical papyrus dating to about 1550 B.C., recommends the use of garlic in the treatment of tumors. More than 3,500 years later, scientists are coming to the same conclusion. Researchers at Loma Linda University reviewed the wealth of studies on garlic and cancer and concluded that this potent plant inhibits the development of abnormal cells, slows the progression of established cancer cells (including cancers of the mouth, digestive tract, breast, liver, and skin), and stimulates the immune system. Garlic might do more than fend off disease; it may lengthen your years. Preliminary evidence shows that garlic extends the life span of cells in culture and has some ". . . youth preserving, anti-ageing, and beneficial effects on human [immune cells]," according to researchers at Aarhus University in Denmark.

Daniel Nixon, M.D., Professor of Medicine at the Hollings Cancer Center at Medical University of South Carolina, says, "There are 30 some odd chemopreventive compounds in garlic, but little conclusive evidence on exactly what does what. So we must rely at this point on the wisdom of the ages."

HOW MUCH OF WHAT?

So how much garlic is enough? Again, disagreement prevails. While some researchers suggest as much as 10 cloves a day, others offer more realistic advice. According to Stephen Fulder, Ph.D., in his book *Garlic: Nature's Original Remedy,* ". . . an appropriate standard medicinal dose of garlic is around three cloves a day." This amount of garlic added to sauces on pasta, stews, soups, casseroles, or baked chicken (to name only a few possibilities), adds flavor to your diet and could provide natural health insurance. Whether more is better remains questionable.

But what about those who tremble at the thought of eating that much garlic? Who want a social life outside of their Wednesday night "Garlic Anonymous" group? Are any of the commercial powders, capsules, or extracts worth their weight? Here the controversy heats up from warm to red hot, because (1) no one really knows what components of garlic should be included in a supplement, and (2) with little or no regulation or standardization, there is little guarantee of a product's effectiveness.

Basically, it's a consumer-beware market for garlic supplements. Analysis of garlic products reveals a 33-fold difference in content from one product to another. Unless the label lists specific amounts (per capsule or tablet) of active ingredients, such as allicin, S-allyl-cysteine, ajoene, and diallyl sulfides, or at least total sulfur content, then assume the product is "condiment grade" and no better, or worse, than garlic powder seasoning.

Cooking with garlic spices up your diet, while possibly adding life to your years. Even if three cloves a day is not a therapeutic dose, if it helps you cut back on salt and fat, then you're a winner either way.

The Garlic Lover's Tool Kit: Part 2

Here are a few suggestions for taming the garlic-breath dragon:

1. Eat fresh parsley or watercress with your garlic.
2. Mix garlic with other strong flavors, such as fennel, dill, aniseed, or caraway.
3. Chew on a coffee bean.
4. Drink lemon juice.
5. Eat lime sherbet for dessert.
6. To remove the scent of chopped garlic from your fingers, rub hands with lemon, followed by salt. Rinse and wash with soapy water.

Calorie Cutback: What the Research Shows

"NEVER EAT ANYTHING AT ONE SITTING THAT YOU CAN'T LIFT."

Miss Piggy

There might be a dietary trick to maximize your life span and avoid most of the age-related diseases, but you're not going to like it. If the abundance of research on animals showing that calorie restriction increases life span can be applied to people, then cutting your food intake by about half for the rest of your life is all it would take to make you the healthiest centenarian on the block.

"Calorie restriction is the only manipulation known in mammals to improve both life expectancy and life span," says Dr. George Roth, Chief of Molecular Physiology and Genetics section of the National Institute on Aging in Baltimore, Maryland. Every mammal the researchers have studied, including mice, rats, hamsters, and monkeys, increases its life span from two- to four-fold when calorie intake is cut to 60 percent of what's called "ad libitum," or 60 percent of what the animals usually eat to feel satisfied and full. Cut the fat at the same time, and the animals live even longer.

The secret is undernutrition, not malnutrition, which means drastically reducing calories while still providing all the vitamins and minerals in optimal amounts for health. Every mouthful must be nutrient-packed, while every mouthful in excess of basic calorie needs increases the risk for disease and aging. The good news is that it's never too late to cut back, since even older animals placed on calorie-restrictive diets live longer and age more slowly than their full-fed friends.

The benefits of semi-fasting far exceed just living longer. The hungry animals also are disease-free. Every age-related disorder—from heart disease, diabetes, and cancer to memory loss and dwindling immunity—seems to vanish. Blood levels of the stress hormones and disease-causing free radicals also drop. In fact, people might reduce their cancer risk by half if they cut calories.

No one is sure why drastically cutting calories boosts longevity. Restricting food might decrease free-radical reactions in the body or alter hormone levels. Another theory states that semi-starving the body lowers the metabolic rate (the rate of life), consequently slowing the aging process. Calorie restriction also boosts growth hormone levels that otherwise drop as a person ages, which might halt or slow many age-related symptoms (see Chapter 4).

The big question is whether or not people are enough like rats to expect the same results. "Calorie restriction has only been studied in animals with short lifespans," warns Jeffrey Blumberg, Ph.D., Professor of Nutrition at the USDA Human Nutrition Research Center at Tufts University in Boston. "It is possible that the lengthened lifespans in these starved animals is a survival mechanism that allows them to live a few extra months, long enough to survive the drought or famine and reproduce." There are no published long-term studies on the effects of semi-fasting on longevity in humans or bigger animals, which live for many decades, not several months. However, studies currently in progress on monkeys show promising results.

There is a wealth of indirect evidence, however, showing that humans could successfully trade a lot less food for a little more life. For example, overweight people die at younger ages than do fit and lean (but not skinny) people. In addition, Seventh Day Adventists, who avoid meat and are leaner than the average American, also live longer. On the other hand, drastic drops in weight or frequent weight fluctuations have been linked to increased mortality, especially in middle-aged and older people.

To maximize the benefits of calorie restriction while minimizing the deprivation and possible harm, a person's best bet is to achieve a lean and fit weight in the early years and then maintain that weight throughout life. As Dr. Blumberg points out, "Either being too skinny or too fat increases a person's risk of dying early." For those beyond their early years, the best bet is to improve fitness (see Chapter 8) and attain a desirable weight by losing pounds gradually and permanently (see Chapter 12).

Move It

"RAISE YOUR SAIL ONE FOOT AND YOU GET TEN FEET OF WIND."
Chinese proverb

If someone said he had a pill that would slow aging, help prevent heart disease and cancer, and help you feel and look younger for the rest of your life, and that it had no side effects other than improved mood and self-image, would you take it? You'd be crazy not to! Well, it may not be a pill, but there *is* something you can do every day that provides all of these benefits: exercise.

You not only can slow the aging process, but you may even be able to reverse it with exercise. A weekly routine that includes some weight-bearing exercise such as walking with some strength-training exercise such as lifting weights helps prevent bone deterioration and even reverses bone loss, reduces the risk of developing heart disease, helps maintain a desirable weight, reduces the risk of losing your independence later in life due to frailty and weakness, might even reduce cancer risk, and is essential to achieving the vitality to enjoy those extra years. In fact, an unfit person at any age can reduce his or her risk of dying prematurely by up to 50 percent by becoming fit, and active people are two decades "younger" than their couch potato counterparts. (See Chapter 8 for a detailed description of why exercise can turn back the hands of time and how to do it right.)

The Anti-Aging Diet in Chapter 7 will explain in detail how to eat for a long and active life. Emphasizing antioxidant- and phytochemical-rich foods and garlic, cutting back on unnecessary calories, and combining these diet strategies with a physically active lifestyle will stack your deck against aging!

Chapter 5

ANTI-AGING POTIONS: DHEA, GROWTH HORMONE, MELATONIN, CARNITINE, AND COENZYME Q10

"Get the facts first. You can distort them later."

Mark Twain

With the largest segment of the population approaching middle age, it is not surprising that anti-aging potions are hitting the market faster than ever. All of these hormone-like products, from DHEA to melatonin, are backed by scanty research at best; their long-term safety is unknown. Hormones have far-reaching effects on the body, many of which are poorly understood. Like the estrogen derivatives, such as DES, given to pregnant women decades ago that resulted in increased cancer risks in offspring, some of these consequences might not surface for decades. While in many cases the research on the "new" anti-aging hormones is promising, anyone who takes these products is playing Russian roulette with their long-term health.

Don't Believe Everything You Hear or Read

"YOU CAN STROKE PEOPLE WITH WORDS."
F. Scott Fitzgerald

Americans' insatiable appetite for nutrition news has spurred the media to amplify its reporting of the hottest topics, but newsworthy is not always factual. Moreover, there is seldom time for reporters to decipher how one study fits into the wealth of information on that topic. Worse yet, important subtleties in the study's findings usually are left on the cutting room floor. In short, we get a truncated tidbit of nutrition news.

How is someone to decipher truth from tabloids? According to Holly Atkinson, M.D. and Editor of *HealthNews,* a consumer health letter from the publishers of the *New England Journal of Medicine,* you should pay attention to how the media report clinical research and how you interpret the stories.

Rule 1: Be wary of overnight breakthroughs. "Science is like a needlepoint, with each study representing one stitch in the tapestry," says Dr. Atkinson. A clear perspective and sound dietary recommendations come only when we weigh the preponderance of the evidence.

Rule 2: Count the legs of the subjects in the study and consider any research on quadrupeds with an interested, but skeptical, eye. "Studies on animals provide the foundation, but these studies only point us in the direction for more research; they can't necessarily be extrapolated to people," warns Dr. Atkinson. For example, caffeine produces birth defects in mice, but there is no evidence that caffeine or coffee has similar effects in humans.

Even in studies on humans, question whether the population being studied is representative of you. Then, select which nutrition changes to make in your life, based on your personal health profile. For example, people who aren't salt-sensitive will do little to reduce their risk for hypertension by cutting back on salt, but cutting back on fat intake might reduce a person's risk of more pressing health concerns, such as weight gain, cancer, and heart disease.

Rule 3: Ask some basic questions about the study, such as who conducted it (is it a reliable group of researchers, such as those conducting the Nurse's Health Study from Harvard who publish ongoing information on women's health?), and where it was published (look for reputable journals such as *Journal of the American Medical Association, New England Journal of Medicine,* or *Annals of Internal Medicine*).

Rule 4: Be wary of any article that thrives on conflict. "The media is very good at structuring stories for controversy by finding people to express the most diverse opinions on an issue," says Dr. Atkinson. Readers would be better served if the reporter discussed the common ground of scientific evidence where researchers agree, rather than disagree.

With these rules in mind, here is a brief look at the truth behind some of the latest headlines.

DHEA: The Mother of All Anti-Aging Tonics

"WHEN YOU ARE RIGHT YOU CANNOT BE TOO RADICAL; WHEN YOU ARE WRONG, YOU CANNOT BE TOO CONSERVATIVE."

Dr. Martin Luther King, Jr.

Since hormones are blamed for everything from moodiness to sterility, it isn't surprising that a hormone should be touted as the cause of the ultimate disorder—aging. And so it goes for DHEA (dehydroepiandrosterone), a steroid hormone produced in the adrenal glands that serves as a building block for the sex hormones, estrogen and testosterone.

DHEA rose to fame in the mid-1980s when researchers at the University of California at San Diego (UCSD) reported that plasma levels of DHEA were linked to all disease-related causes of premature death, from heart disease to cancer. The study showed that low blood levels of DHEA were as important as age in predicting death caused by heart disease. The researchers concluded that low DHEA levels were not a result, but rather appeared to be a cause, of disease and death.

Subsequent research showed that high DHEA levels might increase muscle mass, strength, and immune function, as well as improve mood, energy, libido, mental capacity, memory, and weight loss, while possibly lowering the risk for heart disease, cancer, osteoporosis, diabetes, joint pain, fatigue, high blood pressure, depression, and stress-related diseases.

It also was found that the levels of the hormone drop at a rate of about 3 percent a year; by the time people reach 70 years of age, they have only about 10 to 20 percent of the DHEA they had in their twenties. One study from the University of Bologna in Italy found that old men with high DHEA levels were much more active and vital compared to their same-age colleagues with low DHEA levels.

Why would the body produce so much DHEA early in life and so little later on? Could a DHEA deficit slowly rob people of their youth and health? No one knows the answers to these questions. While DHEA appears to be wasted on the young and dwindling levels in the old go hand-in-hand with disease, it is a major leap in logic to assume that boosting lagging DHEA levels will turn back the clock any more than growing hair on a bald head will erase wrinkles. Critics warn that most studies have been done on rodents. Besides the obvious differences between man and mouse, rodents also have a short life span, which is a major stumbling block when trying to extrapolate data on longevity to humans.

Despite the controversy, the few studies that have investigated DHEA therapy in people are promising. Recent studies at the University of California, San Diego (UCSD), found that DHEA supplements restore the hormone to youthful levels, while raising HDL cholesterol (the "good" cholesterol) and improving immune function in men and women between the ages of 40 and 70 who take up to 50 milligrams daily. Moreover, up to 82 percent of those taking supplements reported they handled stress better, slept more soundly, and rated their general well-being as higher.

THE DOWN SIDE OF DHEA

Reaping the potential benefits of DHEA has a price. Opponents warn that DHEA produces unpredictable results, with side effects ranging from acne and facial hair to greater risks for breast and uterine cancer in women and prostate cancer and aggressiveness in men, birth defects in pregnant women, and liver damage. No one is even sure how DHEA works in the body.

The biggest risk is that no one knows the long-term consequences of taking DHEA. Granted, DHEA-supplemented subjects in the UCSD study reported no side effects after six months; however, whether it is equally harmless to take DHEA for years—which is what someone might need to do to permanently keep disease and aging at bay—is anyone's guess. Many researchers recommend taking DHEA only with physician supervision and routine checks of steroid and cholesterol levels, glucose tolerance, and prostate health in men.

The Food and Drug Administration (FDA) has discouraged the sale of DHEA. Supplements made from wild Mexican yams (claimed to contain the building blocks for DHEA) are available in some health food stores, but scientists say the body can't convert the compound into DHEA. Supplements might not be the only way to boost DHEA levels. One study found that people who meditated daily maintained higher DHEA levels than nonmeditators.

The bottom line? Until there are conclusive studies on DHEA's effectiveness and long-term safety, the best that can be said is that DHEA may not extend life, but it may help a person age gracefully. The question is whether or not you're willing to be the guinea pig for an unproven, but promising, anti-aging hormone.

Growth Hormone

"TAKE CALCULATED RISKS. THAT IS QUITE DIFFERENT FROM BEING RASH."

General George S. Patton

As with most anti-aging quick fixes, this potion started out with a "bang" but is rapidly fizzling as its effectiveness becomes questionable and the cost and side effects mount.

Growth hormone, also called somatotropin, is released by the pituitary gland in the brain beginning in childhood. The hormone enters the bloodstream in pulses, especially during the early hours of sleep. In the liver, it is converted to other compounds that act as growth messengers throughout the body. In childhood, growth hormone aids in strengthening and lengthening bones and stimulating protein synthesis that results in bigger tissues, muscles, and organs, including the heart, kidney, and skin.

A wealth of research shows that levels of the hormone gradually drop by about 14 percent for every decade of adult life. By the age of 60, about four of every 10 persons have 20 percent of the growth hormone that they had at puberty.

Growth hormone levels in some older people, especially couch potatoes, are so low they can't be measured.

More important is that the physical signs of aging mirror the decline in growth hormone. Dwindling levels of growth hormone are associated with reduced muscle mass and strength, increased body fat, reduced resistance to colds and infections, elevated cholesterol, and increased risk for developing high blood pressure and osteoporosis. Research on older animals and humans shows that those who maintain high growth hormone levels naturally or by injecting the hormone sometimes see improvements in many of these conditions.

Growth hormone is not a panacea, since low levels don't cause aging per se. Rather this is one pebble in the avalanche of aging. Raising growth hormone levels may restore some age-related symptoms, but it won't affect many other common aging changes.

THE PROS AND CONS OF GROWTH HORMONE

Growth hormone's biggest claim to fame came in 1990 when a study from the Medical College of Wisconsin in Milwaukee reported that injecting this hormone into older men could turn back the clock when it came to body composition, leaving the men packing denser bones, increased muscle, and less fat. In this study, 21 men between the ages of 61 and 81 with low growth hormone levels injected the hormone three times weekly. After six months, the men taking growth hormone showed an almost 9 percent increase in muscle, a 14 percent decrease in fat, and a 1.6 percent increase in bone density, compared to no changes in the control group. Growth hormone also improved skin tone. Even more exciting, the men taking growth hormone reported improvements in well-being, enhanced vitality, and increased mental alertness. It was the first time any drug had so clearly reversed the signs of aging in humans.

In the next few years, however, the tide would turn against growth hormone. A study from the Veterans Affairs Medical Center in Palo Alto, California, investigated the effects of the hormone on 18 healthy older men, ages 65 to 82, who were on a strength-training program while injecting growth hormone daily. The men on growth hormone showed some improvements in muscle and bone, but there were no differences in muscle strength between the hormone-treated group and a control group. Another study from Washington University School of Medicine in St. Louis reported similar findings.

In a third study, 52 men, ages 70 to 85 years, with initially low growth hormone levels injected the hormone three times a week for six months. While lean body mass increased slightly (4.3 percent) and fat decreased by 13 percent, the men did not show greater strength, endurance, cognitive function, or even mood. Even worse, the men receiving growth hormone were riddled with negative side effects.

THE SIDE EFFECTS AND SOLUTIONS

The more scientists test growth hormone injections, the more adverse side effects surface. Long-term use of growth hormone increases a person's risk for insulin resistance and diabetes-like symptoms, water retention possibly triggering heart failure, enlarged bones and increased production of connective tissue possibly resulting in carpal tunnel syndrome and arthritis, and elevated blood pressure. Men are likely to develop tender, enlarged breasts, while women might be at greater risk for breast cancer. The older people are, the more likely they are to experience side effects. One study on animals found that raising growth hormone levels too high actually shortened life expectancy!

Granted, lowering the dose reduces many of these side effects, but also might limit the hormone's effectiveness. More importantly, any benefits are lost rapidly when the hormone is discontinued. So to see a lasting effect, a person must take growth hormone for the rest of his or her life. It's anyone's guess what the long-term consequences of that might be. Couple the physical risk with the monetary cost of growth hormone injections (estimates range as high as $15,000 to $30,000 a year) and it is clear that the cost of taking growth hormone might outweigh any minor improvements in strength or skin tone.

There is a safer and more proven alternative: daily exercise significantly boosts growth hormone levels, even in older persons. Other growth hormone stimulators include cutting calories, increasing your intake of vitamin A–rich foods such as carrots and spinach, and including more arginine-rich foods such as oatmeal and other whole grains, fish, and cheese in your daily diet.

Melatonin

"LIFE IS SHORT. LIVE IT UP."
Nikita Khrushchev

Melatonin, a hormone secreted in the evening by the pineal gland in the brain, regulates the body's daily time clock—the ebb and flow of wakefulness and sleepiness. Melatonin levels drop with age, so that by age 65 a person has one-third to one-quarter the melatonin levels of a 25-year-old. One can raise melatonin levels by taking a daily supplement.

The theory is that when the daily melatonin cycle deteriorates with aging, other body rhythms are weakened. This gradual loss of function underlies aging and increases a person's susceptibility to age-related diseases. Limited research shows that melatonin supplements might help slow some of the symptoms of aging, but this hormone can't reset the aging clock that underlies these problems, nor can it extend life span.

Melatonin has antioxidant capabilities perhaps more potent than those of other antioxidants, such as vitamin E; consequently, proponents speculate that dwindling melatonin levels expose the body to the free-radical damage that contributes to aging. The brain generates more free radicals than any other organ, so maintaining an active antioxidant system is paramount to maintaining mental acuity as we age. However, while a few studies on aging animals showed that melatonin could increase life expectancy by up to 30 percent and stimulate the immune system, no studies have been conducted on humans.

While no side effects of melatonin supplementation have been identified as yet, the best that can be said is that it helps people get a good night's sleep and glide more easily through jet lag. There is no evidence that it can be counted on as the next anti-aging drug. Moreover, melatonin is not regulated by the Food and Drug Administration, so the purity and dosage of any product is not assured. Scientists urge people to be cautious and to consult a physician before self-medicating with such a compound when so little is known about it.

To boost melatonin levels naturally, try increasing exercise, consuming a low-calorie diet, and consuming more carnitine, which might help stimulate production of melatonin.

Carnitine

"DRINK NOTHING WITHOUT SEEING IT; SIGN NOTHING WITHOUT READING IT."

Spanish proverb

While carnitine might help boost melatonin levels, its effects on aging are not certain. Carnitine is an amino acid (a building block for protein). It can be made in the body when two essential amino acids, lysine and methionine, along with vitamin B_6, niacin, vitamin C, and iron are present. Therefore, carnitine is not theoretically needed from dietary sources, as long as all these building blocks are consumed in ample amounts. Carnitine comes in two forms; only L-carnitine is biologically active, while D-carnitine is not.

Carnitine's primary function is to transport fats into the cells' powerhouses—the mitochondria—for conversion to energy. A deficiency of this amino acid reduces the body's capacity to obtain energy from fats. Consequently, the body turns to glucose and glycogen (the body's storage form of glucose). Since these energy sources are limited, within hours or days the body experiences impaired metabolic function, including muscle weakness, exercise intolerance, and accumulation of fat in muscle.

Maintaining a high carnitine level in the brain also stimulates production of melatonin, which indirectly might aid in the prevention of aging. More serious consequences of long-term carnitine deficiency include heart failure, liver failure, and nervous system disorders. Male organs and fluids essential for reproduction also contain high concentrations of carnitine and probably also are adversely affected by a deficiency.

Levels of carnitine depend on both dietary intake and the amount produced naturally by the body. This amino acid is found in almost every cell in the body, with high concentrations in the adrenal glands, heart, muscle, fat tissue, and liver, and small concentrations in the brain and kidney. Carnitine concentrations in muscle and the heart are especially high, often approaching 20 to 100 times those levels in the blood. This suggests that the tissues richest in carnitine are unable to synthesize this factor and must take it from the blood, making muscles and the heart particularly susceptible to deficiencies.

CARNITINE AND HEART DISEASE

By far, the weight of the evidence on carnitine lies with the prevention of heart disease. Carnitine levels are low in people with heart disorders. In some cases, carnitine supplements can protect oxygen-deprived heart tissue and enhance the stress tolerance of the heart. Carnitine supplementation in patients with intermittent claudication (reduced blood flow in the extremities associated with advanced heart and blood vessel disease) increases muscle carnitine levels and improves the patient's ability to walk. Doses of 500 to 2,000 milligrams also have shown reasonable success in the treatment of high blood triglyceride levels.

CARNITINE AND EXERCISE

Although it regulates when, how much, and how fast the exercising muscle cells burn fat, carnitine remains controversial when it comes to improving a workout. Some studies show that carnitine supplementation (2 to 6 grams daily) increases muscle carnitine levels and improves performance by 6 to 11 percent. Other studies show no effect.

CARNITINE AND AGING

Theoretically carnitine's decline with aging could contribute to some age-related conditions such as muscle weakness, fatigue, memory loss, decreased immunity, and heart disease. A handful of studies (mostly on animals) reports that supplementing with carnitine results in pronounced improvements in brain chemistry, heart and immune functions, and fat metabolism. The elevated carnitine levels help cells recover from damage to the genetic code, thus preventing the cascade of events that leads to cell death and possibly aging.

Although the Recommended Dietary Allowances (RDAs) do not specify a requirement for carnitine, research supports the inability of the tissues to manufacture enough to meet all the body's needs. Consequently, dietary intake of both the dietary building blocks and carnitine is essential. In general, the amount of carnitine in fruits, vegetables, grains, and legumes is low, while foods of animal origin contain higher amounts of this amino acid. Unfortunately, the carnitine content is known for only a limited number of foods and the effects of cooking on carnitine concentrations are unknown.

People who consume limited amounts of carnitine, such as strict vegetarians or those with increased needs for carnitine, might benefit from moderate-dose supplements of 2 to 4 grams daily.

Coenzyme Q10: Myth or Miracle Pill?

"AVOID THE CROWD. DO YOUR OWN THINKING INDEPENDENTLY. BE THE CHESS PLAYER, NOT THE CHESS PIECE."

Ralph Charell

Every cell in the body depends on a fat-soluble substance called coenzyme Q10 to help convert food and oxygen to energy. Without coenzyme Q10, cells cannot perform their essential functions and life would cease within minutes. Numerous studies have found that this vital substance also benefits health in many ways, from improving heart function to boosting immunity and possibly aiding in weight management.

Another name for coenzyme Q10 is ubiquinone, which reflects its ubiquitous distribution throughout the body. Like other coenzymes, coenzyme Q10 assists in metabolic reactions. However, it has a unique ability to aid in the complex process of transforming food and oxygen to ATP, the base fuel required by the body for everything from running a race to digesting food, making new cells, or even pumping blood through the heart.

Virtually every cell of the human body contains coenzyme Q10; however, the mitochondria, the powerhouses of cells where ATP is produced, contain the most. The heart and liver, because they contain the most mitochondria per cell, have the greatest amount of coenzyme Q10 of any tissue or organ in the body.

Coenzyme Q10 levels could be inadequate to meet the body's needs for a number of reasons, including:

- defects in production;
- impaired synthesis caused by nutritional deficiencies;

- greater cellular need resulting from strenuous exercise or from a disease state, such as cardiovascular disease, diabetes, or Alzheimer's disease;
- interference in coenzyme Q10 levels or function from medications;
- advancing age; or
- a sedentary lifestyle.

In addition to its helper role in the release of energy, coenzyme Q10 might act as an antioxidant, neutralizing free radicals that cause potentially irreversible damage to cells, tissues, and organs. Several studies demonstrate that coenzyme Q10 performs many of the same antioxidant functions as vitamin E and selenium in protecting the blood vessels, heart, brain, and other tissues from free-radical damage.

Coenzyme Q10 was first shown to strengthen the immune system almost 25 years ago. Since then, numerous scientific trials have demonstrated that this natural enzyme fights bacteria, increases antibody numbers, resists viral infections, and produces a greater number of immune system cells. Proponents claim that supplementing with coenzyme Q10 might return an impaired immune system to normal or even optimal levels.

But does it prevent aging? Animal studies repeatedly show that maintaining strong immune and antioxidant systems results in a longer, healthier life. If these results are transferrable to humans, coenzyme Q10 might improve longevity by enhancing immune function and deactivating free radicals before they destroy mitochondria and cellular function. Since coenzyme Q10 levels decrease with age, maintaining optimal intake of this natural coenzyme throughout life might delay many age-related changes.

While the research on coenzyme Q10 is promising, dietary supplements of this substance have met with controversy. However, people in other countries, such as Japan and Canada, have long used coenzyme Q10 to protect cardiovascular function, strengthen the immune system, and counteract the aging process—with little or no reported side effects at dosages between 30mg and 90mg.

Coenzyme Q10 should not be viewed as a panacea or a miracle cure. In fact, this substance is an excellent example of how more is not necessarily better. If coenzyme Q10 levels are optimal, ingesting more will not enhance its effects. However, if low coenzyme Q10 levels are contributing to dysfunction, increasing dietary intake could be the "fuel booster" the body needs.

Chapter 6

PRO-AGING FOODS AND SUBSTANCES: WHAT YOU SHOULD AVOID TO STAY YOUNG

"Thou shouldst eat to live; not live to eat."
Cicero

The anti-aging foods are easy to spot. They are the minimally processed, wholesome items that traditionally line the perimeter of your local grocery store. You find them in abundance in the produce section, as whole-grain bread in the bakery, and as nonfat milk and yogurt in the dairy case. Other anti-aging foods include cooked dried beans and peas, soy milk, and canned fruits. In fact, the anti-aging foods far outnumber the pro-aging foods.

There are a few foods or food ingredients you want to avoid, or at least limit, if you're planning to live vitally for a century or more. These include fat (especially saturated fat), meat, and trans fatty acids in processed vegetable oils.

Fat in General

"YOU BETTER LIVE YOUR BEST AND ACT YOUR BEST AND THINK YOUR
BEST TODAY, FOR TODAY IS THE SURE PREPARATION FOR TOMORROW
AND ALL THE OTHER TOMORROWS THAT FOLLOW."

Harriet Martineau

The hands-down best thing you can do diet-wise for longevity is to cut the saturated fat from your diet. Saturated fats in meat and whole-milk dairy products have been linked to an increased risk for a host of age-related diseases, from heart disease to cancer. Not all fats are bad, however. Moderate intake of olive oil and fish oils might actually help extend life and health.

The Mediterranean Menu

Traditional Mediterranean diets are based on foods of plant origin. They also are linked with some of the longest life expectancies in the world. The fat in these diets comes mainly from olive oil. To eat like a Greek and live a long and healthy life, follow these guidelines:

1. Any fat in the diet should come mainly from olive oil.
2. Consume less than one alcoholic beverage daily.
3. Consume daily 3 ounces or more of cooked dried beans and peas.
4. More than half the day's allotment of calories should come from pasta and other starches (i.e., a serving should be mostly pasta and only a little sauce).
5. Consume daily eight or more servings of fruits and vegetables.
6. Avoid meat and meat products, or limit them to no more than 3 ounces daily.
7. Limit intake of fatty dairy products.
8. Eat moderate portions to maintain a desirable weight.

Most people already know they should cut the fat, but many are still consuming far too much. Why? One reason is confusion. Although most people know that fat is bad for them, many can't tell one fat from another, a calorie from a gram of fat, or whether blood cholesterol is different from the cholesterol in an egg yolk. "Knowledge levels are so inadequate that they have to be considered obstacles to successfully implementing effective dietary change," state researchers at the Food and Drug Administration (FDA) who have completed assessments of Americans' fat know-how.

In addition, misinformation is rampant. For example, in the FDA study, only one in every five people knew that a tablespoon of any fat, be it lard, canola oil, or margarine, contains the same amount of calories (approximately 110). Two-thirds of Americans are confused about how cholesterol differs from other fats and therefore might mistakenly assume it can be "burned" as fuel during exercise.

Food manufacturers are partially to blame for this confusion. In this fat-phobic nation, a label that reads "cholesterol free," "light," or "low calorie" gives almost any food the aura of nutritional quality, even if more often than not the food is less nutritious than the label implies. Fast-food restaurants have capitalized on America's fear of fat by touting fish and chicken entrees as healthful alternatives to traditional hamburgers, while many of these dishes, such as some fast-food fish filet sandwiches, derive up to 56 percent of their calories from fat.

Despite the confusion, the fat issue is the most clearly defined topic in nutrition. Yes, most Americans should cut total fat and do it for the rest of their lives. However, everyone needs some fat in the diet to help absorb fat-soluble vitamins, to supply the essential fat called linoleic acid, and just for the pleasure, taste, and aroma of a good meal. Most people should aim for a daily fat-calorie intake of under 30 percent, but no less than 20 percent of their total calories. (People attempting to reduce fat deposits in their arteries should strive for less than 15 percent fat calories.) Stockpiling some fat facts might help you dodge the fat in your diet.

FAT FACTS

The fats that supply calories and texture in foods, that float in your blood, and that accumulate in your thighs and hips are called triglycerides. They can be saturated or unsaturated, and the unsaturated ones can be either monounsaturated or polyunsaturated. All triglycerides supply more than 250 calories per ounce (or 9 calories per gram, equal to the weight of a paper clip or raisin), can contribute to weight gain and elevated body fat, and are associated with numerous diseases, from heart disease to cancer.

All foods contain mixtures of saturated and unsaturated fats with one fat usu-

FAT TRICKS

At a loss on how to cut the fat? Here are a few suggestions that maximize taste, while minimizing unnecessary fat and calories.

Instead of...	Use...
Whole-milk ricotta cheese	Nonfat ricotta cheese.
Cream or whole milk	Low-fat or nonfat milk, evaporated nonfat milk, or nonfat milk mixed with instant nonfat dry milk solids.
Preparing cream sauces with whole milk and butter	Nonfat milk or evaporated nonfat milk thickened with flour or cornstarch.
Using the full amount of hard cheese	Portions in sauces reduced by ⅓ to ½, sprinkled or grated on top of dishes as garnish.
Sour cream	Nonfat sour cream.
Whipped cream	Partially frozen evaporated nonfat milk, whipped into a foam.
Cream cheese	Fat-free or reduced-fat cream cheese.
Whole eggs	Egg whites, two per whole egg.
Chicken with skin	Chicken with skin removed.
Tuna packed in oil	Tuna packed in water.
Preparing 4-to-8 ounce meat servings	2-to-3 ounce servings mixed or served with rice, noodles, and vegetables.
Fatty meats	Ground round, extra-lean chuck, or ground beef or turkey; trim fat from meat.
Frying meat	Baked, roasted, broiled, steamed, or stewed meat, with excess fat drained.

Continued

Instead of . . .	Use . . .
Flavoring soup with ham hocks	Lean pork or one to two drops liquid smoke.
Fatty stock, stews, and gravies	Stocks, stews, and gravies made from refrigerated meat, with hardened fat skimmed from surface. Invest in a defatting cup that pours from the bottom, leaving fat on the top.
Regular salad dressings	Low- or nonfat salad dressings, or nonfat yogurt or buttermilk-based dressings flavored with rice vinegar or lemon juice.
Oil, margarine, and butter for sautéing	Nonstick pans, defatted chicken stock, or nonstick sprays. Hint: vegetable and grain dishes should be less than 20 percent fat calories!
Using the full amount of oil in a recipe	One-third of the suggested amount. Substitute up to half the oil with an equivalent amount of applesauce in quick breads and muffins.
Margarine or butter on toast	Fruit butter, jam, or thick applesauce.
Mayonnaise on sandwiches and in salads	Reduced-fat mayonnaise, nonfat yogurt, or low-fat cottage cheese.
Pound cake	Angel-food cake.
Ice cream	Sherbet, sorbet, or nonfat ice cream.
Preparing French fries by deep-fat frying	Parboiled potato wedges brushed with olive oil and spices (try chili powder and crushed rosemary) and baked until browned.
Popping popcorn in oil	A hot-air popper.

ally predominating, such as saturated fat in meat and monounsaturated fat in avocados. In general, the harder a fat, the more saturated it is. Beef and milk fat (e.g., butter) and stick margarine are mostly saturated fats. Liquid oils are usually unsaturated fats and include the monounsaturated fats in olive and canola oils and the polyunsaturated fats in safflower, corn, soybean, and fish oils. Coconut, palm, and palm kernel oils are exceptions to the hardness rule. These liquid vegetable oils are highly saturated fats.

Cholesterol is a no-calorie fat, so it can't be exercised off, sweated out, or burned for energy. It is found only in animal products, including meats, chicken, fish, eggs, organ meats, and dairy products. It can be attacked and damaged by free radicals either during food preparation or within the blood. These damaged cholesterol oxides can set off a chain of events in the body's cells leading to cell death and possibly contributing to premature aging.

THE PARABLE OF OIL IN WATER

Just as homemade oil-and-vinegar dressing separates into a watery pool with a fat-slick topping, so also would fats if they were dumped directly into the blood. To solve this dilemma, the body transports fats by coating them with a water-soluble "bubble" of protein called a lipoprotein (*lipo* means fat). Low-density lipoproteins (LDLs) carry cholesterol out to the tissues. LDL is known as the "bad" cholesterol, since high LDL levels are linked to increased risk for atherosclerosis and heart disease. High-density lipoproteins (HDLs) carry excess cholesterol back to the liver, where it is processed and excreted. HDLs are the "good" cholesterol; the more HDL you have, the lower your risk for developing heart disease.

All of your blood cholesterol and triglycerides are packed into lipoproteins. Consequently, in a blood cholesterol test, your total cholesterol reading should approximate the sum of your LDL, HDL, and other lipoproteins. That is also why the ratio of total cholesterol to HDL cholesterol is so important. The ideal ratio is 4.5 to 1 or lower; i.e., for every 4.5 milligrams of total cholesterol, 1.0 milligram is packaged in HDLs. According to the National Cholesterol Education Program, a person's total cholesterol should remain below 200mg/dl (unless HDL is high), LDL should be lower than 130mg/dl, and HDL should be 35mg/dl or higher. (People under age 30 may want to shoot for an even lower total cholesterol of 180mg/dl.)

FEAR OF FRYING

A diet oozing with saturated grease from red meat and fatty dairy products raises the bad LDLs and lowers the good HDLs, increasing the risk for heart disease. Cut the saturated fat and blood cholesterol levels and heart disease rates drop. Cancer rates also decrease. A low-saturated, high-polyunsaturated diet (i.e., little meat and fatty dairy products, with a greater proportion of fat coming from salad oil) lowers total blood cholesterol levels but unfortunately also drops HDL levels, so you lose both good and bad cholesterol. Polyunsaturates also have another glitch: they increase a person's risk for cancer.

Olive oil is another story. This oil lowers total blood cholesterol and LDL cholesterol just like the polyunsaturated fats. However, olive oil also maintains HDL levels, thus lowering the total cholesterol-to-HDL ratio and improving heart disease risk. Olive oil also is not as susceptible as are polyunsaturated oils to damage by free radicals that escalate the atherosclerosis, heart disease, and cancer processes. Consequently, olive oil is the oil of choice.

Meat and Potatoes

"CULTIVATE ONLY THE HABITS THAT YOU ARE WILLING SHOULD MASTER YOU."

Elbert Hubbard

With meat linked to everything from heart disease to cancer, some people have taken the plunge and gone vegetarian. Even more have cut out red meat, though they still eat poultry and fish.

Several studies show that women who daily eat meat have a 50 percent higher risk of developing heart disease compared to vegetarian women, and disease risk for both sexes increases as the duration and frequency of meat consumption increases. Consequently, people who adopt a vegetarian diet early in life have a lower risk of disease than do people who wait until after age 50 to switch from meat to beans.

In all fairness to meat, it might not be the harmful effects of a T-bone steak per se, but the protective effects of other foods in the vegetarian diet that is the real boon, according to Paul Mills, Ph.D., Research Epidemiologist at the National Institute for Occupational Safety and Health in Cincinnati. Dr. Mills spent 10 years studying cancer in a group of 35,000 Seventh Day Adventists, a group with a high percentage of vegetarians and a lower cancer rate than found in the general public. "We were surprised to find that meat was not a significant factor in the development of certain types of cancer," says Dr. Mills. "However, we did find that people who ate lots of fruits, legumes, and vegetables were at much lower risk for certain cancers, probably because they simply didn't have as much room in their diets for other fattier foods."

Trans Slam

> "ONE SHOULD BE JUST AS CAREFUL IN CHOOSING ONE'S PLEASURES AS IN AVOIDING CALAMITIES."
>
> *Chinese proverb*

For years we've been told to avoid saturated fat-laden butter and instead spread margarine on our toast. Margarine was heart friendly because it was made from vegetable oil—or so we thought. Now several studies report that margarine might be as bad as, if not worse than, butter.

Margarine and shortening are liquid vegetable oils made creamy when manufacturers convert some of the unsaturated fats into saturated ones. To do this, hydrogens are added to the strings of carbon atoms that make up the fat molecule—hence the terms hydrogenation and hydrogenated vegetable oils.

Hydrogenation hardens a liquid vegetable oil so it looks, feels, and acts like naturally hard fats such as butter, beef tallow, and lard. Consequently, the processed oil doesn't ooze out of cookies or corn chips, spreads on an English muffin, and is the current fat of choice for frying everything from chicken to French fries at most fast-food restaurants. These benefits, combined with improved shelf life, low cost, and the "100% vegetable oil" on the label promising a low-saturated fat alternative to butter, were primary reasons why margarine was selling two-to-one over butter by 1993.

But hydrogenation also leaves a trail of unnatural fats in its wake as it smashes and rearranges the chemical bonds of the molecules, altering the form of up to one-third or more of the remaining unsaturated fats so their natural "cis" shape is transformed into an abnormal "trans" shape. It is these trans fatty acids (TFAs) that have caused all the commotion.

"Partially hydrogenated vegetable oils are a real problem," warns Mary Enig, Ph.D., former Research Associate at the University of Maryland and one of the first researchers to investigate TFAs in our food. What Dr. Enig began uncovering in the early 1980s has been confirmed by numerous studies: TFAs, in amounts typically consumed by Americans, raise total blood cholesterol and LDL choles- terol (the "bad" cholesterol) levels in much the same way as saturated fats. Large amounts also might lower HDL cholesterol levels (the "good" cholesterol). These changes upset the ratio of total cholesterol to HDL, increasing heart-disease risk by as much as 27 percent.

TFAs also might interfere with functioning of a natural fat called linoleic acid, a building block for powerful hormone-like compounds called prostaglandins. The preliminary evidence suggests possible links to cancer, insulin resistance, and obe- sity.

The potential health risks of TFAs wouldn't be an issue if we weren't eating a lot more of them than we think. Until the turn of the century, the naturally occurring TFAs in meat and dairy products comprised a small portion of the diet (approximately 3 percent of total fat intake). That changed dramatically when the food industry introduced hydrogenation into commercial food production. "The worst thing that could have happened is that natural fats were pulled out of our diets and replaced with hydrogenated vegetable oils," says Dr. Enig. Now TFAs account for as much as 25 to 60 percent of the fat in many processed foods. Americans probably average about 10 to 20 grams of TFAs daily, or 15 to 30 percent of the fat in a moderately low-fat, 2,000-calorie-per-day diet. It is easy to consume 20 grams of TFAs just from snack foods alone. Daily intake of up to 100 grams is possible if a person regularly eats potato chips, cookies, crackers, or fried fast foods.

According to the research, as TFA intakes increase, health risks escalate. The Nurses' Health Study, conducted by Walter Willett, M.D., Dr.P. H., and colleagues at the Harvard School of Public Health in Boston, compared dietary intakes to

TRANS-LATING YOUR TABLE

How much trans fatty acids are in the foods you eat? Here are some estimates to help you tally your intake.

Food	TFAs (grams)
Butter (1 Tbsp)	0.40
Mayonnaise (1 Tbsp)	0.55
Dinner roll (1)	0.85
Diet margarine (1 Tbsp)	0.90
Pound cake (1 oz)	0.98–2.15
Vanilla wafers (8)	1.00
Liquid squeeze margarine (1 Tbsp)	1.21
Sugar cookies (2)	1.33
Cookie, chocolate sandwich (3)	2.00
Microwave popcorn, with fat (4 cups)	2.00
Cheese danish (1)	2.24–5.20
Crackers (12)	2.40
Hard stick margarine (1 Tbsp)	2.00–4.60
Vegetable shortening (1 Tbsp)	3.00
Chocolate cake rolls (2)	4.00
Buttermilk biscuit dough (1 biscuit)	4.00
Packaged doughnut (1)	5.00–6.00
Apple turnover (1)	6.50
French fries, 1 large order	4.00–7.90

disease rates in more than 85,000 women and found that as intakes of TFA-containing foods (including margarine, cookies, biscuits, and cakes) increased, so did women's risks for heart disease. Women with the highest intakes had nearly twice the risk of those who ate few hydrogenated fats; women who ate four or more teaspoons of margarine a day increased their risk of developing heart disease by 66 percent, compared to those who limited margarine to less than one teaspoon a month.

Dr. Willett feels that TFAs might contribute to 30,000 heart-disease deaths in the United States each year, even when intake is moderate. Data from the Nurses' Health Study suggest that the risk might be up to five times higher. The evidence against TFAs is so convincing that the Center for Science in the Public Interest (the same group that uncovered the fat in Chinese food and movie-theater popcorn) has petitioned the Food and Drug Administration to require that TFAs be listed on labels, as saturated fats are now.

The claims on processed and fast foods, such as "Cooked in 100 percent vegetable oil" or "No saturated fats," don't offer the protection we once thought. The bottom line: Americans need to bite the bullet when it comes to fat and just eat less of it, period.

Cut the Trans

To cut back on TFAs,

• Read labels and avoid foods that contain "partially hydrogenated vegetable oils." Also avoid foods fried in fast-food restaurants, from doughnuts to French fries, where up to 40 percent of the fats are TFAs.

• If you must use margarine, remember that diet or whipped margarine contains fewer TFAs than tub margarine, and tub margarine contains fewer TFAs than stick margarine. (Look for brands that list water and/or liquid vegetable oil as the first ingredients.)

• Make your own spread by whipping one stick of butter with a half cup of canola oil, then store in the refrigerator. This blend is lower in saturated fat than butter and is trans-free.

• Better yet, switch to olive oil and use it sparingly.

"As far as we know, there is no safe dose for trans fatty acids, but the lower the intake the better," concludes Dr. Willett. One thing we do know: an occasional teaspoon of something spreadable is fine, but the news on margarine doesn't give people a green light on butter.

Don't Smoke

"HE WHO PUTS UP WITH INSULT INVITES INJURY."
Jewish proverb

Next to eating well and exercising daily, the most important habit a person can adopt is avoiding tobacco. Smokers age faster and die younger of heart disease and cancer. They suffer from more age-related diseases, look older, and have thinner skin and more wrinkles, possibly because smoking causes the release of an enzyme that breaks down skin elasticity or restricts the blood supply to the skin. Smoking also escalates cell turnover, the risk of cell mutations, and the development of cancerous cells because of its damaging effects on the lining of the lungs. As mentioned in Chapter 2, anything that speeds up cell turnover, from sunbathing to smoking, sets the aging clock at high gear.

Chapter 7

THE ANTI-AGING DIET

"Keep yourself alive by throwing day by day fresh currents of thought and emotion into the things you have come to do from habit."

John Lancaster Spalding

he Eight Dietary Guidelines for a Long and Healthy Life:

- Eat eight fruits and vegetables each day.
- Eat beans at least five times a week.
- Eat minimally processed foods.
- Drink at least eight glasses of water a day.
- Eliminate excess calories.
- Eat little meals and snacks.
- Enjoy food.
- Supplement responsibly.

Feeling energetic and alive is a byproduct of good health and is fundamental to vitality. What you eat must provide all of the building blocks and fuel to help you attain and maintain that good health. While most people wouldn't dream of putting bad gasoline in their cars, it is common for people to supply their bodies with low-grade fuel and then wonder why their most precious machine is showing wear and tear.

What you choose to eat determines what will happen at the cellular level in your body, where all metabolic processes occur and where life and vitality begin. We have up to 100 trillion cells in our bodies, each one demanding daily a constant supply of 40-plus nutrients in the proper balance in order to function optimally. That's a big responsibility!

You Deserve Better

"To accomplish great things, we must dream as well as act."
Anatole France

What you eat today will determine how you feel in the future. "Aging is not a sudden event," says Robert Russell, M.D., Professor of Medicine and Nutrition at Tufts University in Boston. "You don't wake up one morning to find you are old. It's a continuum, so the same nutrition issues related to the elderly, from osteoporosis to cancer and heart disease, have their roots in the middle years."

A good example of this is vitamin D, a nutrient essential in calcium metabolism and the prevention of osteoporosis. Your body can manufacture vitamin D when the skin is exposed to sunlight, but it gradually loses this ability with age. "People in their 20s can synthesize only 80% of the vitamin D that their bodies made when they were 8 years old. By the seventh decade, that production has decreased to about 40%," says Dr. Russell. That means dietary sources of vitamin D become increasingly more important to prevent osteoporosis. Vitamin D–fortified milk is the only reliable dietary source of this vitamin, and adults must drink two to four glasses daily to reach their recommended intake. Few people are doing that.

In fact, most people aren't getting even adequate nutrition, let alone optimal. They are sacrificing long-term health and their chances for vitality. Gladys Block, Ph.D., at the University of California at Berkeley, reviewed the data from three major national nutrition surveys and found that one in every two women—many of whom think they are eating well—consumes inadequate amounts of just about every vitamin and mineral studied, from vitamin A to zinc. On any four consecutive days, 86 percent of women fail to include even one dark green leafy vegetable in their diets and one in every two women avoids fruit, which explains why women's diets are low in beta carotene, vitamin C, iron, and folic acid—all essential for the prevention of cervical and other cancers, anemia, and possibly heart disease. Most mature women consume about half of the daily recommended 1,200 milligrams of calcium (1,500 milligrams if they are not taking hormone replacement therapy) needed to help offset bone loss associated with osteoporosis. In general, men eat even fewer fruits, vegetables, and whole grains than do women.

The data show nine out of 10 adults need to get much more aggressive about how they fuel their bodies. Keep in mind that you're fueling not only your physical health, mood, and energy level today, but you're setting the stage for your health and vitality tomorrow. You deserve the best, and so does your body!

The Anti-Aging Diet: The Eight Dietary Guidelines

"TO LIVE LONGER AND HEALTHIER, PEOPLE MUST EAT A LOW-FAT, LOW-MEAT DIET THAT CONTAINS AN ABUNDANCE OF FRUITS AND VEGETABLES."

Robert Russell, M.D.

The Anti-Aging Diet has three goals:

1. To supply all of the essential nutrients—including vitamins, minerals, phytochemicals, protein, and fiber—in optimal amounts to ensure that your body is fueled for life. This eating plan also is low in fat, trans fatty acids, sugar, meat, and other harmful substances.
2. To supply these essential nutrients in a steady balance for optimal energy and emotional, mental, and physical function.
3. To assist the body in removing toxic or disease-causing substances efficiently, before they can undermine health and longevity.

The eight guidelines are discussed in detail in the following pages and are put into practice in the week's worth of menus supplied in Appendix A at the back of this book. You should notice a marked improvement in your energy level and

What the Anti-Aging Plate Should Look Like

Eat eight fruits and vegetables each day.

Eat beans at least five times a week.

Eat minimally processed foods.

Drink water, at least eight glasses a day.

Eliminate excess calories.

Eat little meals and snacks.

Enjoy food.

Supplement responsibly.

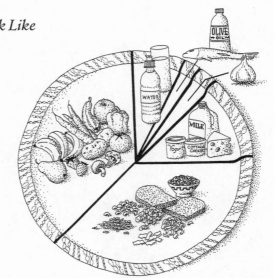

how you feel mentally and physically within one month of following these guidelines and the exercise guidelines outlined in the Anti-Aging Fitness Program in Chapter 8.

GUIDELINE 1: EAT EIGHT FRUITS AND VEGETABLES EACH DAY

"SOME PEOPLE WAIT ALL THEIR LIVES FOR THE OUTSIDE TO CHANGE THEIR INSIDE. BUT IT NEVER SEEMS TO HAPPEN, BECAUSE CHANGE COMES FROM WITHIN US FIRST, THEN THE OUTSIDE BECOMES DIFFERENT."

Elliot Goldwag, Ph.D.

What do the Surgeon General, every major nutrition group, and your mother have in common? They all recommend that you eat lots more fruits and vegetables. From luscious strawberries and crunchy carrots to crispy broccoli and juicy oranges, fruits and vegetables are Mother Nature's most nutrient-packed foods.

The 10 Commandments of the Anti-Aging Diet

1. Base snacks on fruits and vegetables.

2. At least three times a week, plan an all-plant dinner that includes only vegetables, grains, and beans.

3. Limit red meat (even if it's lean) to no more than three servings per week (remember, a serving is 3 ounces). Include baked or broiled fish at least twice a week and cooked dried beans and peas at least five times a week.

4. Consume daily three glasses of nonfat milk or three cups of nonfat yogurt.

5. Choose more whole grains than refined grains, and include at least two servings at every meal.

6. Limit processed or pre-prepared foods (from canned soups to frozen dinners) to avoid excessive salt intake.

7. Cut back or cut out sweets, including soft drinks, desserts, doughnuts and cinnamon rolls, granola bars, scones, and cookies.

8. Drink lots of water and some green tea. Limit alcohol consumption to one 6-ounce glass of wine a day.

9. Cut way back on fat, including added fats in cooking or food preparation, fatty snack foods, fatty dairy and meat products, and hidden fats in prepared foods.

10. Take daily a moderate-dose, multiple vitamin and mineral supplement with extra calcium, magnesium, and the antioxidant nutrients (vitamins C and E, beta carotene and other carotenoids, and selenium).

How many servings daily of fresh fruits and vegetables did you and your family eat yesterday? If you are like many people, you could double that amount and still barely meet the minimum requirements. To fend off the hands of time, you should consume at least eight servings of fruits and vegetables each day. Unfortunately, only one in five Americans eats even five fruits and vegetables each day; more than 40 percent consume three or fewer servings, and 20 percent of adults skip vegetables altogether.

WHAT'S IN A SERVING?

Eight servings may sound like a lot, but a serving size is probably smaller than you think. In general, the U.S. Department of Agriculture specifies one serving as:

- 1 medium-size piece of fruit or vegetable such as one orange or one carrot,
- ½ cup fruit or cooked vegetables,
- ¾ cup juice, or
- 1 cup raw leafy greens.

The following also are considered one serving:

Food	*1 serving*
Apple	One 2" diameter fruit
Apricots, fresh	4 medium
Artichoke	½ medium
Banana	½ of a 9" diameter fruit
Cherries, fresh	12 large
Figs, dried	2 medium
Grapefruit	½ medium
Raisins	2 tablespoons
Tomato	1 medium
Tomato paste	2 tablespoons
Tomato sauce	3 tablespoons

Fresh fruits and vegetables (with the exception of avocados, olives, and coconuts) have no fat, cholesterol, or sodium. They are the most fiber-rich, nutrient-packed foods in the diet, and they are low in calories (a heaping bowlful of greens supplies only 30 calories!). No other food is so closely linked to vitality.

Your daily need for several vitamins, including vitamin C, folic acid, and beta carotene (the building block for vitamin A), can be satisfied almost exclusively from fresh fruits and vegetables, especially citrus fruits, dark green leafy vegetables such as spinach and broccoli, and dark orange vegetables such as carrots. Eight servings of fruits and vegetables daily also supplies approximately 27 grams of fiber, well within the daily target goal of 25 to 35 grams!

Studies repeatedly show that people who consume diets loaded with fresh fruits and vegetables are the healthiest, with significantly lower disease rates, more energy, and less risk for weight gain than those who skip these foods. Many fruits and vegetables supply ample amounts of calcium, iron, magnesium, and many vitamins that prevent age-related crippling diseases. The good news is that it's never too late to enjoy the benefits of these foods; improvements in health risks are noted within weeks of adding more fruits and vegetables to the diet.

How to Make Sure You Get Enough

Making sure you get enough fruits and vegetables takes some planning. Here are the guidelines for meeting the eight-a-day goal:

1. Plan ahead. Include at least two fruits or vegetables at every meal and two more for snacks.
2. Eat your greens. Include at least two servings daily of a dark green vegetable, such as spinach, romaine lettuce, or chard, to ensure optimal intake of beta carotene and folic acid.
3. Grab an orange. Include at least two vitamin C–rich selections, such as citrus fruit, strawberries, or green pepper.
4. Nibble on cabbage. Include at least five vegetables each week from the cabbage family, such as Brussels sprouts, kohlrabi, asparagus, cabbage, broccoli, or cauliflower. These vegetables are chock-full of phytochemicals, which lower your risk of developing cancer.

There's much more to fruits and vegetables than vitamins, minerals, and fiber. Thousands of other disease-fighting compounds in these foods, called phytochemicals, are packed into every spinach leaf, every slice of tomato, and every spear of broccoli. (See Chapter 5 for more information on phytochemicals.)

Are You Getting Enough?

How many fruits and vegetables do you include in your daily diet? If you are like many people, your intake may be short of optimal. Tally your intake on the worksheet below to see how close you come to the eight-a-day goal.

Day: _____ Date: _____

Meal/Snack	# of Fruits	# of Vegetables	Total
Breakfast:	_____	_____	_____
Lunch:	_____	_____	_____
Dinner:	_____	_____	_____
Snacks:	_____	_____	_____
Total for the day:	_____	_____	_____
Goal:	3 to 5	5 to 7	8 or more
How many more should you add to reach the recommended goal?	_____	_____	_____

AND THEY TASTE GOOD

Fruits and vegetables not only protect your heart, your health, and your waistline—they also taste good. Gone are the days of overcooked spinach and limp asparagus. From lightly grilled eggplant to dribble-down-your-chin watermelon, with their rich assortment of flavors, textures, colors, and aromas, vegetables and fruits contribute as much to the visual and sensual appeal of each meal as to its nutritional quality. Peppers, onions, or garlic add flavor to a main course, from pasta to casseroles. Crunchy pea pods, carrots, or jicama add texture to cooked foods and salads, or are tasty appetizers. Luscious kiwi and sweet pears or apples liven up salads. Juicy oranges and strawberries are a low-fat, nutritious sweet treat at the end of a meal. And preparation is a snap: the less you do to fruits and vegetables, the better.

50 + Ways to Get Your Fruits and Vegetables

BREAKFAST

- Drink a glass of 100-percent fruit juice.
- Top cereal with sliced bananas or strawberries.
- Stir fresh fruit into plain, low-fat yogurt.
- Top wholewheat waffles with blueberries and fat-free sour cream, instead of syrup.
- Have a slice or two of fruit pizza (pizza crust baked, then topped with low-fat lemon yogurt and fresh fruit slices). Serve with orange juice.

LUNCH

- Add grated carrots, celery, peas, or jicama to potato salad.
- Eat at a salad bar and load up on greens, rather than fatty toppings.
- Top a baked potato with fat-free sour cream and Parmesan cheese and one or more of the following: steamed broccoli, spinach, mixed vegetables, or mushrooms.
- Top prepared plain pizza crust with sauce, low-fat cheese, and lots of vegetables, including onions, zucchini slices, artichoke hearts, mushrooms, peppers, tomato slices, and/or asparagus.
- Fill tortillas or pita bread with a variety of vegetables, kidney beans, and low-fat cheese.
- Add orange and grapefruit sections to salads or grain dishes.
- Add leftover vegetables from last night's dinner to lunchtime soups and salads, or add frozen vegetables to canned soups.
- Make a tuna sandwich (using low-fat mayonnaise) on wholewheat bread and top it with a sliced tomato. Serve with baby carrots and tomato juice.
- Include cut-up vegetables in your brown-bag lunch.

- Mix pre-shredded coleslaw fixings with apple or pineapple chunks and low-fat coleslaw dressing for a quick salad.
- Fill a thermos with hearty vegetable soup.

DINNER
- Use frozen vegetables when you're in a hurry.
- Have vegetable stir-fry dishes at least once or twice a week.
- Make shish kabobs with more vegetables and less meat (try zucchini, crooked-neck squash, whole mushrooms, cherry tomatoes, eggplant chunks, baby onions, carrots, or red peppers).
- Add broccoli, spinach, or chard to lasagna.
- Add zucchini, grated carrots, green peppers, or mushrooms to spaghetti sauce.
- Add more vegetables, such as peas, carrots, mixed vegetables, beans, or corn, to soups and casseroles.
- Experiment with seasonings: Crush basil over thick tomato slices and broil. Sprinkle dill on cucumbers, allspice on cabbage, chopped chives on broccoli, or tarragon on steamed cauliflower.
- For a quick salad, use pre-cut lettuce and mix with winter pears, apple chunks, and/or shredded carrots.
- Add steamed broccoli or cauliflower florets, green pepper slices, zucchini rounds, and/or pea pods to pasta.

WHEN EATING OUT
- Split an entree and order extra servings of steamed vegetables.
- Frequent the salad bar and focus on the fresh vegetables and fruits.
- Order à la carte and choose vegetable soups, salads (dressing on the side), baked potatos, and fresh fruit.
- If vegetables are not listed on the menu, ask which are available.
- Request that a Chinese vegetable stir-fry or chow mein be prepared with little or no oil.
- At a Japanese restaurant, ask for vegetable sushi.
- At an Italian restaurant, order pasta marinara or primavera.

- Order a fresh fruit platter.
- Order deli sandwiches with extra tomatoes and your pizza with extra helpings of vegetables.
- For an appetizer, choose a fresh melon wedge, gazpacho, fresh fruit medley, or vegetable juice.
- Remember to eat slowly, focus on the company, and eat only until you're comfortably full.

DESSERTS

- Top angel-food cake with fresh berries.
- Top fat-free frozen yogurt with pineapple chunks or papaya slices.
- Bake an apple with cinnamon and nutmeg.
- Nibble on frozen blueberries or grapes.
- Dip fresh strawberries, sliced kiwi, banana chunks, and orange or grapefruit slices in low-fat chocolate syrup.
- Fill a parfait cup with layers of colorful sliced fruit. Top with a tablespoon of low-fat whipped cream.
- Prepare poached pears or baked apples. Make extra and serve cold the next day.
- Cut up fresh fruit and place on the table after dinner.

SNACKS AND MINI-MEALS

- Keep a fresh banana or apple in your desk at work.
- Keep a bowl of fresh fruit on the dining table.
- Keep packages of dried fruit in the glove compartment.
- Use pre-cut vegetables and baby carrots as a crunchy mid-afternoon snack.
- Steam chopped spinach and mix with fat-free sour cream and seasonings to make a vegetable dip.
- Halve squash, such as a large zucchini or crooked-neck squash, scoop out the seeds, bake, then fill the center with steamed broccoli and cheese.
- Stuff vegetables, such as green peppers or large tomatoes, with rice and ground turkey, tuna salad, or beans.
- Mix ⅔ cup orange juice with ⅓ cup sparkling water, ice, and a dash of lime.
- Add grated carrots, zucchini, corn, or green chilies to cornbread batter.

GUIDELINE 2: EAT BEANS AT LEAST
FIVE TIMES A WEEK

"It is not enough to do good; one must do it the right way."
John, Viscount Morley, of Blackburn

People who want to live to 100-plus years might do well to switch from meat 'n gravy to beans 'n rice. Protein in meat is easily damaged by free radicals, which might partially explain why high meat consumption is linked to increased risk of disease and shortened life span. Replacing meat with soy products and other legumes, such as cooked dried beans and peas and lentils, increases life expectancy by up to 13 percent. Strive for at least five servings of beans each week. (See Chapter 6 for more information on meat and longevity.)

Soy products and beans are easily included in the daily menu. Cook dried beans and refrigerate for use in meals throughout the week. Or, toss canned kidney, garbanzo, or black beans into salads, soups, casseroles, and side dishes. Add extra beans to chili. Use fat-free refried beans in burritos, nachos, and other Mexican dishes. Crumble tofu into lasagna, enchiladas, or casseroles. Add chunks of tofu to soups, stews, and stir frys. Use soy milk in place of regular milk on cereals, in smoothies, and in baking. Try some of the soy-based products in the freezer case: look for the words "soybeans," "textured vegetable protein or TVP," or "hydrolyzed vegetable protein" on the label.

GUIDELINE 3: EAT MINIMALLY PROCESSED FOODS

"Let him that would move the world, first move himself."
Socrates

Almost all dietary recommendations can be distilled into one rule: eat food in its most natural form. Choose whole grains more often than refined white breads, rice, cereals, or pasta. Choose plain nonfat or low-fat milk and yogurt rather than highly processed ice creams, sugar-laden frozen yogurts, or cheese spreads. Choose corn or corn tortillas instead of corn oil, fresh fruit instead of candy with fruit added, oatmeal instead of a granola bar, and a baked potato instead of French fries or potato chips.

This guideline will cut your shopping time and food bill in half. Choosing wholesome, minimally processed foods means you shop primarily around the perimeter of the grocery store, focusing on the bakery, produce section, and dairy case.

GUIDELINE 4: DRINK AT LEAST EIGHT GLASSES OF WATER A DAY

"A GREAT SECRET OF SUCCESS IS TO GO THROUGH LIFE AS A MAN WHO NEVER GETS USED UP."

Albert Schweitzer

You regularly wash the outside of your body; well, the inside needs rinsing, too. Your body is mostly water. Men are about 60 percent water and women are about 55 percent water by weight. Most people lose two to three quarts of water daily, even more if they exercise or work in hot climates. That means you need to take in about a gallon of fluid every day to replace these losses.

Thirst is a poor indicator of fluid needs, especially as we age. Consequently, you become more susceptible to mild dehydration, which can sap energy and mental function. The two rules of thumb when it comes to water are:

1. Drink twice as much water as it takes to quench your thirst.
2. Drink at least eight glasses of water daily or one cup of water for every 20 pounds of body weight.

You can count fruit juices and bottled water in your tally, but not diuretic beverages such as coffee or alcohol. Green tea can be counted and is chock-full of cancer-preventing phytochemicals. One tip: fill a pitcher with your daily allotment of water and keep it on your desk at work or on the kitchen table at home. Your goal is reached when the pitcher is empty.

GUIDELINE 5: ELIMINATE EXCESS CALORIES

"SUBDUE YOUR APPETITES, MY DEARS, AND YOU'VE CONQUERED HUMAN NATURE."

Charles Dickens

Cut back or cut out the foods that contribute nothing to your long-term health. These include foods high in sugar and fat. Limiting intake of most alcoholic beverages is also wise. By minimizing these foods in the diet, you save more room for the anti-aging foods: fruits, vegetables, whole grains, nonfat milk, and legumes. In addition, cutting unwanted calories is the best way to attain and maintain a desirable weight, which is essential to a long and healthy life.

SWEET INDULGENCES

Americans' sugar consumption has skyrocketed in the past 150 years. Whereas a person in 1840 sprinkled a scant four teaspoons of sweeteners into home-baked jams and desserts, today the average American heaps 43 teaspoons (or almost one cup) of sugar onto the daily plate. If you include artificial sweeteners, such as aspartame, per capita daily consumption tops 50 teaspoons.

There is evidence that sugar might speed the aging process. Animals consuming high-sugar diets have significantly shorter life spans than do those given more nutrient-packed diets, despite no differences in body weight or blood sugar levels. Researchers speculate that regularly indulging a sweet tooth might alter body mechanisms, which in turn accelerates aging through free-radical damage.

The U.S. Department of Agriculture's Continuing Survey of Food Intakes reported that two of the top three sources of carbohydrates in many adults' diets are not breads and pastas, but regular soft drinks and sugar. Americans consume more than 450 servings per person per year of soft drinks; at five to nine teaspoons of sugar per serving, that equals 2,250 to 4,050 teaspoons of sugar annually from soft drinks alone.

The food industry has capitalized on our sweet tooth. At the turn of the century, sugar was bought directly by the consumer for home use. Today, three out of every four teaspoons are added by industry before foods reach the kitchen. While everyone knows they're eating sugar when they munch on a candy bar, fewer people realize that sugar is added to catsup, dessert wines, cranberry juice, canned soups, salad dressings, peanut butter, fiber bars, baked beans, most cereals, and many other products. Increased use of products sweetened with "white grape or pear juice concentrate" also misleads the consumer, who is unaware that this "juice" is primarily sugar.

In addition, people are not as concerned about sugar as they are about fat. According to Judy Putnam, Ph.D., Agricultural Economist at the U.S. Department of Agriculture in Washington, D.C., "A person may give up butter, but instead spread jam on toast." From fat-free cakes and cookies to the convenience of in-store bakeries, Americans are finding it harder to "just say no" to sugar.

Dental caries and periodontal disease have skyrocketed since people began bathing their teeth in a constant supply of sugar. Although a consistent trend has not yet appeared, many researchers suspect that a sugar-laden diet is a culprit in the development and progression of heart disease, depression and mood swings, lethargy, hypoglycemia, diabetes, kidney disease, gallstones, and ulcers.

When sugar intake increases beyond 9 percent of total calories, people's vitamin and mineral intakes progressively decrease, which compromises their immune systems and might contribute to the development of numerous health problems. Sugary foods added to an otherwise ample diet tip the calorie scale toward weight gain. Animals fed a high-sugar diet, even when fat intake is low, consume more calories and gain more weight compared to those eating more starch and less sugar. In short, excessive sugar intake, with or without a low-fat diet, encourages overeating and obesity. Weight problems, in turn, contribute to the development of cancer, cardiovascular disease, diabetes, and osteoporosis.

HOW MUCH IS SAFE?

Currently, sugar averages more than 21 percent of our total calories. Although exact recommendations have not been set, it is generally agreed people should cut their intake of added sugar in half. People who consume fewer than 2,000 calories a day must depend on nutrient-dense foods to guarantee adequate vitamin and mineral intakes and should consume even less added sugar.

How can you cut back on a sweet thing? Just follow a few simple rules:

1. Avoid sticky, sweet foods, such as processed fruit bars, candy, and caramel, since they are the worst offenders in tooth decay.
2. Limit soft drinks to one serving or less each day.
3. Cut back on doughnuts, pies, cakes, cookies, and ice cream, since these and other sweet foods are doubly harmful because of their high sugar and high fat content.
4. Read labels. Although manufacturers are not required to list the percentage of

sugar calories, you can get an idea of a product's sugar content by reading the ingredients list. A food may be too sweet if sugar is one of the first three ingredients or if the list includes several sources of sugar.

5. Add more spices. Cinnamon, vanilla, spearmint, and anise provide a sweet taste to foods without adding sugar or calories. Aspartame also can be used in moderation.

All added sugar is essentially calories with no redeemable nutrient qualities. A little sugar in the diet adds enjoyment and variety, especially when it comes from natural sources, such as fruit. Going overboard for sweets, however, could undermine your health.

FAT ATTACK

Most people know they should cut back on fat, but our average fat intake is still far in excess of optimal. As mentioned in Chapter 6, high-fat diets subtract years from your life, and they steal quality from the remaining years. Such diets are linked to an increased risk of obesity, most degenerative diseases, and premature aging. Eating too much fat also is likely to crowd out more vitamin- and mineral-rich foods, thus contributing to nutrient deficiencies. Cutting back on fat is one of the most important dietary changes a person can make for health and longevity.

Cutting back on fat means reducing or eliminating obvious fats, such as butter, margarine, salad dressings, mayonnaise, gravies, shortenings, and cream. Use small amounts of olive oil instead. It also means cutting back on hidden fats in processed snack foods like potato chips and granola bars, fast foods like hamburgers and French fries, desserts such as cookies and pies, and convenience foods such as high-fat frozen entrees. It means reducing fat in favorite recipes by substituting nonfat milk for cream or whole milk, low-fat cheese for regular cheese, and baking for frying. It means switching from red meat to fish or beans as entrees. Using fat-free items, such as fat-free sour cream or cream cheese, also can help lower fat intake.

Your fat intake will automatically decrease if you fill your plate with vegetables, legumes, whole grains, and fruit. A rule of thumb is to fill three-quarters of the plate with foods of plant origin, leaving the remaining space for small amounts of fish, nonfat milk products such as yogurt, and nuts or seeds.

ALCOHOL AND LONGEVITY

People who drink too much alcohol, whether it's from beer, hard liquor, or wine, die at a younger age than do teetotalers or people who drink in moderation (less than two drinks each day). In fact, heavy drinking is second only to smoking as the primary cause of premature death. Heavy drinkers also are much more likely to suffer from cirrhosis, high blood pressure, mouth and throat cancer, bronchitis and pneumonia, and liver cancer, and they're at high risk of dying from accidents, suicide, and cardiac arrest. People who consume more than four or five alcoholic drinks daily are likely to develop impaired memory and loss of mental ability as well.

On the other hand, people who have an occasional drink live about two years longer on average than do those who abstain, primarily because of a reduced risk for heart disease. When it comes to the heart, red wine is better than beer, which is slightly better than hard liquor.

THE GREEN LIGHT ON RED WINE

The link between red wine and a reduced risk for heart disease was first identified in France, where people eat a high-fat diet but suffer little from heart disease. The secret might be the French passion for red wine. People who drink a glass or two of red wine daily are much less likely to die from heart disease than people who don't drink or who drink other alcoholic beverages. The benefits might not come solely from the alcohol, but from other beneficial compounds in wine.

Red wine contains a wealth of phytochemicals called phenols that have antioxidant capabilities in protecting the arteries and blood fats from free-radical damage. Phenols are found in most fruits, onions, and tea, but are especially high in grapes. Both grape juice and red wine solids (without the alcohol) lower heart disease and cancer risks in animals, so, while alcohol might offer additional benefits such as possibly boosting the antioxidant potency of the phenols, a person can derive at least some benefits from de-alcoholized wine or even grape juice.

RISKY BUSINESS

But alcohol consumption is not a risk-free deal. Women who consume even one alcoholic beverage daily increase their risk for breast cancer by up to 10 percent. So, a person must weigh the risks and decide whether to drink or abstain.

If you choose to drink, do so in moderation. This means limiting alcohol intake to one drink daily for women, no more than two drinks daily for men, and no more than one drink daily for people over the age of 65, as specified by the National Institute on Alcohol Abuse and Alcoholism. One drink equals 6 ounces of wine, 10 ounces of beer, or 1 ounce of hard liquor.

GUIDELINE 6: EAT LITTLE MEALS AND SNACKS

"IF YOUR DETERMINATION IS FIXED, I DO NOT COUNSEL YOU TO DE-
SPAIR. FEW THINGS ARE IMPOSSIBLE TO DILIGENCE AND SKILL. GREAT
WORKS ARE PERFORMED NOT BY STRENGTH, BUT PERSEVERANCE."
Samuel Johnson

Gone are the days of the "three square meals." Gone, also, is the misconception that skipping meals is a way to control your weight. The best way to stay energized and promote longevity is to eat small meals and snacks regularly throughout the day. Eating more frequently doesn't mean adding more food to your normal intake; it means spreading your food intake more evenly over the course of the day.

Many people overeat or choose the wrong foods not because they are hungry, but because they haven't had a truly satisfying meal all day. Having a little meal—a simple-to-prepare, elegant meal that is bigger than a typical first course, but smaller than a main course—is one way to feel satisfied, not satiated. It also is an excellent way to manage your weight, since research shows that people who eat small, frequent meals, rather than the traditional three square meals, are most likely to maintain a desirable weight and reduce their risk for heart disease and other health problems.

Quick, Easy, and Nutritious Little Meals and Snacks

LITTLE MEALS

- 1 whole-wheat pocket bread filled with ½ cup garbanzo beans, ¼ cup tomatoes, 2 tablespoons sprouts, 1½ ounces grated low-fat cheese, and 2 tablespoons green onions
- 1 serving of Jeanette's Spinach/Raspberry Salad* with a whole-wheat roll and a slice of low-fat cheese
- 1 large tomato stuffed with 3 ounces water-packed tuna mixed with low-calorie mayonnaise and ¼ cup chopped celery, served with fat-free whole-wheat crackers
- 1 whole-wheat tortilla filled with ½ cup beans, 1 ounce low-fat cheese, 1 chopped tomato, and salsa, served with orange juice
- 1 serving of Curried Broccoli Soup*, served with a slice of cornbread
- 1 or 2 Breakfast Crepes*
- 1 slice of Spinach Lasagna Roll Ups*, served with tossed salad and sparkling apple cider
- 1 Salmon Steak with Parsley Sauce*, served with ½ cup rice and 1 cup steamed broccoli
- 1 baked breast of chicken served with Squash on the Rocks* or Mashed Potatoes with Roasted Garlic* and a tossed salad.

SNACKS

- 4 whole-wheat bread sticks and 1½ ounces fat-free cheese
- 1 whole-wheat English muffin with all-fruit jam and fat-free cream cheese, served with 1 cup orange juice
- 1 mini raisin bagel with 1 tablespoon fat-free cream cheese, served with a glass of tomato juice
- 2 ounces oven-baked, fat-free tortilla chips with ½ cup fat-free refried beans and salsa
- 2 tablespoons Refreshing Yogurt Dip* with baby carrots and whole-wheat crackers
- ½ cantaloupe filled with 1 cup vanilla low-fat yogurt and 1 tablespoon raisins

- 1 slice toasted whole-wheat raisin bread dunked in 1 cup nonfat apple-spice yogurt, served with 1 cup pineapple juice
- 1 Fruit-Filled Tortilla Snack*
- 1 cup sliced green pears, apples, cantaloupe, or watermelon dunked in 1 cup honeyed yogurt
- 1 bowl of Santa Fe Sweet Potato Soup* served with orange and kiwi slices
- Low-cholesterol egg salad made with 1 whole egg and 2 egg whites mixed with fat-free mayonnaise, ¼ cup chopped celery, and seasoning on a whole-wheat roll
- 1 slice raisin bread toast topped with ½ cup nonfat ricotta cheese and ¼ cup fresh raspberries, served with orange juice
- Greek salad made with ½ cup nonfat or fat-free feta cheese, 2 chopped tomatoes, ½ cup chopped cucumbers, a dash of olive oil, wine vinegar, and seasonings, served with pita bread
- 1 veggie burrito made with 1 flour tortilla filled with ⅔ cup grated and sliced vegetables, 1 ounce low-fat cheese, and salsa

*Recipes in Appendix B.

Little meals should emphasize nutritious foods—grains, vegetables, fruits, and legumes—and they can do it with flair. They can blend unusual ingredients to tantalize the tastebuds and accent the sensuous side of food—its color, texture, and aromas. Little meals can be anything from a tabbouleh salad with fresh fruit on the side or low-fat cheese, whole-wheat crackers, and baby carrots to an exotic Chardonnay-marinated chicken with grapes or mangoes on flavored rice.

Little meals may be just the ticket for adding a little romance to your life. Often people forget about the romance of home-cooked food and think they must dine out for such luxuries, but sharing fresh fruit dipped in fat-free chocolate on the floor in front of the TV, a backyard picnic of pesto-topped pasta with steamed asparagus, fresh strawberries, and a glass of champagne or a cozy candlelight dinner of several small, tasty dishes can be even more romantic than eating out.

WHAT'S IN A SERVING?

Take a look at people's portions and you'll find that one person's snack could be another person's meal. The moderate servings on which the Anti-Aging Diet is based are in stark contrast to what many restaurants are serving. Here are a few guidelines to keep your portions in line with a fork, rather than a forklift.

One serving of:	*Is the size of:*
MILK PRODUCTS	
8-ounce glass of milk or container of yogurt	Two wineglassfuls
1 ounce of cheese	A large marble or pair of dice
GRAINS	
½ cup rice, noodles, or cooked cereal	A tennis ball
1 slice of bread or ½ small bagel, English muffin, or hamburger bun	A CD case
1 pancake	A compact disk
MEAT/BEANS	
3 ounces of meat, chicken, or fish	The palm of your hand, deck of cards, or cassette tape
VEGETABLES AND FRUIT	
1 cup raw	A baseball
½ cup cooked	Your fist
1 piece	
¾ cup juice	

FATS AND SUGARS

1 teaspoon of butter or margarine	A postage stamp the thickness of your finger
2 tablespoons salad dressing or peanut butter	A standard ice cube or a Ping-Pong ball
2 tablespoons pancake syrup	A shot-glassfull

GUIDELINE 7: ENJOY FOOD

"TAKE PLEASURE OUT OF LIFE . . . AS MUCH AS YOU CAN. NOBODY EVER DIED FROM PLEASURE."

Sol Hurok

Eating is one of life's most pleasurable experiences. Food should taste, look, and smell delicious. It also brings us together with loved ones, is a form of celebration and joy, and accompanies every important tradition and holiday. An extra advantage, according to the National Cancer Institute, is that people who create interesting menus based on a wide variety of wholesome foods are much less likely to die prematurely than those who eat the same few foods day in and day out. Pleasure, health, and vitality are inseparable.

One way to add vitality to your meals is to use spices much as a painter uses paint—to color and texture the masterpiece. Try new or different spices with new foods. Stop depending on salt as your main flavor and sprinkle basil, thyme, cilantro, curry powder, or other herbs instead. Many spices both flavor a meal and contain phytochemicals that help stop the aging clock. Garlic is a perfect example of how vitality and longevity are combined in a spice.

ADD A CLOVE A DAY

As mentioned in Chapter 5, garlic helps lower heart disease and cancer risk and stimulates the immune system. Try some of the following suggestions to maximize the benefits from garlic while enhancing the flavor of meals:

- Chop or mince a few cloves into Italian sauces, vegetable dips, meatloaf, marinades, soups, stir frys, homemade salad dressings, and stews.
- Cook green beans, spinach, zucchini, or other vegetables with garlic in a drizzle of olive oil.
- When cooking pasta, add two to three cloves to the cooking water to impart subtle flavor.
- For fat-free garlic bread, first spray vegetable oil on whole bulbs of garlic with the skin and wrap the bulbs in tin foil. Bake for 45 minutes at 300°F or until soft. Spread the softened baked garlic cloves on French bread.
- Embed several garlic cloves in meat or poultry before roasting.

GUIDELINE 8: SUPPLEMENT RESPONSIBLY

"The way to win a war is to make certain it never starts."
General Omar N. Bradley

In the not-so-distant past, the general consensus was that a person could obtain all the vitamins and minerals in the right amounts by eating a "balanced diet." The reality is, however, that few people actually meet even the minimum standards of a good diet, let alone the optimal standards needed to prevent chronic disease and premature aging.

For example, most women average three servings of fresh fruits and vegetables daily (men do even worse, at only two servings), yet the minimum standard is five servings and the Anti-Aging Diet recommends at least eight. You also should consume at least six servings daily of whole-grain breads or cereals, but, if you are like most Americans, you average less than one serving a day.

Even if people made perfect choices every day, there still is reason to take a supplement. While the antioxidants, such as vitamins C and E and the carotenoids such as beta carotene, might be potent anti-aging nutrients, the amount needed to fend off the ravages of time is far greater than is realistically possible from diet alone. For example, the Alliance for Aging Research recommends that adults consume the following amounts daily:

250 to 1,000mg vitamin C
10 to 30mg beta carotene
100 to 400IU vitamin E

While the Anti-Aging Diet meets the lower levels for vitamin C and beta carotene, a person would need to consume one cup of safflower oil or 21 cups of spinach daily to consume 124IU of vitamin E! In addition, as we age, requirements for other nutrients, such as vitamin D and vitamin B_{12}, escalate to levels not likely to be achieved from food alone. Consequently, for people who cannot always follow the Anti-Aging Diet to the letter or for those who want to ensure optimal nutrition, there is reason to supplement—wisely and moderately.

CAN SUPPLEMENTS HELP PREVENT AGING?

Research repeatedly shows that those who supplement fare better than those who don't.

For example, compared to nonsupplementers:

- People who take antioxidant supplements live longer. A study from Wageningen Agricultural University in The Netherlands reports that seniors with preestablished disease who took supplements reduced their risk of dying prematurely by up to 20 percent, while disease-free seniors who supplemented cut their mortality risk in half. Another study on people over the age of 65 conducted by the National Institute on Aging found that vitamin E supplements lowered mortality rates by 27 percent, reduced the risk of heart-disease deaths by 41 percent, and decreased cancer deaths by 22 percent.
- People who take vitamin C supplements are less likely to develop cataracts.
- Those who take antioxidants or a multiple vitamin and mineral have stronger immune systems and more resistance to colds, infections, and disease.
- People who take vitamin E supplements have up to a 40 percent lower risk of heart disease. Researchers at the National Cancer Institute in Bethesda, Maryland, report that in a six-year study in which 3,318 participants received either a multiple vitamin and mineral supplement or a placebo, the prevalence

of high blood pressure dropped and overall mortality declined in the group who supplemented compared to the placebo group.

- People who maintain high blood levels of several nutrients, including vitamins C and E, beta carotene, and selenium, are less likely to develop cancer.
- Those who maintain optimal tissue and blood levels of B vitamins are less prone to memory loss and heart disease.
- People who take calcium, magnesium, and vitamin D supplements are less likely to develop osteoporosis.
- People who take a multiple vitamin and mineral supplement are less likely to suffer from mood swings and depression. Researchers at the University College Swansea in the United Kingdom measured mood in 129 healthy adults, sent them home with a daily multiple vitamin and mineral supplement, and reassessed mood during the following year. While blood levels of vitamins increased within three months, improvements in mood were noted only after at least one year of supplementation. At that time, the men reported that they felt "more agreeable," while women reported feeling more agreeable, composed, and generally in better mental health when taking a daily supplement.

THE THREE-STEP APPROACH TO SUPPLEMENTATION

Choosing a good supplement program is as easy as one, two, three.

1. Select a broad-range multiple vitamin and mineral supplement. Look for one that contains vitamin D, vitamin K, all of the B vitamins (vitamins B_1, B_2, B_6, B_{12}, niacin, folic acid, pantothenic acid, and biotin), and the trace minerals (chromium, copper, iron, manganese, selenium, and zinc).

Steer clear of "extra" ingredients, such as lipoic acid, enzymes, or inositol; these extras add only cost, not value, to a product since they are either worthless or are supplied in amounts too low to be of use.

In addition, save money by avoiding time-released vitamins, chelated or colloidal minerals, or most "natural" supplements, since they promise more than they deliver.

Some nutrients can be ignored, such as potassium, choline, or phosphorus, since the diet either already supplies optimal levels of these compounds or they are supplied in supplements in amounts too low to be useful.

Read the column headed "Daily Value" on the label. Look for a multiple that provides approximately 100 to 300 percent of the Daily Value for all nutrients provided. What you want is a balanced supplement, not one that supplies 2 percent of one nutrient, 50 percent of another, and 600 percent of a third nutrient.

2. Supplement your multiple with extra calcium and magnesium. Size dictates that one-tablet-a-day multiples can never supply enough of these minerals (the pill would be the size of a Ping-Pong ball!). So, if you don't drink at least three glasses of nonfat milk a day or consume several servings of dark green leafy vegetables, wheat germ, soybeans, and other magnesium-rich foods, look for a calcium-magnesium supplement that provides approximately two parts calcium for every one part magnesium (i.e., 500 milligrams calcium and 250 milligrams magnesium). If your multiple (or your fortified cereal) does not contain vitamin D, make sure the calcium-magnesium tablet also contains 400IU of this vitamin.

3. Consider taking extra antioxidants. If the multiple does not contain extra amounts of vitamin C, vitamin E, and the carotenoids, consider taking an antioxidant supplement that supplies 250 to 1,000 milligrams of vitamin C, 100 to 400IU of vitamin E, and 10 to 30 milligrams of beta carotene. (Smokers should consult their physicians before supplementing with beta carotene.)

CAN SUPPLEMENTS BE TOXIC?

Most popular articles on vitamins caution against vitamin toxicities. But are vitamin toxicities really a threat to most people? Not really. In most cases, raising the red flag of toxicity is making much ado about nothing.

Vitamin A is most famous for its overdose effects, and people in the later years are most susceptible to vitamin A overdose. As people age, their livers become less able to "clear" excessive amounts of this vitamin. Even moderate intake in the later years can raise liver enzymes, an indicator of liver damage.

Ironically, up to 40 percent of all vitamin A overdoses are from food, not supplements. Most people know better than to take too much vitamin A, so reported cases of supplemental overdoses are few. Of course, no one is recommending that anyone take huge doses of vitamin A, especially when there's an even safer option—beta carotene.

Beta carotene is the building block for vitamin A found in vegetables, fruits,

THE BEST SUPPLEMENT

Designing a good supplement program is easier than you might think. You might have to mix and match one to three products, but in the end your total supplement intake should resemble the following:

Nutrient	The Best Form	The Optimal Dose
Beta carotene	Mixture of carotenoids	10mg–30mg
Vitamin E	Alpha tocopheryl succinate	100IU–400IU
Vitamin D		400IU–800IU
Vitamin K		65mcg
Vitamin B_1		2mg–5mg
Vitamin B_2		2mg–5mg
Niacin		20mg–25mg
Vitamin B_6		5mg–10mg
Vitamin B_{12}		3mcg–6mcg
Folic Acid		400mcg
Boron		2mg–3mg
Calcium	Calcium carbonate or citrate	1,000mg–1,500mg
Chromium	Chromium-rich yeast, chromium nicotinate, chromium picolinate	200mcg
Copper		3mg
Fluoride (needed only if drinking water is not fluoridated)		4mg
Iodine		150mcg

Nutrient	The Best Form	The Optimal Dose
Iron	Ferrous fumarate	18mg (premeno-pausal women only)
Magnesium	Magnesium oxide, magnesium citrate, magnesium citrate-malate	350mg–500mg
Manganese		5mg
Molybdenum		250mcg
Selenium	Selenomethionine, selenocysteine	200mcg
Zinc	Zinc gluconate, zinc picolinate	20mg–30mg

and supplements. Americans currently consume 1 to 2 milligrams of beta carotene daily, while supplemental doses up to 180 milligrams have been taken for up to 15 years with no side effects. Unlike vitamin A, beta carotene shows no harmful effects in animals or humans. Other than some yellowing of the skin, a condition called hypercarotenemia, daily doses of 30 milligrams of beta carotene are safe for all adults, except possibly smokers.

Vitamin E is almost safer than water. The current RDA ranges from 8 to 10 milligrams, but doses as high as 3,200 milligrams have been taken for prolonged periods of time with no adverse side effects and doses up to 800 milligrams are safe for older people, according to researchers at the USDA Human Nutrition Research Center on Aging at Tufts University in Boston. The rare reports of toxicity have been letters to the editor about individual case studies or uncontrolled studies, which equate to testimonials and are invalid for making recommendations about toxicity. In general, 100 to 400IU of vitamin E daily are well within the safe zone.

Vitamin C is the most widely used single supplement, with up to 35 percent of Americans taking supplemental vitamin C, often in 500-milligrams daily doses.

Considering the scarcity of reports of any adverse effects in such a large population and the numerous reviews of the research concluding that vitamin C is safe at high doses for prolonged periods of time, the incidence of toxicity for this vitamin must be extremely low. While the evidence is scarce that intakes greater than 250 to 500 milligrams are any more helpful than lower doses, there appears to be little concern with taking up to 1,000 milligrams daily, except in people prone to kidney stones or who are scheduled to take a glucose tolerance test for diabetes (vitamin C supplementation a few days before this test can skew the results).

Granted, there are concerns about vitamin toxicities, especially in high-risk populations such as children, people with liver disease, and pregnant women. But decades of research show that the vast majority of people who supplement do so responsibly. They choose a balanced multiple and may supplement it with extra vitamin C, vitamin E, or calcium. Supplementers also tend to eat better and take better care of their health. They are less prone to disease and premature aging and maintain stronger immune systems than nonsupplementers. Now that's much ado about something!

The Empty Nest Kitchen

"WE MUST NOT STAY AS WE ARE, DOING ALWAYS WHAT WAS DONE LAST TIME, OR WE SHALL STICK IN THE MUD."

George Bernard Shaw

An empty nest brings with it many adjustments. Life previously might have revolved around routines of work and raising children. Probably nowhere was the routine more ingrained than at the dining table, where for years it was your job to make sure the kids ate at least one good meal every day. Many parents find that after the children move out or when a spouse dies, their incentive or interest in cooking dwindles to little or none at all. They may eat the same foods over and over, skip meals, or eat at the kitchen counter rather than prepare a sit-down meal for one.

"People in their 50s and 60s are at a crux. Their physiological reserves begin to dwindle and they will age more rapidly if they don't take care of themselves," says Jeffrey Blumberg, Ph.D., Professor of Nutrition at the USDA Human Nutrition Research Center at Tufts University in Boston. "On the other hand, with the children gone, people have more personal time. If they approach good nutrition with the attitude that it can be fun, they can take advantage of an opportunity to do something good for themselves and their long-term health." In fact, the kitchen may be just the place to foster rediscovery, self-renewal, health, and even romance.

Resurrecting the joy of eating after the kids have left home requires an adventuresome spirit. You must abandon well-worn recipes. Try new fruits and vegetables, such as sliced jicama or radicchio in a salad. Toss sun-dried tomatoes in pasta. Experiment with different combinations: add exotic fruits, such as mangos or papaya, to chicken dishes. Explore the different flavors of "international" cuisine. Try forming a dining club with friends, sampling each other's newest creations. Even discovering new places to shop for groceries can open up alternatives. You may find that variety alone is enough to wake up a sleeping palate.

TAKING NUTRITION FOR GRANTED

While scaling down in the kitchen can add adventure and zest to your life, without a little planning some people may fall short nutrition-wise, at a time when nutrition is more important than ever.

"People at this age are most likely to meet their nutritional needs and maintain a desirable weight if they stop planning traditional meals around meat, which is a main source of fat in the diet. Instead, they should ask themselves, 'What vegetables and grains will I have today?'" recommends Margo Woods, D.Sc., Assistant Professor of Medicine at Tufts School of Medicine in Boston. "Eating well is as simple as preparing a big pot of soup made with lots of vegetables and a little bit of meat. Then, buy a variety of vegetables for accompanying salads and you have several light meals throughout the week." Dr. Woods also recommends that you place sliced fresh fruit on the table every night. "A few bites of fruit after a meal often curb the desire for something sweet. It also gives you something to do that is good for you while your partner is still eating."

Nutritious meals can be easy and quick to prepare if you have stocked your kitchen with nutrient-packed "convenience" foods, such as the following:

- In a can: low-fat soups, tomatoes, tomato sauce, chicken broth, chickpeas, black beans, tuna packed in water
- In a box: nonfat milk powder, cold and hot cereals, dried fruit
- In a bag: an assortment of pastas
- In bulk: flour, rice, bulgur wheat, barley, and other grains
- Breads: tortillas, pita bread, packaged low-fat pizza crusts
- Oil-free, low-sodium condiments: mustard, soy sauce, vinegar including balsamic vinegar, salsa, lemon juice, fruit spreads, salad dressings, sun-dried tomatoes
- In the dairy case: fresh nonfat or 1% low-fat milk and yogurt, cheeses such as Parmesan, part-skim mozzarella and ricotta, or Gorgonzola
- An assortment of fresh and frozen vegetables, including potatoes, jicama, broccoli, onions, garlic, baby carrots, lettuce (anything but iceberg!)
- Fresh fruit, such as mangoes, lemons, oranges, apples, and papaya
- In the freezer: frozen low-fat entrées (purchased or made at home), chicken breasts, fish fillets

PLANNED OVERS

One way to minimize the time you spend preparing food is to cook for more than one meal. Rather than think of the extra portions as leftovers, consider them "planned-overs," or planned ingredients for another meal. Wrap, label, date, and store extra foods quickly. Freeze any portions that will not be eaten within three days.

These foods recycle especially well:

- Pancakes, French toast, muffins, waffles
- Sandwich fillings (tuna, chicken, pureed beans)
- Steamed vegetables: Use in omelets, soups, stews, marinated vegetable salads, for cold stacks, or in burritos.

- Onions and garlic: Chop the whole onion and several cloves of garlic, then store them individually in sealed plastic bags.
- Soups: Add pasta, kidney beans, or more vegetables to change the character.
- Sauces: Tomato or creamed sauces are particularly good, since you can spice the sauce as needed after thawing.
- Chicken breasts: Use as sandwich fillings or tortilla stuffers, add to pasta or rice dishes, or use in a stir fry.
- Fish: Use in fish tacos or pita sandwiches.
- Pasta dishes: These actually taste better when reheated. Add extra sauce to moisten.
- Rice or beans: Add to casseroles, marinated vegetables, or soups.
- Baked potatoes: Mash or puree with milk to make a "cream" soup base.

SEIZE THE MOMENT

The empty-nest kitchen offers a golden opportunity to break free from cooking ruts and explore new tastes, textures, and aromas. This is also a wonderful chance to nurture yourself, your health, your vitality, and your relationships.

Chapter 8

THE ANTI-AGING
FITNESS PROGRAM

"There is no substitute for learning to live in our bodies. All
the tests and all the machines in the world will fail if we do
not first become good animals."

George Sheehan, M.D.

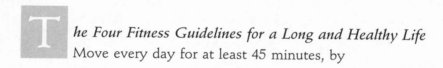he *Four Fitness Guidelines for a Long and Healthy Life*
Move every day for at least 45 minutes, by

1. engaging in some form of aerobic activity, such as walking, swimming, or jogging, at least four hours a week.
2. doing some form of strength training, such as lifting weights or doing calisthenics such as situps, at least twice a week.
3. warming up and cooling down with flexibility exercises.
4. always making it fun.

Are you out of breath after walking up a flight of stairs? Is carrying the groceries from the car more tiring than it used to be? Has your back ever gone out from just leaning over to pick up something from the floor? Does crossing the street to make a green light feel like running the 100-yard dash? Are you stiff in the morning? Tired in the evening? Does an afternoon of gardening leave your muscles sore for days?

If you answered "yes" to any of the above, welcome to the out-of-shape club!

You're not alone. Almost 90 percent of adults don't exercise regularly, and two out of every five are classified as downright sedentary, with heart rates that seldom rise above an idle. Only 15 percent of adults come close to Dr. Sheehan's goal of "being good animals" by exercising at least three times a week for 20 minutes or more. Worse yet, by age 75, a third of all men and half of all women don't exercise at all.

Sitting on your duff won't do you in when you're 10, 15, or even 20 years old. But your muscles will take a nosedive in your thirties. People lose approximately 1 to 2 percent of muscle mass every year after this point, which equates to a 5- to 10-pound loss of muscle for every decade. The loss doesn't become noticeable until your forties, when you notice that pushing a door open takes two hands instead of one or you unconsciously take the elevator to avoid even a two-story climb up the stairs. But that's just the beginning.

As the body ages, it loses muscle and accumulates fat. Fat tissue is like a storage box in your body. Because it is relatively inactive, the more fat you have, the fewer calories you need to maintain a constant body weight. Muscle, on the other hand, is like your car's engine, burning calories when moving and even at rest. Consequently, the fat-for-muscle trade-off results in a lower metabolic rate (called basal metabolic rate, or BMR). It takes fewer calories to keep you going, so if you eat like a 30-year-old, you'll gain weight.

Letting muscle slip away is the first step in the aging process. The gradual loss of fitness also contributes to bone loss and osteoporosis. The increase in body fat is directly linked to increased blood cholesterol and glucose, elevated blood pressure, increased insulin resistance, and loss of bone density, which place a person at increased risk for most age-related degenerative diseases, from heart disease and diabetes to hypertension and cancer.

Where Metabolism Meets Movement

Metabolism is the sum total of all energy-requiring processes in your body. The more you move, the more calories you burn, and the higher your metabolic rate. Metabolism is primarily a combination of basal metabolic rate (BMR) and physical activity. BMR is the calories needed to maintain basic body functions, such as blinking your eyes, sending electrical messages along the nerves, kidney and liver function, and heartbeat.

BMR accounts for about 60 percent of your total daily energy needs. It can account for up to 75 percent of your energy needs if you do strength training. That's because a physically fit body has a higher percentage of muscle to fat tissue compared to an unfit one. Muscle is the body's calorie-burning furnace, so it is called "metabolically active." Fat is metabolically inactive and uses fewer calories. As a person exercises and increases muscle mass, the metabolic rate goes up, more calories are burned during and after exercise, and weight is lost.

The changes don't happen overnight. Body fat increases slowly from 18 to 36 percent in men and from 20 to 44 percent in women between the ages of 20 and 65 years. Between the ages of 30 and 80, breathing capacity gradually declines up to 60 percent, nerve conduction drops 15 percent, and maximum oxygen up-take declines by 70 percent. The changes are so gradual that most people lament their age as the cause, rather than putting the blame squarely where it belongs: inactivity.

As your body becomes less and less fit over time, it takes more effort to do even simple daily tasks; consequently, you do less and less. If you live long enough, you'll reach a point where you can't get up out of a chair without help or even pick up the groceries, let alone your grandchild.

Hold On to Your Youth

" 'KNOW THYSELF' MEANS THIS, THAT YOU GET ACQUAINTED WITH WHAT YOU KNOW, AND WHAT YOU CAN DO."

Menander of Athens

But there's good news. Almost all of the weakness, frailty, and loss of function associated with aging is preventable and even treatable! All you must do is keep moving. The fountain of youth is within you. It's the sweat on your brow after a good workout. It also can be found at the water fountain at the local gym, the water bottle strapped to your bicycle, and the tall glass of iced green tea that refreshes after a brisk walk.

Even better news is that you don't have to rearrange your life or spend hours a day working out. All it takes to rewrite the script for aging at almost any age is a few minutes of brisk walking and a few strengthening exercises to escape the perils of inactivity and aging. Better yet, you'll see results within one month of starting the Anti-Aging Fitness Program in this book.

A recent study from the Harvard School of Public Health found that the risk of dying prematurely from any cause decreased as people increased their participation in vigorous activity. Healthy centenarians exercise more and have more muscle and higher metabolic rates than do 75-year-olds who don't exercise. In short, to avoid the grim reaper, you should not only run away, you should swim, cycle, row, jump, roller blade, or walk.

*B*etter *T*han *A*ny *P*ill

Almost all aspects of aging can be avoided or slowed by moving every day. The single most important habit you can acquire to maintain optimal function throughout life is to stay physically active. Here is a partial list of what to expect as a result of being physically active.

- Decreased risk of developing or dying from heart disease
- Prevention or delay of high blood pressure
- Decreased blood pressure in people with hypertension
- Lowered risk of developing non-insulin-dependent diabetes
- Maintenance of youthful muscle strength
- Improved range of motion of joints
- Improved joint structure and function
- Control of joint swelling and pain associated with arthritis
- Increased general mobility
- Attainment of peak bone mass
- Slowing of the accelerated bone loss associated with aging, thus reducing the risk of developing osteoporosis
- Reduced likelihood of gaining excess body fat and greater ease losing excess body fat
- Improved lean body mass (muscle, organs, and other fat-free tissue)
- Improved digestive function and reduced risk of constipation
- Improved lung and respiratory function

Continued

- Encouragement of other healthful habits
- Improved sleep patterns
- Increased ease in performing daily tasks
- More energy and less chance of suffering fatigue
- Reduced depression, anxiety, and stress
- Improved mood
- Improved psychological well-being
- Improved self-esteem
- Maintenance of physical functioning and independent living
- Reduced risk for falls
- Maintenance of youthful metabolic rate
- Improved recovery from illness

The Aging Muscle

"IF YOU DON'T RUN YOUR OWN LIFE, SOMEBODY ELSE WILL."
John Atkinson

As research findings on active, fit oldsters accumulate, the evidence consistently points to disuse, not age, as the underlying cause of frailty and disease. The older a person is, the more critical this rule of disuse becomes. Weak muscles are more prone to injury and stiffness. The loss of muscle strength in older men and women is a major contributor to disability, osteoporosis, insulin insensitivity and diabetes, and lessened ability to transport oxygen to the tissues (called aerobic capacity or VO_2 max). Older people also are less efficient at burning fat for fuel, which when combined with the lowered metabolic rate results in weight gain and difficulty losing weight.

Anyone, no matter what age, who begins exercising shows increases in strength and metabolic rates. Middle-aged and older persons, however, benefit the most. While 20-year-olds improve their oxygen capacity by about 29 percent after starting an exercise program, people ages 60 to 70 show up to a 38 percent improvement in oxygen capacity. In just 12 weeks of starting a strength-training program, men between the ages of 60 and 72 showed up to a 227 percent improvement in muscle strength. In a study of 96-year-olds, strength improved up to 200 percent. Moderate daily exercise also boosts resistance to both colds and cancer more in older than in younger people.

Moreover, compared to an inactive older person, a 70-year-old who exercises daily has lower blood pressure, lower blood cholesterol, higher HDL cholesterol (the "good" cholesterol), and as much as a 40 percent lower risk of developing heart disease. Physically active men and women have lower body weight and body fat and improved insulin sensitivity, thus lowering their risk of high blood pressure and diabetes. They are less likely to experience colon cancer, stroke, or even back injuries. They have stronger bones and are at lower risk of developing osteoporosis. And they are up to 25 percent less likely to injure themselves or fall compared to unfit older people. Even practicing unconventional physical activities, such as tai chi (an ancient Chinese martial art that combines meditation with rhythmic movements), can reduce the chance of falls and injury by almost 50 percent.

Exercise and Vitality

"THOUGH OUR OUTER NATURE IS WASTING AWAY, OUR INNER NATURE IS BEING RENEWED EVERY DAY."

II Corinthians 4:16

Vitality and a youthful appearance go hand-in-hand with good posture. Standing like an exclamation point, not a comma, takes effort, but you'll feel younger and more vital as a result.

Watch the faces of people out for a brisk autumn walk, or feel the enthusiasm of the runners lined up for a 10K race. Listen to the conversations of middle-aged or older persons at your local gym. You will hear and see the signs of vitality: enthusiasm for life, positive thoughts, and plans for the future. Fitness is the breeding ground for vitality.

The research bears this out. Physically fit people are happier, more satisfied with their lives, and less prone to depression, anxiety, and stress. Exercise becomes their play and brings out the childlike quality inherent in vitality. People who are physically active also think more clearly, concentrate better, remember more, and react quicker than sedentary folks. In short, their physically fit bodies allow them the freedom to do what they want in life.

Staying fit also means living longer. Women who continue to exercise in their second 50 years are as fit as or even fitter than sedentary women who are 20 to 30 years younger. This may explain why they also live longer. Men who take up exercise in the middle years lower their risk of dying prematurely by up to 30 percent. In fact, the more calories a person expends in exercise each week, the longer he or she is likely to live disease-free.

INACTIVITY OR SMOKING: NAME YOUR POISON

Avoiding exercise is the riskiest vice you can choose. A joint statement from the American College of Sports Medicine and the Center for Disease Control and Prevention in Atlanta estimates that 250,000 deaths each year in the United States alone are attributed to physical inactivity. That staggering figure places lethargy in the same high-risk behavior category as smoking, obesity, hypertension, and driving drunk.

Ironically, those who stick with an exercise program for at least six months report that if only they'd known how good they would feel, they would have started exercising earlier! The secret to a long and healthy life filled with vitality is as simple as getting off the couch and moving—every day for the rest of your life.

Exercise: The Natural High

"THAT STILL, AS DEATH APPROACHES NEARER,
THE JOYS OF LIFE ARE SWEETER, DEARER;
AND HAD I BUT AN HOUR TO LIVE,
THAT LITTLE HOUR TO BLISS I'D GIVE."

Anacreon

A daily workout releases brain chemicals, including epinephrine and norepinephrine, that boost alertness. It also raises serotonin levels, which boost mood. At the same time, exercise de-stresses the body by lowering blood levels of the "stress hormones," including cortisol, that prepare the body for "fight or flight." Over time, the body learns to react less intensely to stress, thus providing a built-in coping mechanism. In addition, the rise in body temperature resulting from a vigorous workout has a tranquilizing effect on the body, not unlike that experienced when soaking in a hot bath. Finally, the hour at the gym or pounding the streets might provide a much-needed timeout from a hectic day.

The notorious "runner's high" has been attributed to an exercise-induced release of endorphins, the body's natural morphine-like chemicals that help boost pain tolerance and generate feelings of euphoria and satisfaction. However, the research on endorphins and exercise remains equivocal. "Exercise raises blood levels of endorphins up to ten-fold," says Ed Pierce, Ph.D., Associate Professor in the Department of Health and Sport Science at the University of Richmond in Virginia, "but the key is whether or not brain levels of endorphins are increased."

Endorphins or no endorphins, one thing seems clear: exercise is a great anti-depressant. "There is evidence that exercise relieves depression better than psychotherapeutic medications, counseling, or a combination of the two," says Dr. Pierce. In a study of 357 adults at Stanford University in Palo Alto, California, researchers compared the effects of no exercise and various intensities of exercise on psychological outcomes. After 12 months, the exercisers reported significantly reduced stress, anxiety, and depression compared to their sedentary counterparts, regardless of whether they experienced any changes in fitness or body weight. The level of intensity and even the type of exercise (aerobic activities, such as walking, running, or swimming, or anaerobic sports, such as bodybuilding) doesn't seem to matter; all forms of exercise alleviate depression and improve mood.

"People want to categorize this effect by saying it's biochemical or psychological, but in reality it's probably a synergistic effect of these and, as yet, unidentified factors," says Dr. Pierce. Whatever the cause, one thing is sure: the best mood-elevating effects come from starting and sticking with a daily exercise program.

The Anti-Aging Exercise Program

"EVERYONE IS AN ATHLETE. THE ONLY DIFFERENCE IS THAT SOME OF
US ARE IN TRAINING, AND SOME ARE NOT."

George Sheehan, M.D.

You must be physically active if your goal is a long and healthy life. But you must do it right, which is as simple as 1, 2, 3. That means combining

1. aerobic activity, such as walking, swimming, or jogging;
2. strength training, such as lifting weights, or calisthenics, such as situps; and
3. warm-up, cool-down, and flexibility exercises.

Aerobic activity strengthens your cardiovascular system and helps burn fat. Strength training increases muscle and metabolism. Flexibility activities keep your joints and muscles elastic. This combined program will slow or halt the changes in body composition associated with aging, aid in weight management, help normalize blood sugar and blood pressure, increase muscle, stimulate the immune system, and even possibly stimulate growth hormone release, which in turn might help build more muscle, denser bones, and less fat. The sooner you start the better, but it's never too late for damage control or even reversal.

GETTING STARTED

Whether you are one of the almost 90 percent who are inactive or are an avid exerciser, there are a few important considerations before making a change in your activity level.

First, you need to know where you are before you can decide where you're going. Everyone over the age of 40 should obtain medical clearance from a physician before beginning any exercise program. That includes completing a monitored fitness test to determine where you need to focus your exercise goals. If you're like most people, you'll likely find that you need to work on several goals, such as increasing your cardiovascular fitness level and upper-body strength. Or maybe balance and flexibility will prove high priorities. You also need to determine at what level you should start a fitness program and whether there are any undetected health risks that should be considered, such as high cholesterol or blood pressure. After a thorough physical evaluation, you and your physician can lay out a plan.

THE PLAN

You probably wouldn't host a party or go Christmas shopping without having a plan. But many people jump into exercise, join a fitness club, or purchase exercise equipment without first sitting down and thinking it through. Planning will dramatically increase the odds that you will stick with your exercise routine. Even if it's something as simple as riding your bike to work, you need to decide how you'll carry your briefcase or lunch, how you'll keep mud and grease off your work clothes, and even what route you'll take. You'll also need to repair the bicycle and have an alternate fitness plan for rainy days. Also, you must identify all the reasons you have for not exercising and then devise realistic ways to overcome those barriers.

ESTABLISH A ROUTINE

Exercise will be a priority only if you make it one. So establish a routine by setting aside a time or place every day for exercise, write it on your daily calendar, and don't let anything get in the way. Plan ahead. Bring exercise clothes when traveling. At home, put on your exercise clothes when you get up in the morning or when you arrive home after work; keep them on until you've exercised.

SET GOALS

The biggest mistake most people make when starting an exercise program is that they try to do too much too soon. The resulting soreness, injury, and discouragement can undermine even the best intentions. Devise an exercise program that is well within your capability, knowing that early success will encourage long-term commitment. If you know you can walk 20 minutes at a brisk pace, walk only 15 minutes the first week. That way you won't feel too sore and will be encouraged to stick with your program.

Your Activity Quotient

The first step in starting a lifetime exercise program is to determine where you are now—physically, that is. To calculate your fitness score, determine your rating for each category below. Next, multiply the numbers to obtain a score (Fitness score = Activity Rating × Frequency Rating × Intensity Rating × Time Rating). Retake this self-assessment six months after starting your exercise program to compare how far you've come.

Rating	Type of Activity You Routinely Engage In
3	A mixture of aerobic, strength training, and flexibility. The day also is filled with activity, such as climbing stairs, vacuuming, walking rather than driving, and using nonelectrical appliances, such as a hand-held can opener.
2	Either aerobic or strength training/flexibility, but not both. The day is somewhat active with house or yard work, walking, and climbing stairs.
1	Recreational sports, such as kite flying, bowling, light gardening, archery, canoeing, fishing, volleyball, table tennis, or baseball. Rest of day is moderately inactive, using elevators and escalators instead of stairs or driving whenever possible instead of walking.

	Frequency of planned physical exercise
5	more than 5 times a week
4	4 to 5 times a week
3	3 times a week
2	2 times or less a week

Rating	Intensity of planned physical exercise
5	Very heavy, with sustained heavy breathing and perspiration, as in jogging, aerobic dance, skipping rope, or cycling
4	Heavy, with intermittent heavy breathing and perspiration, as in a vigorous game of tennis or racquetball
3	Moderately heavy, as in continuous bicycling, swimming, calisthentics, shoveling snow, or heavy yard work
2	Moderate, as in brisk walking, golf (carrying bag and walking), leisurely bicycling (5.5mph), rowing, scuba diving, skating, hiking, or horseback riding
1	Light, as in fishing, slow walking, croquet, shuffleboard, horseshoes, billiards, badminton, routine housecleaning, pulling weeds, or planting flowers

	Time Spent Daily
4	More than 45 minutes
3	31 to 45 minutes
2	20 to 30 minutes
1	Less than 20 minutes

PERSONAL FITNESS SCORE

Score	Estimated Fitness Level
144–300	This very active lifestyle sustains a very high level of physical fitness.

Continued

Score	Estimated Fitness Level
54–143	This active lifestyle sustains an above-average level of fitness. You'll experience even more benefits if you boost your score to at least 180!
40–53	This moderately active lifestyle sustains an average level of fitness. You'll see improvements in health and longevity if you increase daily exercise to reach a score of at least 54.
24–39	This borderline active lifestyle sustains a marginal level of fitness. Long-term health and longevity are at risk unless you increase physical activity with physician approval and raise your score to at least 40.
Less than 23	This sedentary lifestyle will contribute to disease risk and shortened life expectancy down the road. Start exercising with physician approval to boost your score to at least 40.

The adage "no pain, no gain" is outdated. Exercise doesn't have to hurt to be good for you. Brisk walking (at a pace that allows you to cover two miles in less than 30 minutes) is one of the best activities for strengthening the cardiovascular system and burning excess body fat. Fitness gains are greatest in those people who go from being sedentary to doing something; the gains are less dramatic for those who move up a notch from fitness to super fitness.

On the other hand, rousing an out-of-shape body off the couch and into the gym won't feel as good as, say, polishing off a bag of Hershey's Kisses—at least, not at first. You must move enough to see benefits (that means you must sweat), but not so much that soreness or fatigue undermine your motivation. As Dr. Sheehan says, "You must listen to your body. [Exercise] through annoyance but not through pain."

You also must answer the question "How fit do I want to be?" It's important that you realistically plan activity so it will fit into your life. For some people, that means getting up a half-hour earlier in the morning to walk. For others, it may mean creating four 10-minute breaks throughout the day to stretch, lift weights, or ride a stationary bike.

You don't need huge amounts of time to exercise. There are 336 half-hours in a week; all you need is five to six of those set aside for aerobic activity such as walking and another two for strength training. If even that sounds monumental, try breaking your activity sessions into several mini-exercise sessions throughout the day. The research shows you can derive the same benefits from two to three mini-workouts as long as the total day's time is still at least 45 minutes.

In addition, you can increase activity throughout the day by using the stairs instead of the escalator or elevator. Park your car at the end of the lot and walk to the store. Better yet, ride your bicycle to the store. Don't let anything interfere with your plan. Remember: failing to plan is planning to fail.

ONE STEP AT A TIME

Develop a progressive exercise program. To see results without feeling miserable, gradually increase the duration, intensity, or frequency of your exercise session— but not all at once. A rule of thumb is to increase time or intensity by 10 percent each week. So, if you're currently walking two miles a day, increase the distance to 2.2 miles the next week and do it in the same amount of time. Also, add activities to the program as you advance. Your ultimate goal is to accumulate 30 to 45 minutes or more every day of moderate-intensity physical activity.

MAKE IT FUN

Physical activity should bring out the kid in you. It should be your playtime during the day, during which you laugh, enjoy the company of friends, love what your body can do, and "lighten up." Doing something physical should be pleasurable, active, freeing, and rewarding. Eventually, exercise can become some-thing you'd do even if it had no benefits other than the joy of doing it.

Rather than calling it exercise, call your daily activity "romping." As Dr. Shee-han notes: "Fitness has to be fun. If it is not play, there will be no fitness. Play, you see, is the process. Fitness is merely the product." That may mean romping with friends if you are a social animal or choosing a solitary sport if you need some quiet time away from the tensions of work. It may mean alternating three or more activities throughout the week to keep your romping fresh and new, or playing sports with the kids. You'll stick with exercise only if it's fun. So ask yourself what you like to do and what is convenient to do, then use your imagination to keep moving interesting.

#1: Cardiovascular Fitness: Your Target Heart Rate

"I'M SIXTY-FIVE AND I GUESS THAT PUTS ME IN WITH THE GERIATRICS, BUT IF THERE WERE FIFTEEN MONTHS IN EVERY YEAR, I'D ONLY BE FORTY-EIGHT."

James Thurber

The first component of the Anti-Aging Fitness Program is to strengthen your cardiovascular system by strengthening the heart and increasing blood and oxygen flow to the tissues. Aerobic exercise achieves this and burns more calories than any other type of activity. It is the best way to burn excess body fat. It also helps relieve stress by tempering the stress hormones and possibly raising brain chemicals called endorphins.

Aerobically fit people are healthier than anyone else, with a lower risk of developing heart disease, hypertension, and diabetes, as well as of being overweight. The more aerobically fit you are, the greater are your chances of living a disease-free, healthy life. Aerobic fitness goes hand-in-hand with vitality. It's as simple as that.

YOUR TARGET HEART RATE

How do you know if your activity is aerobic and if you're doing enough to reap the benefits? Aerobic activities use large muscle groups, such as the legs and arms, in a rhythmic and *continuous* motion. Checking heart rate is the most convenient way to monitor your cardiovascular or aerobic fitness and intensity, since it directly reflects how hard you are working. Your goal is to exercise within your "target heart rate," or THR, which is 60 percent to 90 percent of your maximum heart rate (MHR).

How to Calculate Your Target Heart Rate

To identify your maximum heart rate (MHR), subtract your age from 220. To identify your target heart rate (THR) range, multiply your MHR by .60 and again by .90. For example, a 45-year-old man's THR would be:

220 − 45 = 175 (MHR)

175 (MHR) × .60 = 105 beats per minute for 60% of MHR

175 (MHR) × .90 = 157 beats per minute for 90% of MHR

This man's target heart rate is between 105 and 157 beats per minute. To take your pulse and monitor your heart rate during exercise, lightly place your two middle fingers on your throat, just to the side of center (the carotid pulse). (See illustration below.) Don't press too hard, since this will slow the pulse. You also can use your wrist, placing two fingers on the thumb side (radial pulse). Count the beats starting with the number zero on the first beat. Count for ten seconds and then multiply that number by six, or count for 10 seconds and add a zero to the end of that figure to determine the total heart beats per minute. It is important to count the pulse immediately after stopping exercise, since the pulse rate slows quickly once exercise is stopped.

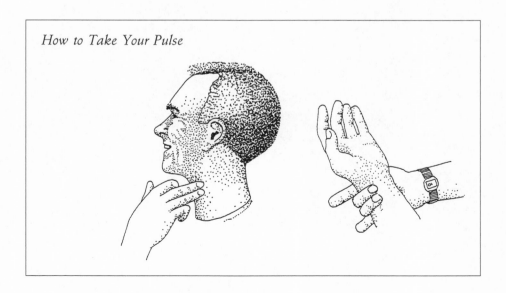

How to Take Your Pulse

It is also important to do a spot check while exercising. How do you feel when you are working at 40 percent of your MHR, at 60 percent, and at 80 percent? How hard are you breathing? Are you comfortable or gasping for air? Are you perspiring? Is your heart pounding wildly or just rhythmically pumping? These spot checks can help you learn the signals of how hard you're working out. Eventually this awareness will be an accurate way to measure exercise intensity.

A general rule of thumb is to exercise at a level that allows you to talk and sweat at the same time. If you can't talk, you're exercising too hard and should slow down, even if you're within your THR. If you are within your THR and can sing or whistle while exercising, you are not working hard enough and should increase your exertion to the higher end of the THR scale.

Guidelines for a Cardiovascular Workout

To maximize the benefits from your workout, follow these guidelines:

1. Warm up for five to 10 minutes before beginning the activity.
2. Be sure the movements are continual and rhythmic, using the major muscle groups, such as the arms and legs.
3. Periodically monitor your heart rate and perceived exertion level during the activity.
4. Do not exceed your THR.
5. Make the workout fun, playful, and enjoyable.
6. Work up to at least 30 minutes of continuous motion.
7. Cool down for five to 10 minutes after the activity, including some stretching and flexibility exercises in your cool-down.

#2: Strength Training

"I AM MORE MYSELF THAN EVER BEFORE."
May Sarton

While aerobic activity will soothe the heart, strength training will put a spring in your step. In fact, strength training may be the most important anti-aging activity there is. The loss of muscle that accompanies aging slows metabolism, contributes to weight gain, and weakens the body, contributing to everything from obesity and heart disease to loss of function, coordination, and the ability to perform everyday tasks. Even highly trained runners will start to suffer from weakened muscles, nagging injuries, and weight gain as they age unless they combine their aerobic workouts with at least two strength-training sessions each week.

Strength training is one of the most important components of a weight-management plan. It preserves or restores muscle tissue and is the only effective way to increase muscle mass as a person ages. The increased muscle boosts calorie burning up to about 7.5 percent for up to 15 hours after the workout. During any weight-loss effort, you will lose more lean tissue and will end up weaker from dieting unless you combine aerobic activity with strength training. Strong muscles also allow you to perform ordinary tasks with less effort, so you can accomplish more and have energy left over!

THE ABCS OF STRENGTH TRAINING

Improving your muscular strength does not mean bulking up like a body builder. It *does* mean developing stronger muscles that prevent needless injury as you age. Nor does strength training mean having to join a gym to use their high-tech equipment. It can be as simple as doing well-designed calisthenics at home and, if you want, adding hand and ankle weights as you progress. Of course, you also can purchase free weights or machines to use at home or join the gym. It's up to you.

Here are the most important rules:

- Include exercises that strengthen major muscle groups, such as the muscles at the back of the thigh (hamstrings), the front thigh muscles (quadriceps), the lower back muscles (erector spinatus), the abdominals, the chest muscles (pectorals), the upper back muscles, the biceps and triceps in the upper arms, and the muscles in the shoulders and neck.

• Include warm-up and cool-down exercises before and after strength training.

• Work each muscle group to near fatigue, which usually takes one to two sets with 10 to 12 repetitions each. Choose weights that are heavy enough that you can't do any more than 12 repetitions at a time. All it may take is lifting the weight equivalent of a jug of milk or a hardbound dictionary. When the last few lifts are too easy, it's time to switch to slightly heavier weights or add another set.

• Take it slow. If you start with eight repetitions of 15 pounds, you might increase to 12 repetitions at the same weight, then increase to two sets of eight repetitions at the same weight, and so forth. The biggest mistake people make is to add too much weight or too many repetitions too quickly, setting themselves up for injury and discouragement.

• Breathe! Inhale before you lift and exhale as you lift a weight. Don't hold your breath.

• Allow at least one day off between sessions to allow muscles to heal and to maximize strength gains, or alternate upper-body and lower-body workouts every other day. You should notice improvements in strength and energy within six weeks of starting a strength-training program.

Meet with a trained exercise physiologist or fitness expert to devise a strength program for your fitness level. Numerous books also are available. Several are listed in the resource section at the end of this book.

#3: Flexibility

"IN THE PAST FEW YEARS I HAVE MADE A THRILLING DISCOVERY . . . THAT UNTIL ONE IS OVER SIXTY ONE CAN NEVER REALLY LEARN THE SECRET OF LIVING."

Ellen Glasgow

As people age, they become more susceptible to falls, injuries, stiff joints, and muscle spasms or pains—not because of their age, but because they haven't kept their bodies limber. After the mid-thirties, subtle changes in muscle and connecting tissues cause joints, ligaments, tendons, and other tissues to become increasingly stiffer and less functional, i.e., more injury prone. But older persons can stay as limber as the young, if they are willing to spend a few minutes daily improving their range of motion.

Flexibility is the ability of the joints to move through their natural range of motion. Flexibility exercises can be part of the five to 10 minutes of your warm-up and cool-down sessions. Stretch slowly, don't bounce, and never stretch to the point of pain. Also, don't forget to breathe while stretching or doing any exercise. Any previous injury to the joints or muscles may require extra precautions. If you are recovering from any injury, consult your physician or physical therapist in designing a safe and effective stretching program.

Why Warm Up?

Warm-up exercises are very important to overall fitness and prevention of injuries. The benefits include:

1. Improved oxygen delivery to the muscles
2. Improved oxygen release in the muscle tissues
3. Stimulation of energy systems within the cell, which improves muscle function during exercise
4. Enhanced transfer of nerve messages to the muscles
5. Increased blood flow to muscles
6. Reduced injuries to muscles, tendons, ligaments, and other connective tissue
7. Improved responsiveness of the heart and blood vessels to sudden or strenuous exercise
8. Increased range of motion in joints
9. Reduced muscular tension and soreness
10. Improved coordination
11. Enhanced sense of well-being

How do you know if you've sufficiently warmed up? The body temperature rises with good warm-up exercises. You've sufficiently warmed up when you break into a mild sweat.

How to Stick with It

*"HE WHO POSTPONES THE HOUR OF LIVING RIGHTLY IS LIKE THE RUS-
TIC WHO WAITS FOR THE RIVER TO RUN OUT BEFORE HE CROSSES."*
Horace

You sign up at the local gym and start lifting weights or taking aerobics four times a week. By the third week, you're down to weekly sessions. By the second month, the gym bag is at the back of the closet.

The promise of longevity isn't enough to induce most people to bounce out of bed at five A.M. for a jog or a workout at the gym. Some immediate reward must reinforce taking time out of the day to sweat, or you're likely to end up back on the couch. It may take up to six weeks for your body to get used to exercising without feeling some degree of fatigue. How do you give exercise a positive spin so you stick with it beyond the initial slump—or even beyond the customary one to six months, after which many people burn out?

DEFINE YOURSELF AS AN EXERCISER

Throw out the old vision of yourself as inactive and start visualizing yourself as an exerciser. Look for excuses to exercise, rather than reasons why you can't. Hang out with other people who exercise in their free time, or join a gym. Nurture your interests in exercise by reading books and magazines, renting exercise or fitness tapes, taking a tennis class, talking about exercise with other enthusiasts, or attending a motivational lecture. The shift in attitude happens gradually, but it slowly will transform how you view yourself and exercise, which in turn will motivate you to stick with it.

DEVELOP A MOTIVATION PLAN

Figure out what motivates you to exercise. Is it a feeling of accomplishment? If so, place stars on a calendar for every day you are physically active, record each day's accomplishments in an exercise log, or place a dollar in a jar for every day you exercise and then use the money to buy something you've always wanted. Reward yourself whenever you reach a fitness goal: purchase clothes in your new smaller size, join a health club, or take a fitness-oriented vacation.

If you crave more time with friends, use exercise as a way to enjoy their company. Write a contract with a fellow worker to walk for 30 minutes before work every day. At lunch, walk with friends and grab a light snack afterward at your desk. Do you and your spouse need more time together? Use exercise as an opportunity to discuss your day and share positive time. Research shows that one in every two people who stick with an exercise program do so because of family and social support.

BEYOND POUNDS

Look for benefits beyond a drop in pounds or inches. Do you notice improvements in your endurance level, your mental focus, or your personal relationships, stress level, or mood? Pay attention to how different life is when you feel good. Maybe the difference is something as simple as not getting angry at the guy who cut you off on the freeway or having the staying power to solve a problem at work. Write down the benefits as you notice them, and tally the results each week.

The Bottom Line

"WHENEVER YOU ARE ASKED IF YOU CAN DO A JOB, TELL 'EM, 'CER-
TAINLY I CAN!' THEN GET BUSY AND FIND OUT HOW TO DO IT."
Theodore Roosevelt

The most important message of this chapter is to MOVE. Move for at least 45 minutes every day for the rest of your life. If thoughts of target heart rates and

Your Workout Journal

The rules for moving are simple: the more consistently you exercise, the better you'll feel. Make a month's worth of copies of this page, or use this sheet as a guidepost and develop your own journal to record your daily activity. Your goal is to move for at least 45 minutes every day, with four to five sessions of aerobic activity and at least two strength-training sessions per week. Review your journal each week and summarize the benefits you experienced. By the end of the month, you will prove to yourself how important exercise is to your physical, emotional, and mental well-being!

Dates: _____

Long-term Fitness Goal: _____

This Week's Goal: _____

Date/Day	Activity ST/Aer.	Time	Intensity*	How Felt Afterward	Other Benefits†

ST: Strength Training / Aer. = Aerobic
*Intensity: 1 = mild, 2 = moderate (broke a sweat), 3 = high
†Did you notice benefits in sleep patterns, energy level, general well-being, ability to concentrate or think, tolerance, stress level, relationships, mood?

stationary bicycles turn you off, forget those guidelines, at least at first. Just start by doing something every day. That will eventually lead to a little more until you will have walked away from recreational couch sitting and started on the road to lifelong fitness. Make physical activity a priority and you'll change the way you grow old.

AVOIDING THE DISEASES OF AGING

Chapter 9

YOUR ANTI-AGING ARSENAL

"Do not go gentle into that good night. . . .
Rage, rage against the dying of the light."
Dylan Thomas

W hile aging is intensely personal, it also is something we all share. That common bond comes with a few inevitables. All women experience menopause where they cease ovulating and menstruating. Men don't experience anything quite so definite (unless a "male menopause" is verified); however, they share with women many age-related changes. The skin loses some of its youthful elasticity and hair color changes. Vision worsens and hearing fails. Just about every other age-related condition, from heart disease and cancer to sleep problems and osteoporosis, is more a matter of lifestyle than time.

It is not years alone that result in old age, but how we choose to live them. The first step in preventing age-related illness is to stockpile your body's natural defense systems, such as the antioxidant system and the immune system.

Your Family Health History: Blueprint for Change

Any disease that runs in your family puts you at risk. The genes your parents passed to you are like links in a health chain; some links are strong and protect you while other links are weak and can break. Knowing your family health history helps you clarify your health chain, identify the weak links, and develop a personalized plan to prevent breaks.

Use the chart below to help identify diseases and health conditions that run in your family. Complete the chart, starting with grandparents. Fill in names, current age or age at death, and any diseases. Discuss the chart with your physician and give a copy to your children.

YOUR FAMILY'S HEALTH HISTORY CHART

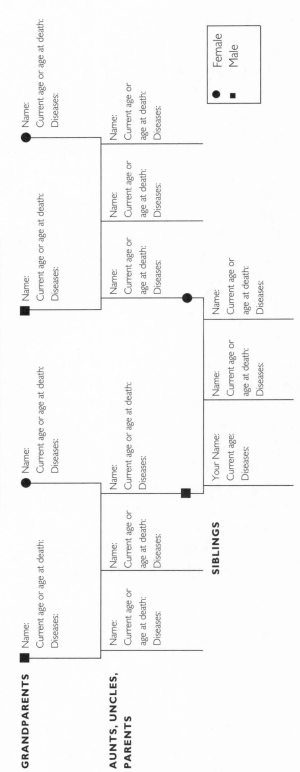

Immune Power

"DESPISE NO NEW ACCIDENT IN YOUR BODY, BUT ASK OPINION
OF IT."

Francis Bacon

Everything in the environment—from the air you breathe to the people you meet—constantly exposes you to bacteria, viruses, and other "germs" that cause infection or disease. In the past, a person was considered a victim of these factors. Researchers now believe the body is more often than not an accomplice, not a victim, to disease.

The condition of the immune system, one of the body's two fundamental defense systems against foreign invaders and renegade cell growth such as cancer, is a critical factor in whether or not a person succumbs to infection, disease, and possibly even premature aging. (Keep in mind that the maximum life span of humans is currently set at 120 years; anything less than this is premature aging!)

A healthy immune system correctly recognizes a foreign substance, multiplies, calls for reinforcements, destroys the enemy, calls off the troops, and creates "memory" cells that file data on subversive invaders. A weakened immune system fails to recognize an invader or mounts a weak attack. The results can be chronic or repeated infections, more serious illnesses such as cancer, and an increased likelihood of dying before your time.

IMMUNITY AND AGING

Antibiotic medications seemed like the answer to people's prayers when it came to fighting infections and the daily onslaught of bacteria. But overuse and misuse of antibiotics during the past four decades has resulted in the growth of antibiotic-resistant strains of bacteria that have "learned" to cope with every attempt humans make to destroy them. Consequently, people are succumbing to, and even dying from, infections that were easily treated before the era of antibiotics, which increases the importance of maintaining a strong immune system at every age.

Until recently, dwindling immune function was considered a natural consequence of aging. Upper respiratory infections, cancer, shingles, tuberculosis, and other immune-related disorders occur more frequently as people age, and older persons with suppressed immunity are the most likely to fall ill, develop complications from surgery, and even die earlier than their healthy counterparts.

It is not age, but the damage caused by years of eating poorly, inactivity, medication use, and/or illness, that destroys the older body's ability to fight disease. The sooner you stop the damage, the less likely you are to become a victim to diseases later in life.

VITALITY AND IMMUNE FUNCTION

People who are optimists have stronger immune systems and are less likely to succumb to disease than pessimists. If a person is stricken with disease, his or her tenacity in fighting the disease can marshal the body's defenses in ways modern medicine cannot equal. Granted, optimism and vitality can't ensure a disease-free life, but embracing these qualities increases the likelihood of health and makes any road you travel a lot more fun!

Boosting Immunity with Food and Supplements

"WORK FOR IMMORTALITY IF YOU WILL, THEN WAIT FOR IT."
Josiah G. Holland

Research shows that seniors who eat well and supplement responsibly can stimulate immune activity, prevent many of the diseases once thought to be age-related, and recover more quickly than someone whose immune system is weakened by inadequate nutritional supplies.

Studies from the USDA Human Nutrition Research Center on Aging at Tufts University in Boston show that supplementing seniors with single nutrients, such as vitamin B_6 or vitamin E, or with broad-range multiple vitamins and minerals boosts immune function. One study from the Memorial University of Newfoundland found that seniors who took multiple vitamin and mineral supplements for one year maintained or enhanced their bodies' natural defenses against disease, while the seniors who took placebos showed a decline in immune function.

All it takes is a moderate-dose multiple vitamin and mineral supplement to see significant improvement in disease resistance. Exceptions to this rule of moderation are vitamins E and C. Taking doses greater than can realistically be obtained from the diet—or approximately 100 to 400IU for vitamin E and 250 to 1,000 milligrams for vitamin C—might be beneficial for adults who want to keep their immune systems in peak performance.

"Unfortunately, you can't just look in the mirror to judge the immune system. A person can look healthy and feel good, but that is not an accurate indicator of a well-functioning immune system," says Adria Sherman, Ph.D., Professor of Nutritional Sciences at Rutgers University in New Brunswick, New Jersey. Dr. Sherman recommends good nutrition to help ensure the immune system remains intact.

IMMUNE SUPPRESSORS

Some components of food, such as fat, interfere with immune function and should be reduced. A low-fat diet stimulates the immune system. The only fats that boost immunity are those found in fish, called omega-3 fatty acids.

The Antioxidants: The First Line of Defense

"YOUR MAN AGES BECAUSE HE LETS HIS BODY RUST."
Tom Robbins, from Jitterbug Perfume

Antioxidants—including beta carotene, vitamin E, and vitamin C—are key players in immunity, preventing the accumulation of free-radical damage to the immune system, much like oiling a cast-iron pan prevents it from rusting. "The gradual accumulation of free-radical damage results in many of the age-related changes we've grown accustomed to, from suppressed immune function to vision loss," states Jeffrey Blumberg, Ph.D., Professor of Nutrition at the USDA Human Nutrition Research Center at Tufts University in Boston.

The antioxidants protect the membranes of immune-related cells, thus strengthening the immune response, increasing resistance to infection, and reducing the risk for developing immune-related diseases such as cancer. Heaping the plate with antioxidant-rich broccoli, spinach, and oranges is one line of defense.

Vitamins E and C are very effective at stimulating immune function and the body's resistance to colds, infections, and disease. Additionally, ample intake of beta carotene-rich foods, such as carrots, apricots, and broccoli, maintains the skin and mucous linings in the nose and lungs, which are the body's first line of defense against invasion.

Snacks That Boost Your Immune System

- Fresh strawberries, blueberries, or blackberries
- Fresh kiwi dunked in yogurt flavored with shredded orange peel, poppy seeds, and cinnamon
- A tortilla filled with shredded carrots, zucchini, low-fat cheese, and salsa
- Fresh fruit stirred into vanilla nonfat yogurt
- Unsweetened fruit juice frozen in ice-cube trays
- Unsweetened fruit juice concentrate mixed with gelatin and chilled to form a "jellied" juice snack
- Blueberry Pancakes à la Lemon*
- A fresh fruit and nonfat milk smoothie
- One-half honeydew melon filled with nonfat yogurt
- One-half papaya filled with cottage cheese
- Jeanette's Raspberry/Spinach Salad*
- Carrots dunked in peanut butter
- Three bean salad with low-fat dressing
- A sweet potato, cut into chunks
- Crisp vegetables dunked in Refreshing Yogurt Dip*
- Nonfat milk blended with fresh fruit, wheat germ, and a tablespoon of frozen orange concentrate
- A glass of fresh-squeezed orange juice

*Recipes in Appendix B.

Beta carotene could be a fountain of youth, at least when it comes to immunity in the later years. As part of the ongoing Physicians' Health Study, researchers at Tufts University and Harvard University in Boston followed 59 middle-aged men

(51 to 64 years old) and 21 seniors (65 to 86 years old) who took 50 milligrams of beta carotene daily for 10 to 12 years. Prior to supplementation, the seniors showed suppressed immune activity. Beta carotene supplementation brought their immune function levels up to that of the younger men, while seniors not taking supplements showed continued low immune activity.

Even marginal deficiencies of one or more of the antioxidant nutrients can compromise the body's defense system. Since typical American diets often are low in the antioxidants, many people are at nutritional risk and don't even know it. In addition, diet alone might not be enough. "Recent evidence shows that a person must consume at least 400IU of vitamin E daily to experience immune-enhancing effects. You must resort to odd eating habits and be the size of a small whale to get that much vitamin E from food," says Dr. William Pryor, Ph.D, Boyd Professor of Chemistry and Biochemistry and Director of the Biodynamics Institute at Louisiana State University. Consequently, some researchers recommend supplements. However, other researchers disagree. "With a proper diet, a person can get all the nutrients needed for optimal immune function," says Robert Jacob, Ph.D., at the Western Human Nutrition Research Center, USDA Agricultural Research Service, in San Francisco. According to Dr. Jacob, it takes approximately 200 milligrams of vitamin C (the amount obtained from one cup of orange juice and two-thirds of a cup of strawberries) to keep the immune system running smoothly. However, many people do not eat even recommended levels of 60mg of vitamin C each day. The key is to combine responsible supplementation with a fruit- and vegetable-rich diet to maximize intake of both antioxidant nutrients and phytochemicals.

Other Nutrients Essential to Immunity

"IF YOU DO THE LITTLE JOBS WELL, THE BIG ONES WILL TEND TO TAKE CARE OF THEMSELVES."

Dale Carnegie

Other nutrients, such as vitamin B_6, zinc, folic acid, vitamin B_{12}, and the phytochemicals in garlic, also are essential for proper immune function in the later years, yet often they are not consumed in optimal amounts.

- At Loma Linda University in California and Oregon State University in Corvallis, researchers report that increasing vitamin B_6 intake enhances the immune response.
- A study from Maimonides Medical Center in Brooklyn found that vitamin B_{12}-deficient elderly were less responsive to vaccines and, thus, were more susceptible to pneumococcus infections that could result in illness or death.
- Folic acid absorption often is reduced as a person ages and poor dietary intake only worsens the deficiency, undermining immunity. In addition, folic acid is easily damaged by many medications, including antacids, diuretics used for high blood pressure, and anti-inflammatory medications.
- Minerals, including iron, selenium, copper, and zinc, also are involved in immunity. "Balance is the key with the minerals," says Dr. Sherman. "These nutrients interact and it is their unified effect on immunity that is important." Dr. Sherman emphasizes that this balance is best found in nutritious foods, not supplements.

    The minerals also are examples of how some is good, but more is not necessarily better. For example, although moderate doses of zinc (15 to 30 milligrams a day) are beneficial, doses of 150 milligrams actually suppress immune function and might increase a person's risk for infection and disease.
- Garlic contains phytochemicals that inhibit the growth of bacteria and might stimulate the immune system.

The Total Picture

"NEVER GIVE UP AND NEVER GIVE IN."
Hubert H. Humphrey

"Whether the attacking organism or the immune system prevails depends on many factors, including a person's nutritional status, general health, stress level, and sleep patterns, as well as the force of the onslaught," says Darshan Kelley, Ph.D., Research Chemist at the Western Human Nutrition Research Center in San Francisco. Consequently, the dietary guidelines outlined in the Anti-Aging Diet can't guarantee protection from all infections and diseases, but, until the last piece in the diet–immunity puzzle is found, they will greatly improve your odds of winning the war.

Medications on the Menu

"ALWAYS CARRY A FLAGON OF WHISKY IN CASE OF SNAKEBITE AND FURTHERMORE, ALWAYS CARRY A SMALL SNAKE."

W. C. Fields

More than 80 percent of older Americans are taking two or more medications every day, but few are aware of the impact some common medications have on nutritional status.

Medications can affect nutritional status in four ways:

1. They increase or decrease appetite, which reduces vitamin and mineral intake or results in overconsumption of nutrient-poor foods. Some medications also produce side effects that affect appetite, such as nausea, heartburn, or altered sense of taste.
2. They interfere with the absorption of nutrients, resulting in marginal vitamin and mineral deficiencies even when dietary intake is adequate.
3. They alter how the body uses or transports a nutrient or might entirely block the body's use of a vitamin or mineral.
4. They increase vitamin and mineral excretion, so nutrients are drained from the body faster than they are replaced.

The best defense against drug–nutrient interactions is to consume a nutrient-packed diet rich in fruits, vegetables, whole grains, extra-lean meat and legumes, and nonfat milk products.

In addition, always read the medication label and consult your physician and pharmacist to learn everything you can about the medications you are asked to take.

The Five Guidelines for Managing Medications

Here is a checklist to ensure your medications are used safely and only when needed.

1. Before you leave the doctor's office, ask the doctor about any possible side effects for any prescribed medications. If you are concerned about any medication being prescribed, say so and discuss your concerns. Ask about alternatives, such as counseling instead of tranquilizers or ice packs instead of anti-inflammatory medications.

2. With any prescription medication, ask the pharmacist:
    a) What is the name of the medication?
    b) What is the medication for?
    c) When is the best time to take it?
    d) Are there any side effects? If so, what are they?
    e) Are there any possible interactions with nutrients or other drugs?

3. Take only medications prescribed for you. Don't take anyone else's medications and don't share your own.

4. People who take more than one prescription medication, especially if prescribed by more than one physician, should take all the medications to a pharmacist to check interactions, dosages, and compatibility.

5. Take all expired medications to the local pharmacy for disposal.

Deprogramming the Biomarkers of Aging

"FOR AGE IS OPPORTUNITY NO LESS
THAN YOUTH ITSELF, THOUGH IN ANOTHER DRESS
AND AS THE EVENING TWILIGHT FADES AWAY
THE SKY IS FILLED WITH STARS, INVISIBLE BY DAY."

Henry Wadsworth Longfellow

The following chapter provides an overview of the latest research on how diet can reduce the risk of many age-related diseases, from arthritis and cancer to aging skin and loss of mental function. In all cases, the foundation for prevention is the Anti-Aging Diet and Fitness Program. Modify these guidelines based on the dietary recommendations for each disorder.

DRUG–NUTRIENT INTERACTIONS

Medication	*Nutrients Affected*	*What to Do/Consequences*
Acetaminophen	Liver damage caused by this pain reliever might be reduced by beta carotene.	Consume several daily servings of beta carotene–rich carrots, apricots, and spinach.
Alcohol	Replaces nutritious food. Increases requirements for B vitamins. Increases need for antioxidants. Inhibits absorption of vitamin C, B vitamins, calcium, and fat-soluble vitamins. Alters metabolism of vitamins D, B_1, B_6, and folic acid. Depletes tissues of vitamins A and E and selenium.	Limit alcohol intake to fewer than five drinks per week. Consume a nutrient-rich diet and take a moderate-dose multiple vitamin daily.
Antacids	Reduce absorption of vitamin A, vitamin B_{12}, iron, and folic acid. All-calcium antacids may upset magnesium balance.	Take antacids between meals and not with supplements. Take extra magnesium.
Antiarthritic medications (d-penicillamine)	Reduce absorption of iron, zinc, and vitamin B_6.	Increase intake of legumes, whole grains, bananas, and wheat germ.

Continued

Medication	Nutrients Affected	What to Do/Consequences
Antibiotics	Alter production and absorption of biotin, vitamin K, and vitamin C.	Consume several dark green leafy vegetables and citrus fruits daily.
Tetracycline	Reduces absorption of calcium in milk products. Reduces tissue levels of vitamins A and C.	Drink milk at opposite time of day from when taking the antibiotic. Consume five or more servings of fruits and vegetables daily.
Arthritis medications (Penicillamine)	Reduce absorption of zinc, iron, and other minerals. Increase requirements for vitamin B_6.	Take medication between meals. Consult physician about drug–nutrient interactions.
Aspirin	Irritates digestive tract, leading to internal bleeding, and consequently reduces iron stores. Large doses can reduce absorption of folic acid, vitamin C, and vitamin B_{12}.	Take aspirin in the morning and supplements at night. Have physician monitor iron status.
Caffeine	Tannins in coffee and tea reduce iron absorption.	Take extra vitamin C. Drink coffee/tea between meals, rather than with food.

Medication	Nutrients Affected	What to Do/Consequences
Cholesterol-lowering medications (cholestyramine and colestipol)	Reduces absorption of vitamin B_{12}, folic acid, iron, vitamins A, D, E, and K, and beta carotene.	Increase intake of chicken, leafy vegetables, and nonfat milk, and/or take a supplement that contains these nutrients.
High blood pressure medications	May increase urinary excretion of potassium, calcium, or magnesium.	Consume potassium-rich fruits and vegetables; magnesium-rich green leafy vegetables, soybeans, and wheat germ; and calcium-rich milk, or take a moderate-dose supplement.
Laxatives	Increase excretion of calcium, potassium, vitamin D.	Deficiencies can result with long-term use. Consult a physician about these effects and the need for supplements.
Mineral oil	Increases excretion of vitamins A, D, E, and K.	Consult a physician about long-term effects of taking this laxative.
Phenobarbital	Reduces absorption of vitamin D, folic acid, and vitamin B_{12}.	Increase intake of nonfat milk, dark green leafy vegetables, and lean meat.
Prozac	May reduce cravings for carbohydrates.	Some people experience a temporary loss of appetite and weight. Eat small meals and snacks throughout the day to sustain energy.

Continued

Medication	Nutrients Affected	What to Do/Consequences
Sulfasalazine	Reduces absorption of folic acid.	Increase intake of dark green leafy vegetables, orange juice, and wheat germ.
Tobacco	Increases requirements for or lowers tissue levels of vitamin A, beta carotene, vitamin E, vitamin C, vitamin B_6, vitamin B_{12}, folic acid, and other nutrients.	Don't smoke. Avoid inhaling others' smoke.

Chapter 10

HOW TO PREVENT THE DISEASES OF AGING

"To know how to grow old is the master work of wisdom, and one of the most difficult chapters in the great art of living."

Henri Frédéric Amiel

Old is what you get if you're lucky. Disease is what you get if you're not. Eating well, exercising regularly, managing stress, avoiding tobacco, maintaining a desirable weight, limiting alcohol, and other positive lifestyle habits can have profound effects on lowering your risk of developing disease in the second 50 years.

Unfortunately, many diseases just happen despite the best intentions. Even then, a healthful lifestyle can help minimize the effects of a disease, shorten its duration, lessen the symptoms, improve the odds for recovery, and help give you the vitality and energy needed to fight for your health.

The Big Four: Heart Disease, Hypertension, Diabetes, and Cancer

"NEVER GIVE IN! NEVER, NEVER, NEVER, NEVER, NEVER, NEVER. IN NOTHING GREAT OR SMALL, LARGE OR PETTY—NEVER GIVE IN EXCEPT TO CONVICTIONS OF HONOR AND GOOD SENSE."

Winston Churchill

Most people would extend their lives if they avoided the four main diseases:

- Ninety-six million Americans have blood cholesterol levels higher than 200mcg/dl, placing them at high risk for heart disease.
- More than 60 million Americans have cardiovascular disease; that's one in every four persons.
- Fifty million people have high blood pressure.
- One person dies every 33 seconds from heart disease.
- Sixteen million people in the United States have diabetes; half are unaware they have the disease.
- Almost one-and-a-half million new cases of cancer, not including skin cancer, will be diagnosed this year.
- More than 1,500 people die from cancer every day, accounting for one in every four deaths.

The statistics on the Big Four are staggering, especially when you consider that two out of every three people whose lives are affected by one or more of these diseases could have prevented the pain, suffering, and loss of life merely by making a few simple changes in diet and exercise.

A COMMON BOND

These diseases have more in common than you might imagine. If you have either hypertension or diabetes, your heart disease risk doubles; if you have both conditions, the risk is four-fold. In fact, 75 percent of diabetes-related deaths are caused by heart disease. Combine either diabetes or hypertension with smoking and your risk for heart disease goes up to eightfold. Smoking also elevates your risk for hypertension and cancer.

Excess body fat, especially if it's around the waist, dramatically increases a person's risk for developing all of the Big Four, as does inactivity. Inactivity leads to weight gain, elevated blood fats, and reduced blood sugar regulation, and sets up a condition called Syndrome X, which will be discussed later in this chapter. Exercising daily, avoiding tobacco smoke, consuming a healthful diet, and coping effectively with stress results in lower body weight, reduced blood cholesterol levels, elevated HDL cholesterol levels, improved glucose tolerance, normalization of blood pressure, and possibly a lowered risk of developing cancer. Heart disease, diabetes, hypertension, and cancer are increasingly found to have free-radical origins, while increased intake of the antioxidant nutrients minimizes the damage.

Most of these diseases are preventable. Up to 70 percent of all cancers are a result of lifestyle; the American Cancer Society estimates that 90 percent of skin cancers could be avoided if people protected their skin from the sun's rays. All cancers, especially cancers of the lungs, bladder, esophagus, and stomach, caused by cigarette smoking or alcohol could be prevented by making healthier choices. Up to 95 percent of many cancers can be effectively treated if diagnosis is made in the early stages of the disease. The vast majority of diabetics could be free from their disease just by losing excess body weight. Heart disease is preventable, curable, and even reversible in some cases by making better food, exercise, and life choices.

Heart Disease and Hypertension

"A MAN IS ONLY AS OLD AS HIS ARTERIES."
Sir William Osler

Heart disease remains the number-one killer disease in this country, but death rates from heart disease have dropped in the past few decades a staggering 42 percent in people under 54 years of age and 33 percent in people between 55 and 84 years of age. On another positive note, heart disease is preventable and treatable in most cases and gives most people fair warning—elevated blood cholesterol levels and low HDL cholesterol (the "good" cholesterol) levels. Keeping total cholesterol at or below 200mcg/dl and the ratio of total cholesterol to HDL cholesterol at or below 4.5:1, maintaining normal blood pressure, and preventing or managing diabetes can lower your risk dramatically.

The development of heart disease and its underlying cause, atherosclerosis (narrowing of the arteries caused by cholesterol accumulation), is often part of a more complex condition called Syndrome X that includes an increased risk for high blood pressure, glucose intolerance and diabetes, excess body fat, and high blood fat levels, including cholesterol and triglycerides. Increased weight elevates blood pressure and cholesterol and places increased stress on the heart and blood vessels. While virtually everyone has some degree of cholesterol accumulation in the arteries by the second decade of life, the condition progresses to disease states for about half the population.

HEART DISEASE BEGINS AND ENDS WITH FAT

The most important dietary change you can make to save your heart is to reduce the amount of saturated fat in your diet. A diet high in these fats increases your risk for developing heart disease by elevating blood cholesterol levels, platelet clumping, and prostaglandin activity. Reducing dietary fat lowers blood cholesterol levels, slows the progression of atherosclerosis, and decreases your risk for heart attack. Even modest changes in the diet can lower blood cholesterol as much as 10 percent, with a subsequent reduction in heart disease risk of 20 percent.

The oil in fish and olive oil are exceptions to the fat–heart disease connection. Inclusion of either olive oil or fish in the diet not only decreases blood fat levels and lowers blood pressure, but reduces platelet clumping and prostaglandin release, which in turn lowers the risk for atherosclerosis and heart disease. As little as 4 ounces of salmon can benefit the heart if consumed on a regular basis. These oils lower the risk for heart disease, but only if combined with a low-fat diet.

FIBER AND HEART DISEASE

The second most important dietary change a person can make is to increase fibrous foods in the diet. The soluble fibers in oats, cooked dried beans and peas, fruit, guar gum, and alfalfa lower blood cholesterol and low-density lipoprotein cholesterol (LDLs), the type of blood cholesterol most closely linked to heart disease risk. A high-fiber diet helps decrease the production and increase the excretion of cholesterol and helps reduce blood pressure, all of which lower a person's risk for heart disease.

SALT SENSITIVITY

The Anti-Aging Diet doesn't specify guidelines for salt intake, but anyone at risk for developing hypertension should limit salt to no more than 6 grams per day, or slightly more than a teaspoon. Further reduction to 4.5 grams or less is best for people who are "salt-sensitive" and develop high blood pressure when they consume excessive amounts of salt. Salt (sodium chloride) is 40 percent sodium, so this recommendation is the equivalent of 2.4 grams of sodium.

To prevent or treat hypertension, include several servings a day of calcium-rich foods. Numerous studies show that it is the combined effect of too much salt and too little calcium that might predispose a person to hypertension. You should consume the equivalent of three to four glasses of nonfat or low-fat milk or yogurt each day.

BEYOND FAT AND FIBER

Even the most carefully designed diet can fall short of optimal when daily calorie intake is below 2,000 or when disease or medication use increases nutrient needs above normal requirements. In addition, some nutrients, such as vitamin E, are needed in amounts far greater than are realistic from diet alone. Consequently, a moderate-dose multiple vitamin and mineral plus an extra dose of vitamin E should be considered.

Several B vitamins are important in the prevention of heart disease or hypertension. Nicotinic acid (a form of niacin) lowers both total cholesterol and LDL cholesterol while raising high-density lipoprotein cholesterol (HDLs), the beneficial form of blood cholesterol. Pharmacological doses (doses greater than are typically consumed from foods) of niacin in conjunction with cholesterol-lowering medications are effective in the management of heart disease. Niacin therapy can cause adverse side effects, however, and should be monitored by a physician.

Optimal intake of vitamins B_6, B_{12}, and folic acid also are associated with a reduced risk for heart disease. These B vitamins are essential in controlling a compound called homocysteine. Levels of this compound rise when the diet is low in these vitamins, thus increasing a person's risk for developing heart disease even if other factors, such as blood cholesterol, remain low. "It appears that the amount people need are amounts slightly greater than current recommendations," states Robert Russell, M.D., Professor of Medicine and Nutrition at Tufts University in Boston. "People may not need to take a supplement, if they obtain five to nine servings of fresh vegetables every day and a total of at least 400 micrograms of folic acid, 3 micrograms of vitamin B_{12}, and 2 milligrams of vitamin B_6."

Adequate intake of the antioxidants (vitamin C, vitamin E, and beta carotene) might lower the "bad" blood cholesterol levels while elevating the "good" HDL cholesterol. Vitamin C also helps remove cholesterol from the arteries, encourages the formation of prostaglandins that lower atherosclerosis risk, and aids in the regression of heart disease. Vitamin E, in doses of at least 100IU and possibly as much as 800IU a day, helps prevent and treat heart disease, improves prognosis and recovery after open-heart surgery, and might even aid in the regression of atherosclerosis, the underlying cause of heart disease.

Some people with heart disease show improvement when the chromium content of their diets is increased. A daily intake of 200 micrograms of chromium reduces total blood cholesterol, increases HDL cholesterol, and helps normalize blood sugar levels.

Magnesium relaxes artery walls and the heart muscle. A deficiency of this mineral results in hypertension, irregular heartbeat, chest pain associated with reduced blood and oxygen to the heart, atherosclerosis, and damage to the heart. Supplementing with magnesium might return the heartbeat and blood pressure to normal and reduce the chances of experiencing a heart attack. In addition, the doses of many heart and blood pressure medications can be reduced when magnesium intake is optimal. Some hypertension medications increase urinary loss of magnesium and increase the risk for marginal deficiency of this essential mineral.

THE BOTTOM LINE

The guidelines for a healthy heart are simple: reduce fat to no more than 30 percent of total calories (i.e., choose nonfat dairy products and lean meats and use little or no fat in food preparation); reduce cholesterol to no more than 300 milligrams a day (one egg contains 220 milligrams of cholesterol; whole milk contains 34 milligrams of cholesterol per cup; one ounce of Cheddar cheese contains 28 milligrams); increase daily fiber intake to between 25 and 45 grams by choosing whole-grain products, cooked dried beans and peas, and fresh fruits and vegetables; use olive oil rather than other oils or butter (though sparingly); and include at least three servings of fish in the weekly diet. Make sure that three out of every four foods you eat are plant derived, including vegetables, fruit, grains, and legumes. In addition, even a modest weight loss of 10 to 20 pounds can reduce blood pressure, cholesterol levels, and heart disease risk, while improving glucose tolerance and other indicators of Syndrome X.

Diabetes—Under Control

"DON'T FIGHT FORCES, USE THEM."
Richard Buckminster Fuller

Diabetes is a disease characterized by the body's inability to produce or properly use insulin, the hormone that converts blood sugar and other fuels into energy needed by cells. One form of diabetes, insulin-dependent diabetes, is an auto-immune disease that usually develops in children and young adults; it can be controlled through diet, exercise, and daily insulin injections. Up to 95 percent of diabetics have the other form, non-insulin-dependent or adult-onset diabetes, which results from the body's inability to make enough or efficiently use insulin. Non-insulin-dependent diabetes is usually caused by inactivity, poor eating habits, and excess body weight. Try to avoid this debilitating disease by maintaining a desirable weight.

WHAT GOES WRONG?

Energy is obtained from food by the release of insulin in response to carbohydrates as they enter the bloodstream after a meal. The pancreas secretes the hormone insulin to help transport the rising blood glucose into the cells of the muscles, brain, liver, and other organs. This provides fuel for the tissues and returns blood glucose levels to normal. In some people, however, the body's cells are insensitive to insulin, so blood glucose levels remain high. The pancreas tries to overcompensate by secreting more insulin and the result is a condition called insulin resistance or hyperinsulinemia. Left unchecked, this condition can progress to diabetes, where both insulin and glucose levels remain high. In people with diabetes, elevated insulin levels also promote the conversion of glucose into fat. Insulin resistance is part of a larger metabolic condition called Syndrome X that is associated with above-the-belt fat accumulation, high blood fats, diabetes, hypertension, and an elevated risk for developing heart disease and possibly some forms of cancer.

Excess body weight precedes hyperinsulinemia, while weight loss, especially when combined with a regular exercise program, normalizes insulin levels. In people who exercise, less insulin is needed to move more glucose into the cells, so less of the hormone is secreted by the pancreas in response to food intake. Consequently, more incoming carbohydrates are burned in the muscles for energy and fewer are stored as fat. Exercise also protects against insulin resistance by improving the body's ability to mobilize fat from storage for fuel, which prevents fat accumulation. The leaner cells also respond more quickly and efficiently to insulin, so less of the hormone is needed to transport glucose out of the blood.

To prevent non-insulin-dependent diabetes:

1. Attain and maintain a desirable weight by following the Anti-Aging Diet and Exercise Program. Daily exercise reduces diabetes risk even in the absence of weight loss.
2. Emphasize fiber-rich foods in the diet, especially cooked dried beans and peas, oats, and fruits. These foods help normalize blood sugar levels.
3. Keep sugar, fat, alcohol, and unnecessary calories in check.
4. Take a moderate-dose multiple vitamin and mineral that contains 200 micro-

grams of chromium, the antioxidants including vitamins E and C, and the B vitamins. Make sure you consume ample amounts of magnesium-rich foods, such as bananas, dark green leafy vegetables, nuts, and wheat germ, or take a magnesium supplement.

Cancer Cures

"IF I'D KNOWN I WAS GOING TO LIVE SO LONG, I'D HAVE TAKEN BETTER CARE OF MYSELF."

Eubie Blake

Today, fewer people over age 50 are dying from heart disease, but more are dying from cancer. By far the greatest contributor to cancer is smoking, with women being five to six times more likely to die from tobacco-related cancers than their grandmothers who didn't smoke. In fact, if lung cancer is excluded from the statistics, the cancer-death toll has dropped 15 percent in this country since the 1930s. Unfortunately, however, breast cancer is on the rise and is twice as common today as it was in women a hundred years ago. One in every nine women today will develop breast cancer.

The good news is that you can decrease your risk. The National Academy of Sciences' report "Diet, Nutrition, and Cancer" states that lifestyle is responsible for up to 60 percent of cancers. While women can lower their risks by not smoking, exercising regularly, and (in the case of breast cancer) breastfeeding their babies, by far the biggest impact might come from a few simple dietary changes that reduce fat, increase fiber, replace meat with tofu, and limit or eliminate alcohol.

HORMONES, FAT, AND CANCER

The causes of cancer have evaded researchers for years. One link, at least with breast cancer, seems clear-cut: women in cultures with a low breast cancer incidence, such as Japan, also have significantly lower levels of a group of female hormones called estrogens. Women in the United States, where breast cancer risk is high, have 30 to 75 percent higher levels of two estrogens—estrone and estradiol—than do women in Japan.

The lower hormone levels might have more to do with diet than with genetics. Studies show that when Japanese women migrate to the United States and adopt a Western lifestyle, their risks and their children's risks of developing breast cancer rise to match those of American women. One possible explanation is that breast cancer rates soar as Japanese women abandon their low-fat diets in favor of high-fat American cuisine. Other epidemiological studies (studies that investigate disease rates across countries) report similar findings. In fact, one study found that a woman's risk for breast cancer increases as much as 30 percent for every 10 percent increase in fat calories.

The fat issue also is firmly documented in studies on animals. Animals fed high-fat diets get cancer, while those fed leaner fare don't; no other nutrient is as strongly tied to this disease.

Research is contradictory, however, when the fat–cancer link is studied in people living in the same country. For example, the Nurse's Health Study conducted by Walter Willett, M.D., Dr.P.H., and colleagues at the Harvard School of Public Health in Boston collected dietary intake information and monitored disease rates on more than 80,000 women living in the United States and found no link between fat intake and breast cancer risk. Critics of this study argue that the data collected had potential inaccuracies. In addition, the variance in fat intakes might have been too small; even the "low-fat" group still consumed approximately 30 percent of calories as fat, while women in Japan consume closer to 11 to 15 percent of calories as fat. However, without consistent findings, the effect of dietary fat on cancer remains controversial.

"Regarding breast cancer, there is a huge amount of data showing that the large amounts of fat in the US diet are doing something and it's not good," warns Leonard Cohen, Ph.D., Section Head of Nutrition and Endocrinology at the American Health Foundation in Valhalla, New York. According to Dr. Cohen, dietary fat is a promotor, not an initiator, of the cancer process and probably exerts its effects by altering expression of the genetic code within cells, affecting regulatory processes in cell membranes, and upsetting estrogen balance. The effects of fat on estrogen also make it reasonable to assume that a high-fat diet of hamburgers and French fries during puberty, when these hormones kick in to initiate breast development, could set the stage for cancer later in life. Dietary fat also shows harmful effects when it comes to other cancers, such as colon and rectal cancers.

Another theory highlights the type, not the amount, of fat in the diet. "Just like people have different personalities, different fats also have different effects on cancer risk and shouldn't be lumped together as all bad," says Dr. Cohen. For example, polyunsaturated fats in safflower and other vegetable oils raise levels of hormone-like compounds called prostaglandins, which in turn promote some types of cancers, such as prostate and breast cancer. Saturated fats in meat also escalate risk for several types of cancer including colon cancer, while olive oil and the oils in fish might suppress cancer growth.

"There is more evidence that monounsaturated oils [such as olive and canola oils] lower cancer risk, than there is evidence that total fat intake raises risk," says Dr. Willett of the Nurses' Health Study. Unfortunately, no one knows exactly how much olive oil or fish oil is best, but most agree that cutting back on total fat, with more coming from olive oil and fish and less coming from meat, dairy, and vegetable oils, is a safe and potentially healthful start.

Another advantage of switching to a low-fat diet is that this eating style might help a person maintain a desirable body weight. Obesity is related to several cancers, from colon to breast cancer. You don't have to be obese to develop cancer; however, the risk escalates with increasing body weight and the chances of surviving the cancer are worse if you are overweight.

People who store more fat above the belt, compared to those who carry their extra weight in the hips and thighs, also are more likely to have higher estrogen levels and higher risks of developing cancer. This link between "belly" fat, disease, and estrogens might explain why cutting calories and increasing exercise, two ways to reduce fat tissue, also lower estrogen levels and disease risk.

CALORIES AND CANCER

Studies on animals consistently show that severe calorie restriction lowers cancer rates. "But we're not talking a moderate cut back in calories," warns Dr. Cohen. "These animals are very hungry, to the point that they become aggressive and irritable." Dr. Cohen believes it is unrealistic to expect people to cut calories enough to reduce risk; however, modifying what we eat by consuming less fat and more fiber is very viable.

SOY GOOD

Fat is not the only link to low estrogen levels in Japanese women. These women also consume 30 to 50 times more soy than do women in the United States, foods that contain an arsenal of anti-cancer compounds called phytoestrogens, of which genistein and diadzein appear to be the most potent.

The protective effects of genistein have been substantiated in studies on animals. Only 60 percent of newborn female rats exposed to chemicals known to cause breast cancer actually develop cancer when their diets are supplemented with genestein, while 100 percent of unsupplemented rats develop cancer.

How do phytoestrogens work? According to Johanna Dwyer, D.Sc., R.D., Professor of Medicine and Community Health at Tufts University Medical School in Boston, phytoestrogens might bind to receptor sites on breast cells that otherwise bind to estrogen, which reduces the cell-altering effects of the hormone.

Soy Solutions

In a quandary over how to add tofu to your diet? Here are a few tasty suggestions.

1. Add tofu to enchiladas, pasta primavera, lasagna, and stir frys.
2. Blend tofu to a make a creamy base for soups, salad dressings, and sauces.
3. Crumble tofu into salads (it picks up the flavor of the dressing).
4. Use soy milk in preparing packaged pudding mixes, on cereal, in cream sauces, or as a coffee creamer.
5. Replace hamburgers with textured vegetable patties (made from soybeans) from the frozen food section.
6. Add isolated soy protein (ISP) powder to baked goods such as breads and muffins, pancakes and waffles, cookies, and meatloaf.

Soy products also are an excellent source of fiber, which might lower estrogen and cancer risk in its own right. One study from the American Health Foundation in New York reported that estrogen levels dropped significantly within two months when people increased their fiber intake from 15 to 30 grams a day.

The optimal daily or weekly dose of soy products has not been established. However, two or more servings weekly would provide a low-fat, high-fiber alternative to meat and should benefit overall health as well as possibly aid in cancer prevention.

JUST SAY ''NO'' TO ALCOHOL

More than a dozen studies have consistently found that moderate alcohol intake (three or more drinks a week) increases cancer risk by 20 to 70 percent. "Alcohol may raise estrogen levels, which would help explain its underlying connection to breast cancer," says Dr. Willett. Alcohol alters both hormone balance and the menstrual cycle in patterns similar to those characteristic of aggressive cancer progression. It also has been linked to an increased risk for esophageal and bladder cancers.

WHAT SHOULD YOU DO?

We don't have firm answers yet about what factors—dietary or otherwise—affect cancer risk. What we do know is that cancer is a multi-stage process, so a person's best bet is to block that process with a host of healthful foods at as many steps along the way as possible.

1. Limit your intake of potential initiators or promoters of cancer by cutting back on fat and alcohol.
2. Eat lots of foods that contain cancer-fighting compounds, such as fiber-rich fruits, vegetables, and whole grains. Make sure some vegetables come from the cabbage family, such as broccoli, asparagus, Brussels sprouts, and cauliflower. These vegetables are rich in phytochemicals called indoles that reduce cancer risk.
3. Consume a diet rich in calcium and vitamin D (nonfat milk is the most reliable source), since these nutrients combined with a low-fat diet show promise in lowering the risk for developing colon cancer.

4. Consume moderate amounts of monounsaturated fats, such as olive and canola oils, as a substitute for other fats.

5. Include several servings weekly of soybean products.

6. Don't smoke or expose yourself to other people's smoke.

7. Exercise daily and for life. As little as a one-mile walk each day throughout life can cut your risk in half for developing several types of cancer.

8. Take a supplement that includes additional antioxidant nutrients, including vitamins C and E and beta carotene.

9. Drink tea, green or black, decaffeinated or regular. Phytochemicals in tea help lower cancer risk. The same does not hold true for herbal teas.

Dr. Dwyer is right when she says, "There isn't a magic or miracle food that will cure or prevent cancer." However, there might be many health-enhancing compounds in a variety of wholesome foods that could do the trick.

Arthritis: Staying Limber

"LET ME TELL YOU THE SECRET THAT HAS LED ME TO MY GOAL. MY STRENGTH LIES SOLELY IN MY TENACITY."

Louis Pasteur

You can tie Vyrillian tubes around your neck, wrap your wrists in copper bracelets, drink vinegar and honey, chug Dr. Smedley's miracle potion, take shark cartilage capsules, or inject snake venom, but don't expect any of these quick-fix remedies to cure arthritis.

No one knows exactly the cause of, let alone how to cure, arthritis in the 40 million Americans who currently suffer from the disease (the numbers are predicted to increase to 60 million by the year 2020). What we do know is that arthritis is probably as old as the human race, with the bones of Java Ape Man and mummies from ancient Egypt showing signs of joint damage.

Arthritis is an umbrella term for hundreds of conditions that cause pain and discomfort in the joints and the surrounding tissues. The most common forms of arthritis are osteoarthritis and rheumatoid arthritis. Osteoarthritis develops after a lifetime of use and abuse to the joints, which roughens and wears away the cartilage (the material that cushions the surface of the joints). As a result, the joint—especially the weight-bearing joints in the back, hips, knees, and the bones in the hands and wrists—becomes stiff and painful. With rheumatoid arthritis, the joints are inflamed and swollen, rather than worn, with stiffness and pain. Compared to osteoarthritis, rheumatoid arthritis usually affects the whole body and can range from mild discomfort to severe crippling.

OLD OR ABUSED BONES?

Osteoarthritis (from now on called arthritis) is easily confused with aging, since its incidence increases as people get older. One in eight people under the age of 50 years have arthritis, while 25 percent of people over 50 and one in every two people age 65 and older have one or more stiff joints. Arthritis is often more a matter of time and use than age. You have some control as to whether or not you develop arthritis, how serious the condition is, and at what rate it progresses. Since developing a reliable, effective cure remains elusive, your best bet is to prevent the disease in the first place.

FEEDING YOUTHFUL JOINTS

Since abusing the joints contributes to the development and progression of arthritis, it makes sense that excess body weight, or more specifically fat weight, is directly linked to arthritis. Even a modest weight gain of 25 pounds equates to constantly carrying a backpack of that weight; over time the extra burden damages cartilage.

A study from the Centers for Disease Control and Prevention found that men and women who are overweight are 30 percent more likely than lean adults to develop arthritis, regardless of age. Shedding weight also can help relieve symptoms in people already afflicted with arthritis. In contrast to body fat, extra muscle strengthens the bones and joints and maintains good posture, and both help prevent arthritis. Strength training is essential to the prevention of the disease.

To maintain a desirable weight, focus on the fruits, vegetables, cooked dried beans and peas, nonfat milk, and whole grains in the Anti-Aging Diet. People who develop arthritis often consume too few of these foods and miss many essential nutrients. Whether or not this contributes to the development of the disease is not clear, but why take the chance?

For example, consuming too little calcium, selenium, and zinc from foods such as nonfat milk, cooked dried beans and peas, and fresh vegetables contributes to skeletal damage in humans. Preliminary research shows that some nutrients, such as vitamins E, B_2, and C, inhibit the development of arthritis, while vitamins E, B_1, B_6, and B_{12} improve joint function in some animals. Bioflavonoids in oranges and other citrus fruits and vitamin D in milk also might help prevent the disease. Since the only reliable dietary source of vitamin D is milk, anyone not drinking at least two to three glasses daily should consider taking a moderate-dose supplement.

The cumulative damaging effects of free radicals on joints and surrounding tissues are suspected to contribute to arthritis. Boost antioxidant intake by supplementing with vitamin E and consuming several servings daily of vitamin C- and carotene-rich fruits and vegetables. These antioxidant nutrients counteract free-radical damage to tissues and might help prevent the disease and/or slow its progression. Researchers at Boston University state that consuming a vitamin C–rich diet slows the rate of progression of arthritis threefold. Consuming ample amounts of beta carotene reduces risk by 60 percent, and supplementing with vitamin E reduces risk by 30 percent. (See Chapters 2 and 9 for more on free radicals and antioxidants.)

*R*heumatoid Arthritis: A Research Update

Although no evidence exists that rheumatoid arthritis is caused by diet or that diet can cure the disease, several studies show a reduction in symptoms from a few dietary changes.

1. *Eat primarily vegetarian.* Numerous studies show that switching to a vegetarian diet reduces pain, morning stiffness, the number of joints affected, and the number of swollen joints in people with rheumatoid arthritis.

2. *Include fish in the weekly menu.* Fats in fish oils called omega-3 fatty acids reduce lev-

els of hormone-like compounds in the body called prostaglandins and leukotrienes that aggravate the inflammation associated with rheumatoid arthritis. Eating fish or taking fish oil capsules might reduce morning stiffness and joint tenderness in some arthritis sufferers. The effects appear to be dose-related, with greater improvements at higher doses.

3. *Take a moderate-dose multiple vitamin and mineral.* Numerous studies report that people with rheumatoid arthritis consume insufficient amounts and have low blood levels of several nutrients, including vitamin E, beta carotene, folic acid, vitamin B_{12}, selenium, zinc, iron, vitamin B_6, and niacin. These deficiencies undermine general health and aggravate the arthritis.

4. *Consume three to four servings daily of nonfat milk.* Bone loss associated with rheumatoid arthritis is linked to poor intake of calcium and vitamin D.

MOVE IT

Consider the following two scenarios:

Cathy started feeling some stiffness in her joints at age 65. When her joints hurt, she moved less. She spent more time sitting, while her muscles became weaker and her joints became stiffer. After several years, she was in constant pain and seldom left her easychair.

Jeanette is 80 years old and has had arthritis for years, but she doesn't let it slow her down. She walks or swims daily, in spite of the discomfort. By staying active, she has maintained strong muscles, maximum joint flexibility, a positive attitude, and an active life.

While the two women have the same disease, its effects on their lives, vitality, and longevity are very different, for two simple reasons: attitude and exercise. Cathy's "give up" attitude hastened the progression of arthritis. Jeanette's "never give up" optimism motivated her to keep moving when she learned she had arthritis. As a result, her disease has progressed slowly, allowing her to live a full and active life.

In the past, it was mistakenly thought that long-term exercise increased a person's risk for arthritis. Today, research shows that exercise is vital for both the prevention and the treatment of arthritis. Runners who pound the pavement actually have a lower rate of arthritis and less overall disability than their couch-potato friends. To reduce your risk of developing arthritis later in life, start moving today.

Times also have changed when it comes to exercise for the treatment of arthritis. When our parents developed arthritis, they were told to "take it easy." Today, the recommendation is to MOVE. Exercise is essential to keep the disease under control once it has developed. Staying physically active stretches the joints, helps move fluids and chemicals through the surrounding tissues, and reduces stiffness. Exercise also keeps the bones, muscles, and tendons strong around the joint. One study found that walking, stretching, and strength training in patients with arthritis in the knees lowered their pain by 27 percent and improved their movement by 30 percent.

If you have joint pain or stiffness, first consult a physician to confirm that arthritis is really the problem, since some joint problems other than osteoarthritis are better treated with physical therapy, not exercise. If arthritis is the cause, discuss with your physician the exercise options, including walking, swimming, water walking, water aerobics, or other nonjarring exercise. Remember to always warm up prior to exercise.

Eyesight Survival Skills

" . . . IF EYES WERE MADE FOR SEEING, THEN BEAUTY IS ITS OWN EXCUSE FOR BEING."

Ralph Waldo Emerson

Life is filled with unforgettable sights, pictures we hold in our mind's eye that give meaning and joy to our daily lives. Not so long ago, loss of sight was considered an inevitable consequence of aging. That belief is changing as evidence shows that vision is as much a matter of lifestyle as age, which means that many of the over one million cataract procedures performed each year in the United States might be needless if people made a few changes in what they ate and how they supplemented. Age-related eye diseases that once led to blindness, such as cataracts and macular degeneration, might be prevented if you make a few simple changes in what you eat today.

YOU CAN PREVENT CATARACTS

For good vision, the eye lens must collect and focus light on the retina, and to do so, it must remain clear. With age, many people suffer clouding or "opacification" of the lens, a condition called cataracts and one of the leading causes of blindness.

Cataracts are an excellent example of how lifestyle is the problem in disorders once thought to be the natural consequence of aging. While only 4.5 percent of people under the age of 45 develop cataracts, the statistics increase tenfold with age, with almost one in every two persons over 75 suffering from vision loss caused by cataracts. (If pre-cataract changes in the lens are included, the incidence is twice as high.)

Research shows that long-term exposure to free radicals, not aging per se, is the underlying cause of cataracts. Repeated exposure to sunlight and/or tobacco smoke generates oxygen fragments or free radicals that attack and damage proteins within the lens. Damaged proteins clump together and, over a lifetime, cause clouding and cataracts. The greater the exposure to ultraviolet (UV) light, the higher the incidence; people who work outdoors or who live close to the equator or at high elevations are at highest risk.

ANTIOXIDANTS, SUPPLEMENTS, AND CATARACTS

The development of cataracts indicates that the body's protective antioxidant system isn't keeping pace with the damaging onslaught of free radicals. Consuming ample amounts and maintaining high tissue levels of the antioxidant nutrients, such as vitamin C, vitamin E, and the carotenoids, and counteracting sun damage to the lens might delay development of cataracts and prevent vision loss.

Studies show that people with cataracts have low tissue and blood levels of the antioxidants, while people who consume ample amounts of antioxidant-rich foods or supplements and maintain optimal tissue levels of these nutrients reduce their risk by up to 70 percent. Researchers at Harvard Medical School in Boston report that of the more than 17,000 men they studied, those who took supplements reduced their risks of developing cataracts by more than 25 percent.

Diagram of the Eye

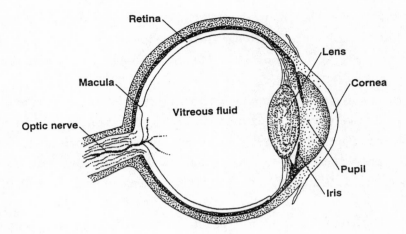

When researchers at the University of Wisconsin Medical School in Madison investigated the development of nuclear sclerosis (cloudiness and discoloration in the lens of the eye characteristic of pre-cataracts) in 1,919 people and compared that incidence to dietary habits during the preceding 10 years, they found that the people who supplemented with vitamins A, C, E, B_2, B_1, and niacin and who also consumed lots of vegetables rich in folic acid, beta carotene, fiber, and the phytochemicals lutein and zeaxanthin cut their risk for developing cataracts by half compared to people who did not supplement. These dietary habits also might protect the eyes from other age-related disorders, such as macular degeneration.

WHAT IS MACULAR DEGENERATION?

The number-one cause of vision loss is age-related macular degeneration, or ARMD. The term refers to an area of the eye called the macula, the light-sensitive portion of the retina that is responsible for central vision. When the macula is working well, a person can read fine print, drive a car, work on hobbies, thread a needle, or recognize a face. Damage to the macula, however, causes gradual vision loss, creating a blur or blind spot in the center of vision. In the early stages of ARMD, the person may see shapes, but can't see well enough to read. Then objects become blurry, and finally they disappear.

Not everyone in the early stages will progress, but there is no way to know who will and who won't develop ARMD. While surgical procedures and clot-busting medications are useful treatment in a small number of cases, by far the best strategy is to prevent the damage in the first place.

Antioxidants, Pro-Vision

Long-term exposure to air and light, not age per se, generates free radicals that damage the macula. Fortifying the eye with the antioxidants vitamin C, vitamin E, selenium, beta carotene, and zinc should help protect against the development of ARMD. People with high levels of antioxidants are at low risk of developing ARMD.

Vitamin C is the antioxidant found in oranges, strawberries, and other fruits and vegetables. The eye naturally stockpiles vitamin C to levels 20 times and higher than those found in the blood. Interestingly, vitamin C levels in the eyes of nocturnal animals are very low in comparison. Dr. Donita Garland at the National Eye Institute in Bethesda, Maryland, theorizes that the high concentration of vitamin C in our eyes might be an adaptation that protects them from solar radiation.

Popeye Wouldn't Get ARMD

A host of health-enhancing phytochemicals in fruits and vegetables have been identified as sight savers. The potential benefits of phytochemicals were discovered after studies showed that people with ARMD consumed significantly fewer fruits and vegetables than did those who maintained healthy eyesight. In contrast, people who consume diets rich in fruits and vegetables, particularly tomatoes and dark green leafy vegetables like spinach, maintain higher blood levels of phytochemicals (such as lycopene, lutein, and zeaxanthin).

Researchers at Florida International University in Miami report that when people consume 30 milligrams of lutein daily, serum lutein levels rise tenfold within 20 days. Macular pigment densities also increase. As a result, people are less likely to develop ARMD; and if they do, the disease is less likely to progress to advanced stages.

What's Good for the Heart Is Good for the Eyes

Researchers at the University of Wisconsin surveyed more than 2,000 people age 45 and older and found that those who ate the most saturated fat and cholesterol had an 80 percent greater risk of developing ARMD compared with those who ate little fat. At this time, it's not clear whether consuming a diet high in saturated fat contributes to vision loss, or whether filling up on vegetables and whole grains instead of fat protects the eyes.

THE VISIONARY DIET

The secret to preventing age-related vision loss is to start the prevention program immediately and to continue throughout life:

1. Consume daily at least eight servings of fresh fruits and vegetables (including two servings of dark green leafy vegetables and two servings of vitamin C–rich citrus fruits).
2. Take a moderate-dose multiple vitamin and mineral supplement (see Chapter 7 for guidelines on choosing a supplement).
3. Take an antioxidant supplement that contains 250 to 1,000 milligrams vitamin C, 100 to 400IU of vitamin E, and a mix of carotenoids including beta carotene, lutein, and zeaxanthin.

In addition to following these dietary guidelines, wear protective sunglasses year-round that filter out 95 to 100 percent of the sun's ultraviolet rays.

Radiant Smile, Beautiful Teeth

"THIS BREAD OF LIFE DROPPED IN THY MOUTH DOTH CRY:
EAT, EAT ME, SOUL, AND THOU SHALT NEVER DIE."
Edward Taylor

Until recently, gum disease (called periodontal disease and characterized by swollen and tender gums, bad breath, and a bad taste in the mouth) was considered an inevitable consequence of aging. While infections of the gums and loss of calcium from the jawbone still contribute to dental problems in the second 50 years, the vast majority of gum disease could be prevented. In fact, with proper care and good diet, dentures could become obsolete.

HAVE YOU BRUSHED YOUR TEETH TODAY?

The first step in caring for your teeth is proper daily and yearly care. That includes brushing at least twice daily with a quality toothbrush (most dentists recommend replacing your brush every three months), flossing once a day, and getting a professional cleaning twice yearly. Fluoride helps neutralize acid formation and strengthens the enamel, making it more resistant to decay. Consult your dentist about the possible need for fluoride supplements or rinse.

Hormonal changes during menopause can trigger a condition called menopausal gingivostomatitis, characterized by dry or bleeding gums, a burning mouth, abnormal taste sensations, and/or a sensitivity to hot or cold foods. Hormone replacement therapy (HRT) alleviates this condition. If you suffer from these menopausal symptoms and are not on HRT, try a saliva substitute for dry mouth, which can be purchased from most local pharmacies, or drink plenty of water and chew sugarless gum to keep the mouth moist and stimulate saliva. Also, floss and brush gently, using a soft-bristle brush, and use toothpaste especially formulated for sensitive teeth. Consult your dentist if the sensitivity persists or worsens.

SWEET TOOTH

Virtually all Americans have some decayed teeth by the time they reach adulthood, not because their teeth wear out, but because they eat too many sweets. In cultures where refined sugar is nonexistent, cavities are an oddity, even in the oldest of the old.

While children are warned to limit their sugar intake to avoid cavities, little attention is paid to the sugar consumed by adults. Yet studies show that 53 percent of men and 47 percent of women over 65 consume more sugar-containing foods than do younger adults. (See Chapter 7 for more information on sugar.)

The bacteria that normally live in the mouth break down sugar to form acid, which wears away tooth enamel. Sugar also fuels the growth of plaque, the colonies of bacteria that cause periodontal disease. The cure is easy. Follow the guidelines outlined in the Anti-Aging Diet, and

1. cut back on sweets, from desserts and candy to honey and soda pop;
2. eat sweets only with meals;
3. avoid sticky sweets, such as dried fruits, toffee, and caramelized desserts; and
4. keep the exposure short, e.g., avoid sucking on candies or cough drops or sipping soft drinks throughout the day.

Since Americans consume twice as much sugar as is generally recommended for health, or up to 20 to 25 percent of their daily calories, a general rule is to cut your current sugar intake by half. Nonnutritive sweeteners, such as aspartame, don't fuel acid-forming bacteria, so are a safe way to sweeten your day.

Snacking also can be a problem, since even natural sugars from fruit, yogurt, or grains can stimulate oral bacteria. Rather than not snack, combine some anti-cavity foods, such as a small amount of cheese or a few peanuts that help neutralize acids, with the more problematic foods that tend to stick to teeth, such as crackers and raisins. Chewing on sugarless gum after a meal produces saliva, which helps neutralize tooth-decaying acids. Brushing after every meal and snack is the best option.

ANTIOXIDANTS AND A HEALTHY SMILE

The cells lining the mouth have short life spans and require a constant supply of energy and nutrients for repair and replication. Optimal levels of coenzyme Q10 are needed to provide this energy. Diseased dental tissues often have low levels of coenzyme Q10 compared to healthy gums. Several studies on patients with gum disease show that this antioxidant helps speed the healing process of the gums and even reverses the signs of gum disease in some patients.

SWEET TEASERS

Food	Serving Size	Teaspoons of Added Sugar	% Calories from Sugar
Pecan pie	1 slice (4.6 ounces)	12.0	35
Orange soda	12 ounces	11.8	100
Coca Cola	12 ounces	9.3	100
Strawberry shortcake, w/whipped cream	1 slice	8.4	57
Low-fat fruited yogurt	1 cup	8.8	54
Cranberry juice cocktail	8 ounces	6.4	73
Sherbet	½ cup	6.7	80
Apple pie	1 slice (4.6 ounces)	4.9	22
Applesauce, sweetened	½ cup	4.3	60
Instant oatmeal: cinnamon/spice	1.5 ounces	4.3	40
Peaches, in heavy syrup	½ cup	4.0	64
Beans & franks	¾ cup	3.3	19
Dessert wine	3.5 ounces	3.0	35
Sugar cookies	9 or 1 ounce	3.0	40
Frozen yogurt	½ cup	2.8	50
Peaches, in light syrup	½ cup	2.3	50
Chewing gum	1 stick	1.5–0.6	92
Peanut butter	2 tablespoons	1.3	11
Ketchup	1 tablespoon	0.6	63

OF DAIRY CASES AND PRODUCE SECTIONS

Replace sugar calories with more nonfat milk, fruit, and vegetables. Milk supplies calcium, vitamin D, magnesium, and phosphorus, which are needed to build and maintain strong teeth and the jawbone (also called the alveolar bone). Fruits and vegetables supply antioxidants, such as vitamin C and beta carotene, which reduce the risk for gum disease and oral cancer.

Dental problems might be a signal for osteoporosis later in life. One study of

329 postmenopausal women found those who needed dentures before age 40 also were at highest risk for the depleted bone density in the spine, wrist, and hip indicative of a high risk for osteoporosis later in life. Consuming three to four calcium-rich foods each day, including nonfat milk or yogurt, calcium-fortified soy milk, or canned salmon with the bones, helps remineralize tooth enamel, buffer acids that otherwise would contribute to tooth decay, and maintain strong bones throughout the body, from the jaw to the hip.

One study from the National Cancer Institute found that oral cancer was cut by two-thirds in people who consumed the most fresh fruits and vegetables. Numerous studies support this link between a high intake of antioxidant-rich foods or supplements and the prevention of oral cancers. Antioxidants also reduce the risk by up to 71 percent of developing oral leukoplakia, a precancerous condition characterized by white patches in the mouth. Consuming lots of fruits and vegetables, while cutting back on or eliminating alcohol, fatty meats, and tobacco, could reduce oral cancer rates by more than 80 percent!

Maintaining a radiant smile is within your grasp. The health of your mouth, teeth, and gums depends a great deal on what you eat and whether you take a few moments each day for proper dental care.

Battling the Blues

"DRAG YOUR THOUGHTS AWAY FROM YOUR TROUBLES—BY THE EARS, BY THE HEELS, OR ANY OTHER WAY, SO YOU MANAGE IT: IT'S THE HEALTHIEST THING A BODY CAN DO."

Mark Twain

Depression, once thought to be "all in a person's head," is now recognized as a common problem caused by a multitude of factors ranging from the physical, dietary, or lifestyle-induced to the psychological. While serious depression requires medical attention, in many cases how you feel is a result of what you're eating and how you're living.

If you have ever used food to soothe a bad mood or found yourself craving sweets when your energy is low, join the club. Many people at one time or another have turned to food to feel better. An occasional indulgence is harmless and comforting. However, some people unknowingly choose foods that make them feel worse and that set up a vicious cycle of depression and overeating.

SWEET DELUSIONS

People crave carbohydrate-rich foods when they feel down in the dumps. These foods have a profound effect on the body chemicals that regulate how a person feels and acts.

Drs. Richard and Judith Wurtman at Massachusetts Institute of Technology in Cambridge propose that carbohydrates raise brain levels of a nerve chemical called serotonin, which regulates both mood and appetite. When serotonin levels are low, people feel blue and crave carbohydrates. Within an hour or so of eating a carbohydrate-rich snack (such as crackers and fruit, candy or a granola bar, a bagel, or a handful of jelly beans), serotonin levels rise and the person feels better. The catch is that some carbs are a quick fix that can leave you feeling worse in the long run, while others help you rise above the blues.

The two offenders in the food/mood link are sugar and caffeine. These "quick-pick-me-ups" actually are likely to bring you down. Research conducted by Larry Christensen, Ph.D., Chair of the Department of Psychology at the University of South Alabama in Mobile, shows that depression often vanishes when sugar or caffeine is removed from the diet. "For the person who is sensitive to sugar or caffeine, simply removing these substances from the diet may be all it takes to reduce or even eliminate depression," says Dr. Christensen. "The person suffering from depression who turns to sugary foods may relieve the depression and feel better for a short while, but the depression returns." The person then often reaches for another sugar fix, which sets up a spiral that can last for months, years, and even decades where food choices fuel the depression. In contrast to the temporary sugar high, eliminating sugar and/or caffeine ("Seldom are people sensitive to both," says Dr. Christensen) from the diet and replacing it with pasta, bread, or other complex carbohydrates might be a permanent solution to depression for some people.

Early reports that sugar substitutes, such as aspartame (Equal or NutraSweet), might cause depression have not been substantiated. The majority of evidence

Is Your Diet Affecting Your Mood?

Rate how often you practice the following dietary habits. Then total your score for a quick check on how your diet might be contributing to your mood.

	Always	Often	Seldom	Never
	3	**2**	**1**	**0**
1. Do you eat four or more meals and snacks throughout the day, including breakfast?				
2. Do you limit sugar intake?				
3. Do you limit caffeinated beverages to three five-ounce servings or less each day?				
4. Do you consume at least 2,000 calories each day of fresh fruits and vegetables, whole grains, low-fat milk products, nuts, and extra-lean meats or legumes?*				
5. Do you take a moderate-dose multiple vitamin and mineral supplement on days when you do not eat "perfectly"?				
6. Do you drink at least six to eight glasses of water each day?				
7. Do you avoid tobacco and limit alcohol intake to five drinks or fewer each week?				
8. Do you get at least seven hours of restful sleep each night?				

	Always	Often	Seldom	Never
	3	**2**	**1**	**0**
9. Do you practice daily some form of relaxation?				
10. Do you exercise regularly?				

Totals: *more than 23:* Your diet and lifestyle support a good mood. If you still suffer from depression, consult your doctor.

15 to 23: Your diet and lifestyle might be contributing to depression, irritability, or mood swings. Select two changes from the above list that you will make to improve your diet.

less than 15: Your diet and lifestyle are major contributors to your doldrums. Select four or more changes, based on the above list, to get yourself back on track. After you have successfully implemented the dietary and/or lifestyle changes, expect at least three weeks before your mood improves.

*It is very difficult to consume optimal amounts of all vitamins and minerals on a daily intake of fewer than 2,000 calories. For example, a well-balanced diet supplies approximately 6mg of iron/1,000 calories. Women (of childbearing age) must consume at least 2,500 to 3,000 calories daily to meet their iron needs of 15 to 18 milligrams. Postmenopausal women not taking hormone replacement therapy need the calcium equivalent of at least four glasses of milk each day; most consume two glasses or less.

shows that moderate intake of these sweeteners is safe. A study from Kansas State University reported that women showed no changes in mood (including tension, depression, anger, fatigue, and confusion) one hour after drinking either water or aspartame-sweetened beverages.

WHAT'S WRONG WITH SUGAR?

How sugar affects mood is poorly understood. One theory is that concentrated sugars in the diet affect blood sugar levels, sending them from too high to too low. This leaves a person feeling depressed and lethargic. A second theory states that the taste of sugar on the tongue releases morphine-like chemicals in the brain called endorphins, which produce an immediate, but temporary, pleasurable feeling followed by "withdrawal" symptoms of fatigue, mood swings, and cravings for more sweets. Finally, the more sugar you eat, the more likely your diet will be low in vitality-giving vitamins and minerals.

VITAMINS, MINERALS, HERBS, AND DEPRESSION

Research conducted by Iris Bell, M.D., Ph.D., at the Department of Psychiatry at the University of Arizona Health Science Center in Tucson shows that more than one in four patients with depression are deficient in vitamins B_2, B_6, and B_{12} and folic acid. Supplementing their diets often improves their moods. In addition, when your diet is low in vitamin B_6 or if you take medications, such as birth control pills, that upset vitamin B_6 levels, your nerve cells are unable to manufacture adequate amounts of serotonin and other nerve chemicals. The result might be insomnia, depression, irritability, and nervousness. In fact, vitamin B_6 deficiency is reported in as many as 79 percent of people with depression, compared to only 29 percent of other people. Marginal dietary intakes of vitamin C, calcium, iron, magnesium, selenium, and zinc also might cause depression, irritability, or mood swings.

The research on herbs and mood is sketchy. However, one herb shows promise in boosting mood. According to a study from the University of Munich and the University of Texas in San Antonio, an herb called Saint-John's wort might help curb mild depression if taken regularly in doses of 600 to 900 milligrams.

BLUES-FREE

If you frequently skip meals or turn to sweets, colas, or coffee for a quick pick-me-up, then making a few changes in your diet could be all it takes to feel better. The Anti-Aging Diet outlined in Chapter 7 will supply all the vitamins and minerals in the right proportion and spaced evenly throughout the day to fuel your spirits. In addition, the following six dietary rules are the guideposts for a better mood:

Rule 1: Make sure every meal contains some complex carbohydrate-rich foods.

Breakfast can include French toast, waffles, pancakes, cereal, toast, or an English muffin. Lunch and dinner can include pasta or rice dishes, bagels and cheese, or vegetable soup and a sandwich. Snacks should include fruits, crackers, bread, or starchy vegetables, along with yogurt or slices of lean meat. Plan a carbohydrate-rich snack, such as whole-grain crackers and peanut butter, an onion bagel with low-fat cheese, or baked tortilla chips and low-fat bean dip, to curb mid-afternoon snack attacks.

Rule 2: Cut back on sugar-filled desserts, cereals, candy, beverages, and snack foods such as granola bars. Replace these foods with nutrient-packed foods such as fresh fruit, crunchy vegetables, whole-grain bagels, or low-fat yogurt.

Rule 3: Cut back on or eliminate coffee and other caffeinated beverages, foods, and medications. That includes tea, chocolate, cocoa, colas, and certain medications. Keep in mind that it may take three weeks or more after you have eliminated sugar and caffeine from your diet before you notice an improvement in mood.

Rule 4: Increase dietary intake of vitamin B_6 by including several servings daily of chicken, legumes, fish, bananas, avocados, and dark green leafy vegetables. Whole grains are preferable to refined, enriched grains, since more than 70 percent of the vitamin is lost during processing.

Also, consume at least two folic acid–rich foods daily by scrambling an egg substitute with spinach for breakfast, complementing a sandwich at lunch with a plate of raw broccoli spears and low-fat dip, drinking a glass of orange juice, mixing steamed collard greens into mashed potatoes, or using Romaine lettuce for salads.

Rule 5: Review your eating habits over the past few months. Have you made dramatic changes in your normal eating patterns? Are you dieting, frequently skipping breakfast, indulging a snack attack in the evening, or limiting your daily food intake to less than three snacks and meals? Any of these habits will alter brain chemistry and might contribute to mood swings.

Rule 6: Make changes gradually. Select two or three small changes and practice these until they are comfortable. This will assure long-term success in sticking with your plan and will allow your brain chemistry time to adjust to the new eating style.

12 High-Powered Snacks to Fuel Your Mood

1. One slice toasted whole-wheat bread topped with ¼ cup fat-free cottage cheese and 3 tablespoons crushed pineapple.
2. One corn tortilla filled with ½ cup black beans and 1 ounce low-fat grated cheese. Heat for 1 minute in microwave and top with ⅛ cup cilantro, avocado slices, and salsa to taste.
3. Six graham crackers topped with peanut butter and sliced banana.
4. 6 ounces low-fat kiwi/strawberry yogurt mixed with one sliced kiwi. Serve with fat-free cinnamon-flavored crackers.
5. ½ papaya or cantaloupe filled with low-fat lemon-flavored yogurt. (Optional: Serve with a bran muffin.)
6. Raisin bread dipped in nonfat apple-spice yogurt. Serve with a piece of fruit.
7. One slice Vegetable Pizza* served with a glass of orange juice.
8. A bowl of low-fat minestrone soup, 1 ounce low-fat cheese, and a French roll.
9. One cup broccoli florets, baby carrots, and other crunchy vegetables dipped in fat-free sour cream dip. Serve with a glass of milk.
10. Mix 1 tablespoon wheat germ, 2 teaspoons honey, and 2 tablespoons peanut butter. Spread on a toasted raisin bagel. Serve with a banana.
11. Chicken and Grape Salad*
12. A smoothie made with ½ cup nonfat milk, six canned apricot halves, 2 tablespoons orange juice concentrate, ¼ cup pineapple chunks, and ⅛ cup wheat germ. Blend in blender.

*Recipes in Appendix B.

CHIN UP

What you eat is only part of the blues battle. Regular exercise, effective coping skills, a strong social support system, and limiting or avoiding alcohol and cigarettes that compound an emotional problem also are important considerations. Depression can be a symptom of other problems as well, so always consult a physician if emotional problems persist or interfere with your quality of life and health.

Fatigue Busters

"Be master of your petty annoyances and conserve your energies for the big worthwhile things. It isn't the mountain ahead that wears you out, it's the grain of sand in your shoe."

Robert Service

Fatigue is one of the most common complaints voiced by both men and women, and it's the most likely to undermine vitality. But before you blame your lack of "oomph" on your busy schedule or the fact that you're getting older, think again. The answer to waning energy could be as simple as your diet.

THE CALORIE CRISIS

Any eating habit that interferes with a steady supply of carbohydrates to the body—from erratic eating habits to skipping meals—will undermine your energy level. Blood sugar levels begin to drop within four hours of eating, so frequent small meals and snacks, rather than two or three big meals, are your best bet for maintaining a constant energy supply and avoiding fatigue. Complex carbohydrates in grains and starchy vegetables—from breads, rice, and pasta to lima beans and yams—are the fuels of choice, since they are digested gradually, maintain an even blood sugar level, and provide a constant fuel supply for the body and the brain.

Dieting is a common cause of fatigue. "Cutting calories at breakfast and lunch to lose weight is likely to leave most people in an energy drain that interferes with the daily routine, exercise, or even enjoying life," says Nancy Clark, M. S., R. D., author of *Nancy Clark's Sports Nutrition Guidebook: Eating to Fuel Your Active Lifestyle*. For example, a 120-pound woman needs between 1,800 and 2,200 calories daily (men and larger or more active women need even more), but the average intake for young women in the United States is under 1,600 calories (women 55 and older average only 1,360 calories a day). That means many people force their bodies to run on "fumes"!

Rather than drastically cut calories to maintain a desirable weight, people should increase exercise, which burns calories, boosts energy levels, and decreases fatigue-related moods, such as depression and despondency.

Fatigue Fighters

Too busy to rest and too tired to fix a big meal? Energizing snacks can be quick and easy. For example, try some of the following:

• Whole-wheat fig bars with a glass of nonfat milk
• A raisin bagel topped with fat-free cream cheese and served with baby carrots
• Vegetable Medley Platter*
• A bran muffin spread with apple butter
• A soft microwaved pretzel with honey-mustard dip and a glass of V8 juice
• Crunchy Chinese Salad*
• Pita bread stuffed with shredded jalapeño cheese and grated zucchini
• A crepe filled with fat-free ricotta cheese and fresh fruit
• Sunrise Salad*
• Cheerios, raisins, nuts, and a cup of nonfat yogurt
• Pear, cantaloupe, strawberry, and banana slices dipped in vanilla-flavored nonfat yogurt

*Recipes in Appendix B.

BREAKFAST BASICS

Skipping breakfast is a big mistake. Eight or more hours have passed since your last meal. Demanding that your body shift into full gear without stopping to refuel is like expecting a car to run on an empty tank. You may feel fine at first, but people who skip breakfast struggle more with fatigue later in the day than do those who take time in the morning to eat. People often skip breakfast in an attempt to cut calories, but research shows that breakfast skippers are more likely to overeat later in the day.

The breakfast rules are simple: avoid sugar, limit caffeine, and choose foods with a mix of protein and starch to maintain blood sugar and energy levels throughout the morning. Examples include egg substitutes, whole-wheat toast, and juice; a whole-grain bagel or English muffin with low-fat cheese and fruit; or a bowl of instant oatmeal with low-fat milk and a banana. Or try nontraditional foods, such as leftover pizza, toast and soup, or a sandwich. Other five-minute meals include:

- A toasted frozen whole-wheat waffle topped with fat-free sour cream and fresh blueberries
- A whole-wheat tortilla filled with cottage cheese and fresh fruit, warmed in the microwave
- A low-fat bran muffin with applesauce and yogurt
- A bowl of low-fat whole-grain cereal with low-fat milk and fresh fruit

MIDDAY ENERGY BOOSTERS

"IN THE DEPTH OF WINTER, I FINALLY LEARNED THAT WITHIN ME THERE LAY AN INVINCIBLE SUMMER."

Albert Camus

What and how much you eat at lunch can make or break your energy level for the rest of the day. First, keep it light (a light meal of 500 calories or less will fuel your energy without leaving you drowsy). A tossed salad and crackers might sound nutritious but can leave you short on energy and hungry again too soon. Add some kidney beans or grilled chicken to the salad, go light on the high-fat dressing, and complement it with a glass of nonfat milk and a slice of whole-wheat bread.

Second, keep lunch low in fat. Fatty meals will prime you for a nap, rather than a get-things-done afternoon.

Third, combine protein-and carbohydrate-rich foods. An all-carb meal, such as pasta with marinara sauce, raises brain levels of a chemical called serotonin, which leaves you feeling relaxed and drowsy. In contrast, a turkey sandwich and a bowl of minestrone or a bean-cheese burrito with rice and spicy carrots (the protein-carb combination) raises brain levels of another chemical called norepinephrine, which increases alertness and mental clarity.

IN-BETWEEN-MEAL BOOSTERS

Your body's high performance requires frequent stops for fuel and nutrients, which means eating a small meal or snack every three to four hours. Here are the rules for energy-boosting snacks:

Rule 1: Keep it simple. A nutritious snack must be convenient, i.e., it must be readily available and take little time to prepare.

Rule 2: Include at least one fruit, vegetable, or whole grain at every snack, plus one or more of the following:

1. nuts and seeds
2. nonfat dairy products, such as yogurt or milk
3. cooked dried beans and peas

Rule 3: While cookies, candy, colas, and other sugary treats are quick fixes for dwindling energy levels, they may produce a short-acting response. According to Robin Kanarek, Ph.D., Professor of Psychology at Tufts University in Medford, Massachusetts, "Sugar leads to a release of insulin, which results in an increase in sugar uptake and use by the cells. It is possible that once the sugar is used, feelings of fatigue will follow."

Instead, snack on bagels, fat-free crackers and cheese, fresh fruit and cottage cheese, or low-fat tortilla chips and bean dip. "Our research shows that a snack in the late afternoon improves performance, especially on tasks that require sustained attention and alertness," says Dr. Kanarek.

One cup of coffee can kick start your day, but more than three cups and you're likely to spiral into needing more coffee to fend off fatigue from caffeine withdrawal, yet sleep poorly and awake tired the next morning.

Rule 4: Plan ahead. Pack your purse, briefcase, glove compartment, desk drawer, and office refrigerator with fresh fruit, bagged baby carrots, pita bread, dried fruit, boxed juice, and yogurt. Eat a nutritious snack at the first signs of hunger; a starving body is likely to grab anything to curb the hunger pangs—and usually that means candy from the vending machine!

FLUID FUELS

Water is the most available and inexpensive way to boost your energy, but we often don't drink enough of it. Over the course of days or weeks you can become mildly dehydrated, with a common symptom being fatigue. People who choose soda pop, iced tea, or coffee instead of water further dehydrate their bodies, since caffeinated beverages have a diuretic effect.

Drink six to eight glass of water, fruit juice, and other noncaffeinated beverages every day. Since thirst is a poor indicator of fluid needs, a general rule is to drink twice as much water as is needed to quench thirst. That means about one glass of water every other hour during the day. Also, sip on a glass of water while preparing meals, which will help replenish fluids and curtail nibbling. Exercisers need even more water and should drink at least a glass of it prior to, during, and following all training and sports events, as well as regularly throughout the day.

IRON AND ZINC: THE FATIGUE FIGHTERS

If your energy level is in perpetual low gear, your problem could be lack of iron. While only 8 percent of premenopausal women are anemic, as many as 80 percent of active and up to 39 percent of premenopausal women are iron deficient, a pre-anemic condition that results in fatigue and other energy-related problems. For these women, a moderate-dose iron supplement (18 milligrams) and iron-rich foods will boost lagging iron stores. Seldom do men or postmenopausal women need to supplement with iron.

Fatigue also could be a sign of zinc deficiency. Monkeys fed zinc-poor diets are lethargic and apathetic, with short attention spans. These findings have not been confirmed in people; however, people often consume suboptimal amounts of zinc as they age. Excellent sources of this trace mineral include extra-lean meat, oysters, lima beans, yogurt, and wheat germ. If you don't consume enough of these foods, make sure your daily multiple supplement contains between 15 and 30 milligrams of zinc.

KEEP TRACK OF YOUR ENERGY

Exercise also is essential in the battle against fatigue. Physically active people have more energy to accomplish routine tasks and ample energy left to enjoy life. The energy-boosting effects of exercise become increasingly important as a person ages. (See Chapter 8 for more information on exercise and energy.)

Learn to recognize the mental or physical symptoms of fatigue and what time of day they usually occur, i.e., are you a lark or an owl? Keep a journal to identify when you are most energized, tired, or in the best and worst moods. What precedes your periods of high and low energy, including sleep, stress, diet, and exercise patterns? (Remember, fatigue can be a symptom of something more serious, so always consult a physician if it persists.) Then, develop a plan that works with your natural energy cycles and combats the blahs.

Listening Well

"IT TAKES TWO TO SPEAK THE TRUTH—ONE TO SPEAK, AND ANOTHER TO HEAR."

Henry David Thoreau

Without hearing, we'd miss the sound of our loved ones' voices, the splash of water over rocks, the emotions stirred when listening to symphony music, the warning signal of a fire alarm, and the millions of other noises that enrich and protect our lives. Loss of hearing robs us of our interaction with the world and others, which brings loneliness and speeds the aging process.

Hearing is the most likely of the five senses to be lost with age. Approximately one in three people age 65 and older, and 50 percent of those age 85 and older, report hearing loss ranging from mild to severe. Presbycusis (derived from two Latin words meaning "old" and "hearing") is a gradual, progressive loss of high-frequency hearing. As people age, they are still likely to hear the deep tones of a man's voice, but struggle with the higher-pitched voice tones of children and women.

Noise abuse is the most likely cause of presbycusis, with exposure to 85 decibels or higher being enough to damage the ear. (For example, a firecracker at 10 feet is 160 decibels, a stereo headset at volume number 6 is 115 decibels, and a car horn is 100 decibels.) A rock concert can permanently damage the ear in less than half an hour! The damage becomes worse as a person ages. Medications, such as antibiotics and diuretics, also can affect hearing.

When it comes to cures for hearing loss, there are a few nutrients that might be useful.

VITAMIN D, FLUORIDE, AND CALCIUM

A deficiency of vitamin D is associated with progressive cochlear deafness. (The cochlea is the spiral-shaped bone in the ear canal that converts sound waves into electrical impulses to be sent to the brain.) Poor intake of vitamin D might produce calcium loss from the bones—including this fragile bone within the ear, which would affect the cochlea's ability to conduct impulses. Whether or not deafness caused by changes in the cochlea is responsive to vitamin D supplementation is not clear.

Optimal intake of vitamin D, fluoride, and calcium also shows promise in reducing the symptoms of hearing disorders, such as tinnitus (ringing in the ears). So consume 200 to 400IU of vitamin D, either from fortified milk or cereal, or from supplements, throughout life.

VITAMIN B_{12} AND ZINC

Low intake of vitamin B_{12} and zinc might contribute to the development and progression of tinnitus and hearing loss. Increasing intakes of zinc-rich foods, such as turkey, lima beans, wheat germ, and yogurt, or taking a moderate-dose supplement might be effective in preventing hearing loss or in restoring hearing.

MAGNESIUM

Magnesium supplements might prevent hearing damage from loud noises. In one study, more than 300 healthy volunteers were monitored during two months of military training with frequent exposure to firearm noise. Those soldiers who took magnesium supplements showed significantly less hearing loss than the control group. Although this study is interesting, it does not provide conclusive proof of magnesium's effectiveness in preventing hearing damage. In general, avoid loud noises and wear protective hearing devices when loud noises are unavoidable.

Sleepless Nights?

"FOR FAST-ACTING RELIEF, TRY SLOWING DOWN."
Lily Tomlin

Do you enjoy about eight hours of uninterrupted sleep each night?
Do you awaken easily and feel refreshed without the aid of an alarm clock?
Does it take you at least 10 minutes to settle down before you fall asleep?
Do you feel awake and alert all day long?

If you answered "no" to any of these questions, you might not be getting enough sleep.

Busy lifestyles have reduced the average night's sleep by 20 percent. While most adults used to sleep at least nine hours a night and need at least eight hours, most average closer to seven; seniors do even worse, and average five to seven hours a night. This chronic sleep debt impairs memory, logical reasoning, decision-making, and the immune system. It also undermines vitality and your sense of humor. Most people would be more productive, healthier, happier, and vital if they slept more.

While sleep deprivation is sometimes self-imposed, in many more cases it is caused by some form of insomnia. Up to 95 percent of adults experience some form of insomnia during their lives. Many people assume that insomnia refers only to chronic sleeplessness, but they are wrong. Insomnia is any sleep problem, from occasional difficulties falling asleep or waking in the middle of the night to awakening too early or sleeping too lightly. While insomnia is a complex issue with numerous causes, sometimes the answer to sleep problems starts at the dining table, not in the bedroom. The most likely dietary culprits that undermine sleep include caffeine, alcohol, spicy or gas-forming foods, and some additives, such as MSG.

CAFFEINE AND SNOOZE CONTROL

"People eat chocolate or drink coffee during the day and then wonder why they can't sleep at night," says Robert Sack, Ph.D., Professor of Psychiatry and Director of Adult Sleep Disorder Medicine at the Oregon Health Sciences University in Portland. "Even small amounts of caffeine can affect sleep architecture, especially in caffeine-sensitive people." If you are a coffee drinker troubled by sleep problems, try eliminating caffeine for at least two weeks and see if your sleep habits improve.

NO NODDING OFF WITH ALCOHOL

A nightcap might make you sleepy, but actually it will undermine a restful night. Alcohol and other depressant drugs suppress a phase of sleeping called REM (Rapid Eye Movement), during which most of your dreaming occurs. Less REM is associated with more night awakenings and restless sleep. One glass of wine with dinner probably won't hurt, but stop drinking alcohol within two hours of bedtime, and *never* mix alcohol with sleeping pills!

SNACKING BY THE LIGHT OF THE MOON

"If you don't consume enough calories throughout the day, you're likely to wake more frequently during the night because you're hungry," warns Gary Zammit, Ph.D., Director of the Sleep Disorders Institute in New York City and author of *Good Nights*. If dieting is causing your sleep problems, increase your calorie intake throughout the day and include some protein-rich foods at the evening meal to help fend off hunger at midnight.

Midnight snacking also can signal underlying medical conditions. For example, if you are eating in the middle of the night in an effort to relieve digestive discomfort, you might have an undiagnosed ulcer that should be checked by your physician. Hypoglycemia, although relatively rare, might be causing your night eating. A common symptom is frequent hunger in the middle of the night as the body attempts to boost lagging blood sugar levels. Eating regularly throughout the day and including some protein at the evening meal and at the bedtime snack (cheese and crackers or nuts and raisins) will help decrease these snack attacks. In addition, avoid snacking on sugary foods, such as cookies, cake, candy, pie, or sorbet, especially in the evening.

FROM GARLIC TO BEANS

Spicy or gas-forming foods can cause nagging heartburn or indigestion that disrupt sleep. Eating too fast (too much air is swallowed when you gulp food) also can cause abdominal discomfort, which interferes with sound sleep. Avoid spicy foods at dinner, limit your intake of gas-forming foods to the morning hours, and thoroughly chew food to avoid gulping air.

MSG: SLEEP ROBBER OR INNOCENT BYSTANDER?

People have been concerned about MSG (monosodium glutamate) since the 1970s, when research found that this additive used to enhance flavors in processed foods might cause brain damage and other serious side effects in animals. While these serious consequences have not been reported in humans, some people are sensitive to MSG. The most common symptom in people is numbness in the back of the neck that can radiate down the arms and back. Other people report insomnia and vivid dreams, mild to severe headaches, tightness in the chest, pressure around the cheeks or jaw, or mild mood changes.

A safe dose of MSG has not been established and probably varies from person to person. Generally, the higher the dose, the more people develop symptoms. "The average American consumes between one-third and one-half gram of MSG each day," says Margo Wootan, D.Sc., a Senior Scientist at the Center For Science in the Public Interest. "But it is easy to consume two grams in one meal at a Chinese restaurant." Fortunately, most foods don't contain this much MSG.

If you suspect you might react to MSG, check with a physician who specializes in allergies or test yourself by eliminating all MSG-containing foods for at least two weeks. (This will take a bit of sleuthing, since MSG comes in a variety of names and in many foods, so it is difficult to avoid all the sources.) If symptoms disappear, then slowly add one food at a time to your diet and monitor your sleep patterns. In addition, frequent only restaurants that promise to serve MSG-free food.

EAT TO SLEEP

"Big dinners, especially high-calorie meals, make you temporarily drowsy, but they can cause stomach discomfort and prolong digestive action, which keeps you awake," cautions Dr. Zammit. Dinner should be low in fat, light in calories, and consumed at least two hours before bedtime.

An evening snack might be the best alternative to sleeping pills. A carbohydrate-rich snack triggers the release of a brain chemical called serotonin that aids sleep. Serotonin-enhancing snacks include low-fat popcorn, one-half of a toasted English muffin topped with jam, or graham crackers and honey. The traditional glass of warm milk, a protein-rich beverage, probably doesn't affect serotonin levels, but the warm liquid soothes, relaxes, and fills you up, which might help you fall asleep.

WHAT ABOUT MELATONIN?

Melatonin has been touted as the latest cure for America's 60 million insomniacs. The hormone is naturally manufactured in the pineal gland of the brain at night. Melatonin's job is to tell the body that it is rest time by synchronizing its internal biological clock.

While the gland pumps out melatonin throughout life, it secretes less and less as people age, which might partially explain why sleep problems increase as people get older. Research at MIT in Cambridge, Massachusetts, in 1994 showed that melatonin supplements, in doses as low as 1 milligram, reduced the time it took to fall asleep from 25 minutes to six minutes.

Not everyone is convinced that this hormone-in-a-pill is safe or effective long term. Researchers at Oregon Health Sciences University in Portland caution that taking melatonin orally alters the sleep cycle and reduces the amount of deep sleep a person gets, at least in young people.

Moreover, the brain naturally secretes melatonin in a wave pattern that causes melatonin levels to rise early in the night, peak around two A.M. to four A.M., then gradually taper off by dawn. In contrast, melatonin supplements boost blood levels like a flash flood, leaving the user high and dry at two A.M. Researchers at Tel Aviv University in Israel might have a solution to this problem. In their studies, time-released melatonin supplements improved sleep quality even in seniors.

The biggest concern is not with "pure melatonin" used in well-controlled research studies, since this high-quality melatonin is assured of purity and safety, but with the unregulated products on the market. The long-term effects of ingesting commercial melatonin are unknown, especially with regard to women, as the hormone's effect on the female reproductive system is unexplored territory.

YOUR WAKE-UP CALL

Sleepless nights can be caused by stress, emotional problems, hormone changes during the premenstrual period, menopause, medical conditions, smoking, a busy lifestyle, or a snoring bed partner. Often solving these troubles or tensions eliminates sleep problems.

A major difference between good sleepers and poor sleepers is not what they do at bedtime, but what they did all day. Good sleepers exercise and use every opportunity to move. Physical activity helps a person cope with daily stress and tires the body so it is ready to sleep at night. Older people who battle sleep problems report they fall asleep faster and sleep longer after starting a daily exercise program. (Beware of exercising too hard or too fast, however, since strenuous exercise stresses the body and disrupts your sleep.) Sleeping pills are a temporary fix, while a few simple dietary and lifestyle changes could do wonders for your snooze control.

Tricks of the Sleep Set

A day filled with good eating, exercise, little stress, and healthy habits leads to a good night's sleep. You also can maximize your sleep quotient by following these seven rules:

1. Go to bed and get up at the same times each day.
2. Don't take naps.
3. Establish an evening ritual that relaxes your body and signals your brain that it's time to sleep. At the same time each night, take a warm bath, read or listen to music, sip a cup of hot herbal tea, or have a light all-carb snack.
4. Use the bedroom for sleeping only, not for working or reading in bed or for watching TV.
5. Get out of bed and the bedroom when you can't sleep.
6. Dim the lights in the evening, and keep the bedroom dark at night.
7. Don't depend on sleeping pills.

Kidney Stones: Avoiding the Big Chill

> "GOD IS SEEN GOD
> IN THE STAR, IN THE STONE, IN THE FLESH, IN THE SOUL
> AND IN THE CLOD."
>
> *Robert Browning*

Kidney stones come in all shapes and sizes. The small ones usually pass with the urine, but 20 percent of stones are large enough to require medical attention and surgery. Stones also are composed of different substances including uric acid, oxalate, struvite, and cystine, but by far the most common—accounting for up to 85 percent of all kidney stones—are calcium oxalate stones. Nine times out of 10, it's a man passing the stone.

The evidence shows that kidney stones are a product of lifestyle. Millions of research dollars are spent investigating treatments, but surprisingly little effort has focused on prevention. Consequently, dietary guidelines to avoid kidney stones are rudimentary.

How to Avoid a Kidney Stone

1. Base the diet on fresh fruits and vegetables, whole grains, and cooked dried beans and peas.
2. Consume daily at least three servings of calcium-rich foods, such as nonfat milk or yogurt.
3. Drink daily at least eight 8-ounce glasses of water, even more if you exercise or work in hot climates. Also drink fruit juices.
4. Include several servings of magnesium-rich foods in the daily diet, such as bananas, beet greens, cashews, nonfat milk, and wheat germ.
5. Limit daily intake of meat and fatty or salty foods, and use little or no fat and salt in cooking.
6. Ask your physician about reducing oxalates in the diet.

HOW TO AVOID GETTING STONED

People who consume too much meat and salty foods and not enough fruits, vegetables, legumes, calcium, and water are at the highest risk for kidney stone formation. Since the turn of the century, Americans have doubled their intake of animal protein compared to vegetable protein from a ratio of 1:1 to 2:1 and—not coincidentally—the incidence of kidney stones also has increased.

Meat: Although some studies show that vegetarians have a lower incidence of kidney stones than do meat-eaters, curtailing meat to one small (3-ounce) serving daily and filling the plate with lots of fresh vegetables and other foods of plant origin could substantially cut your risk. In addition, eating more beans and less meat will automatically reduce fat intake, which also lowers kidney stone risk.

Fluids: Everyone agrees you should drink lots of fluids, enough to produce at least two liters of urine each day. The rationale is that stones are less likely to crystalize in diluted, as compared to concentrated, urine.

While drinking at least eight glasses of water is the foundation of an anti-stone-forming diet, there might be additional protection in including other beverages in the daily menu. Researchers at the Harvard School of Public Health in Boston prepared to answer the question of types of fluids by comparing the intake of 21 different beverages and the incidence of kidney stones in more than 45,000 men ages 40 to 75. They found that drinking fruit juices daily reduced kidney stone formation by up to 37 percent. However, coffee increases urinary excretion of calcium. Whether or not this predisposes a person to kidney stones is unknown.

Calcium: People used to be warned to limit their intake of calcium and oxalate-containing foods based on the false assumption that by not consuming the main constituents of a kidney stone, they would avoid its formation. Research has proven just the opposite. People who consume too little calcium are at higher risk for developing kidney stones than are those who consume at least 800 milligrams a day, or the amount of calcium found in 2½ cups of nonfat milk or yogurt.

Research is sketchy when it comes to limiting oxalate-containing foods. The largest contributor to oxalate levels is not from the diet, but from the body's manufacture of this compound. Limiting intake might or might not have a significant impact on stone formation. In addition, a low-oxalate diet is complex and difficult to follow, requiring elimination of an unpredictable assortment of foods, from spinach and rhubarb to nuts and chocolate. Since low intake of calcium increases intestinal absorption of oxalates, it is likely that too little calcium, rather than too much oxalate, is the dietary risk factor for kidney stone formation. Until the controversy is resolved, anyone at risk for kidney stone formation should discuss with a physician the usefulness of switching to a low-oxalate diet.

Vitamin C: A handful of studies report that large doses of vitamin C might encourage the formation of oxalate-containing kidney stones in people prone to stone formation. Other studies show that up to 8 grams of vitamin C consumed daily has no effect on kidney stone risk, even in adults prone to stone formation. Consequently, the link between vitamin C and kidney stones remains controversial.

Vitamin B₆: A vitamin B_6 deficiency might increase the risk for developing oxalate-containing kidney stones. Supplementation with the vitamin reduces the amount of oxalate in the urine and reduces a person's risk for developing kidney stones or kidney damage.

Magnesium: Magnesium inhibits the formation of crystals in the urine, possibly by improving the ratio of magnesium to calcium in the urine. The magnesium content of the urine of those who form stones and those who don't is similar; however, stone formers excrete greater amounts of calcium, making their urinary ratio of calcium to magnesium very high. Increased intake of magnesium alters the ratio of calcium to magnesium in the urine to resemble that of stone non-formers and reduces the formation of kidney stones.

THE BOTTOM LINE

The treatment of all kidney diseases, including kidney stones, should be designed and monitored by a physician and dietitian and include dietary, medication or medical, and lifestyle components.

Osteoporosis: The Silent Thief

"LIKE AS THE WAVES MAKE TOWARDS THE PEBBLED SHORE,
SO DO OUR MINUTES HASTEN TO THEIR END."

William Shakespeare,
from "Sonnet 60"

Osteoporosis is a silent condition that slowly robs the body of its strongest and most durable tissues, the bones, much like ocean waves erode the shoreline. Neither the patient nor the physician may notice the damage until a bone fractures, showing the disease is in its final stage. The lifelong loss of bone minerals also brings the threat of disability from a hip fracture, the loss of mobility and independence, stooped posture from collapsing vertebrae, pain, anxiety, and sometimes death.

More than 1.5 million bone fractures are caused by osteoporosis each year and more than 25 million Americans, 80 percent of them women, live with the daily fear that a simple movement, such as sneezing or stepping off a curb, will result in a serious bone break.

DISPELLING THE MYTHS

Bones are the body's bank account for calcium, containing 99 percent of all the calcium in the body. Every minute of life, our bones are releasing calcium into and absorbing it from the blood to maintain a constant blood concentration of calcium.

Up until a person's mid-thirties, more calcium is absorbed and deposited into bone than is removed. The more calcium is consumed in the first third of life, the larger the calcium bank account and the less likely a person will develop osteoporosis later in life. After age 35, bones slowly lose calcium faster than they absorb it. Recent evidence suggests that dwindling levels of growth hormone contribute to this calcium drain from the bones.

Consuming ample amounts of calcium after age 35 can delay calcium loss and diminish the seriousness of fragile bones later in life. Most people consume too little calcium; consequently, the bones become increasingly porous and brittle, and the result is osteoporosis. Although it is potentially more hazardous, administering growth hormone in the later years might boost bone density as well.

Brittle bones are largely the result of lifestyle choices, not aging. Robert Heaney, M.D., a calcium expert at Creighton University in Omaha, estimates that women can reduce their risk for bone fractures by up to 60 percent if they consume diets rich in calcium and vitamin D.

MILK BONES

Low-fat dairy products, especially milk and yogurt, contain more calcium than any other food regularly consumed in the diet. Women need the calcium-containing equivalent of at least three glasses of milk daily. However, milk is not without controversy.

One belief is that the protein in milk interferes with calcium metabolism. "Parts of the world where milk consumption is highest also have the highest incidence of hip fractures," says Walter Willett, M.D., Dr.P.H., Chairman of the Nutrition Department at Harvard. "Although it's clear we need to conduct more studies, it could be that the type of protein in milk increases urinary calcium loss."

"This statement is partially true and mostly wrong," says Dr. Heaney. A high-protein diet does increase urinary excretion of calcium. "Sulfur-containing amino acids in all dietary protein act much like acid rain on limestone in flushing some calcium out of the body," says Heaney. However, these amino acids are found in all protein foods, from milk and meat to beans and grains.

According to Dr. Heaney, it is the ratio of calcium to protein that is important. A cup of milk supplies 300 milligrams of calcium for only 8 grams of protein (a ratio of 37 to 1), while a 3½-ounce hamburger supplies up to 32 grams of protein but only 5 milligrams of calcium (a negative ratio of 1 to 6.4). A cup of black beans contains twice the protein but only one-sixth the calcium of milk, for a ratio of 3 to 1.

"Protein's effect on calcium metabolism is primarily theoretical; no one has shown that the amounts typically consumed in this country cause bone loss," says Bess Dawson-Hughes, M.D., Chief of Calcium and Bone Metabolism Laboratory at the USDA Human Nutrition Research Center at Tufts University in Boston. If protein is a factor in osteoporosis, it is more likely our high meat intake that is to blame, not milk.

TO DRINK OR TO SUPPLEMENT, THAT IS THE QUESTION

Many women think they are getting enough calcium, when in fact their calcium intake is low enough to place them at high risk for developing osteoporosis later in life.

Researchers at the University of Illinois surveyed women's attitudes about, and intakes of, calcium. They found that calcium intake averaged only 591 milligrams per day and only 25.1 percent of the women met RDA levels, or 800 milligrams. The latest Dietary Reference Intakes (DRIs), which replace the RDAs, recommend that adults consume even more calcium, or 1,200 milligrams. Postmenopausal women might need up to 1,500 milligrams daily.

"Women's calcium needs are greater than we previously thought and might be as much as four to five times higher than they are getting from their diets," says Dr. Heaney. Research shows that high calcium intakes protect against age-related bone loss and prevent fractures. "The effect is most strongly associated with calcium," says Heaney, "however, since milk is the best dietary source of calcium, the weight of the evidence comes down on the side of including [two to three servings of] milk in the diet."

Getting Your Milk Without Drinking It

Can't bring yourself to down three glasses of milk each day? Try these tricks for sneaking calcium-rich nonfat milk into your diet.

1. Use canned nonfat evaporated milk in creamed sauces instead of heavy cream.
2. Use nonfat milk instead of water when preparing packaged hot chocolate mixes.
3. Instead of regular coffee, drink a caffè latte made with nonfat milk.
4. Cook rice, oatmeal, or any hot cereal in nonfat milk instead of water.
5. Use nonfat milk or dry nonfat milk powder instead of water when preparing canned creamed soups or tomato soup.
6. Use nonfat milk instead of water when preparing baked goods, such as cookies, muffins, or pancakes.
7. When making mashed potatoes, add extra dry nonfat milk powder to the nonfat milk and cut back on the butter or margarine.
8. Make a morning smoothie with nonfat milk, concentrated orange juice, and fresh fruit such as a banana or a peach.
9. Make a sweet whipped topping by mixing one-half cup dry nonfat milk powder in one-third cup water and chill. Whip until the milk stands in soft peaks; then add one tablespoon lemon juice and whip. Add three tablespoons of powdered sugar and whip until blended. Refrigerate until ready to use.
10. Add dry, nonfat milk powder to meat loaf, muffins, meatballs, or other menu items.
11. Top crackers with Refreshing Yogurt Spread*. One tablespoon supplies 130 milligrams of calcium!

*Recipe in Appendix B.

You can take several calcium pills each day instead of drinking milk, but this goes against all dietary recommendations. "There is no evidence that calcium supplements are superior to milk [in preventing osteoporosis] and food always should be a person's first choice when it comes to obtaining optimal nutrition," says Dr. Dawson-Hughes.

Milk contains other factors that enhance calcium absorption and help prevent osteoporosis. The most important of these is vitamin D, a deficiency of which results in poor calcium absorption and rapid bone loss. Dr. Dawson-Hughes' research shows that increasing vitamin D intake, even without extra calcium, can help reduce bone fractures and slow the progression of osteoporosis. Aging reduces vitamin D absorption by up to 40 percent and using sunscreens also inhibit vitamin D production. Several studies show that adding 1,200 milligrams calcium and 800IU vitamin D to the diets of older women reduces the number of hip fractures by 23 percent or more. Vitamin D–fortified milk is the only reliable source of this vitamin, so your diet could be inadequate if you snack on yogurt or cheese.

Many nutrients are important in maintaining overall health and preventing osteoporosis, including boron, copper, magnesium, zinc, manganese, vitamin A, vitamin K, and some B vitamins. These nutrients are found in milk and other foods, but would be lacking if a person supplemented only with calcium.

However, for both the young and old who cannot meet the two-to-three daily servings goal for low-fat milk and other calcium-rich foods, supplements are a must. "It's prudent to take a 1,000 milligram supplement of calcium, since most women average only 500 milligrams of calcium from their diets," says Dr. Heaney. In addition, avoid the "natural source" calcium pills, such as oyster shell and bone meal, since they might contain the toxic metal lead.

BEYOND MILK

Preventing osteoporosis involves more than just consuming enough calcium and other vitamins and minerals. Lowering your intake of salt to improve your blood pressure also could help protect your bones. Researchers at the University of Western Australia found that cutting sodium (salt) intake in half was as effective as increasing daily calcium intake to 891 milligrams in slowing bone loss and preventing osteoporosis.

Alcohol abuse and smoking escalate bone loss, so drink in moderation, if at all, and don't smoke. Compounds in coffee increase urinary loss of calcium, but the research has not confirmed a direct link between this beverage and osteoporosis. Until the controversy is settled by well-designed studies, it is best to drink coffee in moderation and with milk.

Exercise also is essential to maintaining strong muscles. Researchers at the University of Cincinnati Medical Center in Ohio report that people can exercise or consume more calcium, but they're not likely to maximize bone density unless they do both. A careful review of 17 trials of physical activity that also reported calcium intake showed that the benefits of exercise on bone density were apparent only when calcium intake was high. Both weight-bearing exercise, such as walking or jogging, and strength training are essential to maintaining strong bones for life. If you already have osteoporosis, work with your physician to develop a safe activity program.

Bone loss escalates rapidly after menopause, when the protective effects of estrogen on maintaining bone mass are lost. Hormone replacement therapy (HRT) significantly slows the rate of bone loss after menopause and reduces a woman's risk of developing osteoporosis. In addition, many new drugs for the treatment of osteoporosis are now available, including alendronate, which slows mineral loss and might build new bone and prevent fractures.

Skin and Hair: Turning Back the Hands of Time

"FOR AGE IS OPPORTUNITY NO LESS
THAN YOUTH ITSELF, THOUGH IN ANOTHER DRESS.
AND AS THE EVENING TWILIGHT FADES AWAY.
THE SKY IS FILLED WITH STARS, INVISIBLE BY DAY."
Henry Wadsworth Longfellow

A person's skin is an outer reflection of his or her inner health. Those who are healthy and vital also are radiant—with clear, moist, glowing skin. The skin is a sensitive timeline for aging. Youthful skin is soft, moist, and smooth, while wrinkles and sagging gradually develop over time as the skin's elastin and collagen fibers deteriorate. The process begins around age 30 and progresses throughout life. Heredity and gravity influence how and when the skin ages, but by far its greatest enemy is sun exposure.

Because the cells of the skin have a short life span, signs of poor nutrition show up quickly in the skin.

HEALTHY SKIN FROM WITHIN

Radiant, youthful skin requires a steady supply of all nutrients, including protein, calories, fat, vitamins, minerals, and water. Maintaining an optimal blood supply is critical to delivery of oxygen and nutrients to the skin and the hair and for removing waste products from these tissues. Red blood cells and the blood supply depend on ample amounts of protein, iron, folic acid and other B vitamins, copper, vitamin C, selenium, and vitamin E. An iron deficiency alone can leave the skin looking pale and drawn.

Some nutrients directly affect the health of the skin and hair. An essential fat in vegetable oils called linoleic acid helps maintain smooth, moist skin. Very low-fat diets often are low in this fat and cause dry, scaly skin. Adding a little safflower oil, a handful of nuts or seeds, or a tablespoon of wheat germ to the daily diet can reverse the condition within a few weeks.

Vitamin C helps build collagen, the "glue" that holds the body's cells together. Poor intake of this vitamin results in bruising, loss of skin elasticity, poor healing of cuts and scrapes, and dry skin. A glass of orange juice or a bowl of strawberries daily provides enough vitamin C to ensure adequate collagen formation, although more might be better if you want to protect the skin from sun damage.

ANTIOXIDANTS AGAINST SKIN AGING

With free radicals accused of being the dark force behind aging, it's no surprise that antioxidant nutrients have hit the market with a vengeance. Major cosmetic companies are spiking their face creams with everything from vitamin C to green tea extract.

The antioxidant nutrients help neutralize free radicals generated in the skin from sun exposure before they can irreversibly damage the skin. Basically, antioxidants prevent free radicals from destroying the fats that form a protective moisture barrier in the skin and prevent the dryness, loss of elasticity, and wrinkles caused by sun damage. Free radicals also are suspected of attacking the skin's collagen, which keeps the skin firm and supple. If antioxidants can prevent the breakdown of this spongy material, then a person could expect to see fewer deep wrinkles over time. Antioxidants also might act as a weak sunscreen, comparable to an SPF 3.

HEALTHY HAIR

As with skin, the health of your hair is a reflection of internal health. Shiny, flexible, vibrant hair signals an optimally nourished body, while dry, dull, or lifeless hair is a gauge for nutritional deficiencies.

However, nutrition cannot work miracles. It can't reverse graying or balding caused by heredity. And while hair loss caused by a nutrient deficiency is reversed when the nutrient is added to the diet, consuming extra nutrients in hopes of regaining lost color, hair, or length is likely to end in disappointment. The following is a summary of how deficiencies and toxicities of certain nutrients can affect hair.

Symptoms	*Could result from . . .*
Hair loss/baldness	Vitamin A deficiency or overdose
	Biotin deficiency
	Iron deficiency
	Zinc deficiency
	Protein deficiency
	Molybdenum overdose
Dandruff	Vitamin A deficiency
Dry or dull hair	Vitamin A overdose
	Vitamin C deficiency
	Linoleic acid deficiency
	Protein deficiency
Hair lacks luster	Deficiency of vitamin B_6 or B_{12}, or folic acid
Premature graying/loss of color	Pantothenic acid deficiency
	Copper deficiency
Itchy scalp	Vitamin A overdose
Poor hair growth	Vitamin D overdose
Hair splits and breaks and tangles easily	Vitamin C deficiency

Interesting Facts About Hair and Skin

1. The use of hair dyes is linked to an increased risk for developing non-Hodgkins lymphoma and leukemia.

2. Hair analysis is useful for determining long-term exposure to toxic metals, such as lead, but is unreliable for assessing nutritional status.

3. Although they are touted as "hair tonics," there is no credible evidence that inositol, PABA, or vitamin E prevent hair loss or restore color to hair.

4. Herbs such as jojoba oil, nettle, and royal jelly do not prevent hair loss, according to Varro Tyler, Lilly Distinguished Professor of Pharmacognosy in the School of Pharmacy at Purdue University.

5. Does using sunscreens that block ultraviolet light increase a person's risk for vitamin D deficiency? Apparently not, according to a study from the University of Melbourne in Australia. Blood vitamin D levels remained within the normal range even in 70-year-olds who used sunscreen lotion.

6. If you get a sunburn despite using sunscreen, try pouring cold tea over your aching skin. Tannins in tea help take the sting out of a sunburn, and researchers at the University of Arizona report these compounds also help curb the sun's cancer-causing effects.

7. A study from the University of Texas Medical Branch in Galveston reports that topical application of aloe gel to sunlight-exposed skin helps prevent ultraviolet light damage associated with immune suppression and disease.

Unfortunately, the body's antioxidant supply is often caught short when bombarded repeatedly by large doses of ultraviolet (UV) light. "Concentrations of the antioxidants, such as vitamin E, are reduced following exposure to UV radiation, which implies that these nutrients protect the skin," states Helen Gensler, Ph.D., Associate Professor in the Department of Radiology/Oncology at the University of Arizona Cancer Center. For example, as much as 70 percent of the vitamin C in skin is destroyed after a single UV exposure. Stockpiling the antioxidant nutrients theoretically should reduce skin damage caused by environmental pollutants and sunlight.

Preliminary research supports this assumption. A study from Cornell University showed that chronic exposure to sunlight lowered blood levels of beta carotene.

The researchers concluded that repeated sun exposure might increase daily requirements for this antioxidant. Other studies showed that diets enriched with antioxidant nutrients, including selenium, beta carotene, vitamin E, and vitamin C, inhibit the formation of UV-induced tumors.

These findings suggest that UV damage to the epidermis affects deeper layers of the skin and even blood and other tissues. Antioxidants obtained from the diet probably are stored in the deeper subcutaneous layer of the skin, leaving the corium and outer epidermis only partially protected. To compound the problem, blood vessels that supply the skin with antioxidants become constricted over time. Even if an older person has high blood antioxidant levels, that doesn't mean the skin is getting its fair share.

Studies show that topical application of vitamin C, vitamin A, vitamin E, or a mixture of antioxidant nutrients in the presence of UV light might reduce skin cancer risk, premature aging, and liver spots. Because UV-induced skin damage continues for hours or days after sun exposure, application of vitamin C after sun exposure also might help repair long-term damage. In one study, delaying application of vitamin E for up to eight hours after UV exposure still offered protection.

Douglas Darr, Ph.D., Director of Technology Development at the North Carolina Biotechnology Center, has conducted several studies showing the effectiveness of vitamin C in preventing sun damage to the skin. In one study, the forearms of volunteers were treated with a 10 percent vitamin C solution or placebos and then exposed to UV light. The sites treated with vitamin C showed significantly less sun damage compared to that experienced by the untreated group.

"Antioxidants are not a panacea because not all UV damage to the skin can be attributed to [free radicals]; however, antioxidants plus sunscreens might be much better together than either one alone," recommends Dr. Darr. Dosage is important here. Many commercial creams contain 3 percent vitamin C or less, while the research shows at least a 10-percent mixture is needed.

Water-soluble vitamin C is not the only antioxidant that promises relief from premature aging. Researchers at the Dermatology Clinic in München, Germany, state that vitamin E is the primary fat-soluble antioxidant in protecting the skin from photoaging. They conclude ". . . vitamin E occupies a central position as a highly efficient antioxidant, thereby providing possibilities to decrease the frequency and severity of pathological events in the skin."

Researchers at the University of Leuven in Belgium report that other carotenoids, in particular lycopene, also might protect the skin from damage. Supplementation with beta carotene in healthy women raised serum and skin concentrations of the carotenoid; however, when a patch of skin was exposed to UV light, skin beta carotene levels did not change, while skin lycopene levels dropped 31 to 46 percent compared to levels in an adjacent nonexposed area. The lowered lycopene levels suggest that this carotenoid is essential in inhibiting oxidative damage to tissues.

Antioxidants might not turn back the hands of time and reverse the damage already done by too much sunbathing, but combined with a daily sunscreen lotion, they might help slow the future ticking of that clock.

Feeding Your Skin

The dietary guidelines for healthy, youthful skin are simple.

1. Consume daily at least 2,000 calories of low-fat foods, including fresh fruits and vegetables, whole-grain breads and cereals, and cooked dried beans and peas, with two to three servings of nonfat milk and no more than 4 to 5 ounces daily of fish, chicken, or very lean meat.
2. Include several servings daily of antioxidant-rich foods, such as citrus fruits for vitamin C, dark green leafy vegetables for beta carotene, and wheat germ for vitamin E.
3. Include in the daily menu at least one tablespoon of linoleic acid–rich safflower oil.
4. Drink six to eight glasses of water daily to maintain the skin's moisture.
5. Avoid repeated bouts of weight loss and regain, since weight cycling can result in premature sagging, stretch marks, and wrinkling.
6. Take a moderate-dose vitamin and mineral that contains extra amounts of the antioxidant vitamins.
7. Try mixing vitamin E (the natural form, called alpha tocopherol, is best, but should be refrigerated) with your sunscreen. Vitamin E oils and creams are already available on the market. Many cosmetics, skin creams, and even sunscreen lotions also contain vitamin C.

MIRROR, MIRROR ON THE WALL

Healthy, radiant skin is beautiful regardless of a person's age. With a nutrient-packed diet, no smoking, a combination of sunscreen and antioxidants, and an appreciation of the experiences that formed a few wrinkles here and there, a person can feel at peace with nature and the mirror.

THE NUTRITION AND HEALTHY SKIN CONNECTION

All nutrients are related to healthy skin. Here are a few examples why.

Nutrient	The Skin Connection	Sources
Protein	Maintains underlying muscles and skin structure, elasticity, and resiliency; maintains hormones that regulate skin moisture; regulates skin pigments.	Milk, meat, fish, chicken, legumes
Fat	Essential fatty acid maintains skin moisture. Deficiency results in scaly, dry skin.	Safflower oil, nuts, seeds, whole grains
Water	Maintains skin moisture; helps maintain normal oil secretion.	Water
Vitamin B_2	Deficiency causes blisters and cracks at corner of mouth, oily and flaky skin.	Milk, dark green vegetables, mushrooms
Niacin	Deficiency causes dermatitis.	Chicken, peanut butter, green peas
Vitamin B_6	Deficiency causes itching, dry skin, and anemia.	Bananas, meat, fish, chicken
Folic Acid	Deficiency causes anemia and pale skin.	Dark green vegetables, orange juice
Vitamin B_{12}	Deficiency causes anemia and pale skin.	Milk, meat, fish, chicken
Pantothenic acid	Deficiency causes dry, flaky skin.	Milk, chicken, peanut butter, vegetables, rice

Nutrient	The Skin Connection	Sources
Vitamin C	Maintains oil-producing glands, collagen, and skin elasticity and resiliency; is an antioxidant against premature aging and skin cancer.	Citrus fruits, vegetables
Vitamin A (beta carotene)	Maintains outer layer of skin; protects against skin cancer and premature aging.	Dark green or orange vegetables
Vitamin E	Antioxidant against premature aging and skin cancer.	Safflower oil, nuts, wheat germ
Copper	Prevents anemia.	Oysters, avocados, potatos, fish, soybeans
Iron	Prevents anemia.	Dark green vegetables, red meat, legumes, dried apricots
Selenium	Antioxidant against skin cancer.	Organ meats, seafood, whole grains
Zinc	Maintains collagen and elastin; might prevent stretch marks; helps heal cuts; deficiency causes dry, rough skin.	Oysters, turkey, pork, wheat germ

Chapter 11

THINKING CLEARLY, REMEMBERING WHEN

"For as I like a young man in whom there is something of the old, so I like an old man in whom there is something of the young; and he who follows this maxim, in body will possibly be an old man, but he will never be an old man in mind."

Cicero

Aging is on everyone's minds after we pass the 40-year milestone. Wisdom often flowers in the later years, but brainpower starts to dim in the middle years. Rather than blame the loss of swift thinking on your genes or your age, take a look at your diet. Research is finding that what you eat and how you live affect how well you think.

From each nerve cell and the chemicals (called neurotransmitters) that relay information between these cells to the circulatory system that carries oxygen to the brain, the entire system depends on a constant supply of nutrients to function properly throughout your life.

As the years pass, your mental function is affected long before you notice physical problems. Consequently, vague yet profound changes, such as cloudy thinking, mental fatigue, or impaired memory, can progress undetected because you otherwise feel fine.

Smart Foods

"THE TEST OF A FIRST-RATE INTELLIGENCE IS THE ABILITY TO HOLD
TWO OPPOSED IDEAS IN THE MIND AT THE SAME TIME, AND STILL
RETAIN THE ABILITY TO FUNCTION."

F. Scott Fitzgerald, from The Crack-up

Most people recognize that what they eat will affect their physical health. Yet the link between brain function and food, while not visible, is more immediate. What you eat (or don't eat) for breakfast, or even whether or not you snack during the day, can affect how clearly you think or how well you can recall information by mid-afternoon.

STOPPING TO REFUEL

Skipping meals is a big mistake, especially if one of those meals is breakfast. Breakfast restocks dwindling glucose stores, the brain's sole source of fuel. Keeping glucose levels in the optimal range enhances learning, memory, and thinking.

Breakfast should be light and comprised of complex carbohydrates and a little protein, such as a bowl of shredded wheat, nonfat milk, and a banana; oatmeal topped with wheat germ and nonfat milk and served with a glass of orange juice; or a whole-wheat English muffin with peanut butter, an orange, and a glass of nonfat milk.

Provide your brain with a constant supply of high-quality fuel by spreading food intake into four to six mini-meals and snacks evenly distributed throughout the day. Keep these mini-meals light. Avoid high-fat or "heavy" meals that contain more than 1,000 calories, which divert the blood supply to the digestive tract and away from the brain, leaving you feeling sluggish and sleepy.

EAT TO THINK

It's not only when but what you eat that could undermine thinking. The eight servings of fruits and vegetables in the Anti-Aging Diet are there for good reason. These foods are loaded with the antioxidants—vitamin C, vitamin E, beta carotene, and the hundreds of phytochemicals—that help prevent premature aging of the brain and nervous system. Excellent antioxidant sources include green or red bell peppers, orange juice, grapefruit juice, carrots, sweet potatoes, spinach, apricots, wheat germ, and broccoli.

Several minerals are essential for clear thinking, including iron, boron, and zinc. Iron helps transport oxygen to and within the brain's cells and works closely with the nerve chemicals that regulate all mental processes. Low intake of this trace mineral results in shortened attention span, lowered IQ, lack of motivation, inability to concentrate, poor educational achievement, and reduced work performance. Premenopausal women should include at least four, and men and postmenopausal women should include two to three, iron-rich foods in the daily diet, including extra-lean meat, cooked dried beans and peas, oysters, dried apricots, dark green leafy vegetables, and lima beans. Also, cook in cast-iron pots and drink orange juice, not milk, with high-iron meals to facilitate absorption of this mineral.

Dr. James Penland at the USDA Agricultural Research Service in Grand Forks reports that boron is essential to mental function, hand–eye coordination, attention span, perception, and both short-term and long-term memory. He concludes that boron "... plays a role in human brain function and cognitive performance ... and is an essential nutrient for humans."

Learning and memory slow in the presence of even a mild zinc deficiency. Low zinc intake is common in people—especially women—as they age. Include in the daily diet several zinc-rich foods, including wheat germ, yogurt, almonds, cooked dried beans and peas, and dark green leafy vegetables.

Choline is a vitamin-like component of acetylcholine, a nerve chemical that facilitates memory. Choline-rich foods include whole-wheat bread, peanut butter, cauliflower, egg yolks, liver, and leaf lettuce.

B vitamins are essential in the development of the nervous system. They help maintain the insulating sheath around nerve cells that speeds nerve communication, convert energy to a useable form for the brain, and regulate the chemicals that allow brain cells to communicate. Consequently, a deficiency of any one of the several B vitamins—including vitamins B_1, B_2, B_6, and B_{12}, or folic acid—can impair thinking, concentration, memory, reaction time, and mental clarity.

According to a study from the University College Swansea in Wales, people who take a moderate-dose multiple supplement show improved attention skills, reaction times, and cognitive functioning. Researchers at the University of New Mexico School of Medicine in Albuquerque report that seniors who consume a diet rich in vitamins B_1, B_2, B_6, C, niacin, and folic acid score higher on tests measuring memory and thinking ability than do people who eat poorly. Good sources of B vitamins in the Anti-Aging Diet include nonfat milk and yogurt, wheat germ, bananas, seafood, and green peas.

Finally, drink coffee in moderation. Caffeine in coffee and a related compound called theobromine in tea directly stimulate the nervous system and can sharpen your reaction time and improve concentration, alertness, and short-term memory. But more than about three 5-ounce cups of coffee can give you the "coffee jitters" and muddle your concentration and thinking.

The Dumbing Effect of Diet

"IF YOUR HEAD IS WAX, DON'T WALK IN THE SUN."
Benjamin Franklin

Cutting calories might boost brainpower or make you dumber, depending on how you cut. Paring down your calorie intake, while still eating a nutrient-packed diet, and doing it for life is the only dietary habit known to increase life span in every animal that has been tested. Paring calories also prevents age-related mental and memory decline. While testing thus far has been restricted to animals, there is every reason to believe humans would get the same mental jolt from a low-calorie, well-balanced diet.

Jump on any quick-fix diet bandwagon and you're sure to come out dumber as a result. Michael Green, Ph.D., Senior Research Psychologist, and colleagues at the Institute of Food Research in the United Kingdom have been studying the dumbing effect of diet for several years. In one study, 55 women between the ages of 18 and 40—some of whom were currently on a diet while others were not—were seated in front of computer terminals where a continuous stream of single numbers were displayed. The women were asked to press a response button whenever they detected a sequence of three odd or three even numbers. A total of 40 such groupings were presented in random fashion over the course of five minutes.

"The women who were currently dieting to lose weight displayed poorer reaction speeds, immediate memory, and ability to sustain attention," concludes Dr. Green. They processed information slowly, took longer to react, and had more trouble remembering sequences compared to their nondieting counterparts.

Evidence that dieting makes us dumb dates back to the 1950s, when Ancel Keys and colleagues at the University of Minnesota evaluated men who volunteered to eat approximately one-half their normal food intakes (the equivalent of a 135-pound woman cutting her daily intake to under 1,200 calories). After six months, the men had lost approximately 25 percent of their original body weight, but at high emotional and mental costs. They were more irritable, anxious, and lethargic. The men also showed increased signs of depression, fatigue, insomnia, impaired judgment, inability to concentrate, poor memory, and agitation. Many of these same symptoms are noted in women with eating disorders or on fad diets.

Common sense tells us that any drastic reduction in calories will cut off the brain's main fuel supply—carbohydrates. Starved nerves, in turn, relay messages halfheartedly, which means that thinking and emotions suffer. Restricting carbohydrates and calories also upsets the production of nerve chemicals, such as serotonin, that regulate both appetite and mood.

Dieting also wreaks havoc with other appetite-control chemicals, such as neuropeptide Y (NPY), galanin, and the endorphins. This disruption can undermine the best weight-loss intentions, while also potentially affecting mood and mental state, according to research conducted by Sarah Leibowitz, Ph.D., Professor of Neurobiology at Rockefeller University in New York.

While glucose levels dwindle, blood levels of fat fragments called free fatty acids are on the rise during restrictive dieting, which is a clear indicator of stress. The stress of dieting, in turn, would contribute to the heightened emotions, increased distractibility, and clouded thinking. "The degree of impairment . . . is similar to that found with other types of extreme preoccupying worry," says Dr. Green.

Finally, cut back too far on calories and you also jeopardize nutrient intake. In fact, it's virtually impossible to guarantee optimal vitamin and mineral intake on less than 2,000 calories. The dumbing effect is limited only to quick-fix diets. In contrast, "Weight loss in a slow, steady fashion (about 2 pounds a week) will lead to a more permanent weight reduction and also will be less likely to lead to feelings of frustration and anxiety," concludes Dr. Green.

Is There a Dietary Cure for Alzheimer's Disease?

"THE HEART DOES NOT GROW OLD, BUT IT IS SAID TO DWELL AMONG THE RUINS."

Voltaire

Alzheimer's disease seems like the most sinister of all the incurable diseases. This degenerative brain disorder first kills a person's identity by slowly erasing all memories, names, dates, places, and personality. Only after the simplest tasks, such as chewing or swallowing, are lost in the fog of confusion does the disease take the body. The process is excruciatingly slow, unfolding over the course of six to 10 years.

Age is a contributor to Alzheimer's, but not a decree. In some cases, age works in a person's favor. While 40 percent of people over the age of 85 have Alzheimer's, the numbers drop in people in their nineties. In fact, as few as 25 percent of people over the age of 93 years have symptoms of this debilitating disease. This suggests that the oldest old are in better shape mentally than their children. Whatever helps these people reach a ripe and active old age also enables them to avoid or delay the diseases that commonly are linked to aging.

A WEAK LINK WITH DIET

Early onset of Alzheimer's is probably a result of genetics. However, environmental factors also contribute to the disease, especially if it occurs later in life. Early studies reported an increased accumulation of aluminum in the brain of Alzheimer's patients, which led to speculation that the use of aluminum cookware, antacids, or even deodorant could trigger the disease. However, subsequent studies have found little to link aluminum with the onset of Alzheimer's.

Poor nutrition is probably related to Alzheimer's disease, but it is unclear whether it is a cause or an effect. Early damage to brain cells located in the region of appetite control might explain changes in food intake. A poor diet resulting in low vitamin and mineral intake might encourage a predisposition to the disease. Once the disease has reached advanced stages, the patient loses interest in or the ability to choose or consume nutritious foods, which only speeds the loss of memory and function.

Consuming enough of certain nutrients, such as the B vitamins and vitamin E, might at least slow the progression of Alzheimer's. Vitamin E and other antioxidants protect brain cells from free-radical damage associated with memory loss, while vitamin B_1 is essential for the synthesis and release of acetylcholine, the neurotransmitter involved in memory. A study conducted at the Medical College of Georgia found that high doses of vitamin B_1 (three to eight grams daily) slightly improved dementia symptoms in Alzheimer patients. However, vitamin B_1 therapy does not halt the progression of Alzheimer's disease, and doses this high should be taken only under the supervision of a physician.

Poor intake and low blood levels of vitamin B_{12}, folic acid, and vitamin B_6 also are linked with Alzheimer's disease. Scores on cognitive-function tests are lowest in Alzheimer patients with the lowest vitamin B_{12} blood levels. In addition, older persons with low vitamin B_{12} levels are at highest risk of developing the disease. It is unknown whether the vitamin deficiency causes or results from deterioration of brain tissue. One of the functions of vitamin B_{12} is to maintain healthy nerve tissue, which might explain how a deficiency of the vitamin contributes to the progression of Alzheimer's disease. Poor intake of any or all of these B vitamins results in elevated levels of a nerve toxin called homocysteine, which impairs memory and mental alertness.

Choline, a vitamin B–like compound, and its dietary source lecithin have shown varying effectiveness in the treatment of memory loss and Alzheimer's disease. A neurotransmitter called acetylcholine contains choline, suggesting that memory might be enhanced with oral intake of choline.

Supplementing with choline or lecithin (containing 90 percent phosphatidylcholine) sometimes has improved brain function in patients with memory loss.

Unfortunately, both choline and lecithin have been ineffective in other cases; they raised blood levels of choline, but had no affect on acetylcholine levels or brain function. If choline and lecithin are effective in the treatment of memory loss, they are probably useful only in the beginning or mild stages and are then useful only in prolonging the onset of more advanced stages of the disease. According to researchers at Duquesne University in Pittsburgh, caffeine and choline administered together might be more effective for enhancing memory than either one alone.

More Than Diet

"THE OLD MAN KEEPS ALL HIS MENTAL POWERS SO LONG AS HE GIVES
UP NEITHER USING THEM NOR ADDING TO THEM."

Cicero

Hormones, medications, lack of sleep, and disease can undermine mental clarity. Lagging estrogen levels in menopausal women can cloud thinking, while women on hormone replacement therapy (HRT) or people who manage their high blood pressure report improvements in mental function. HRT also reduces a woman's risk for developing Alzheimer's disease. Many commonly prescribed drugs, including antihypertensives and antidepressants, can slow memory. If you're taking any medication and notice changes in your mental abilities, ask your pharmacist or physician if there could be a connection. Anything that disturbs sleep, from arthritis pain and prostate problems to worry or caffeine, can undermine mental function.

The herb ginkgo biloba shows promise in boosting cognition in older folks. Avoid exposure to mercury, lead, and other toxic metals that damage brain and nervous tissue and are associated with subtle neurological and psychological disorders, including learning disabilities, reduced attention span, poor reasoning and concentration skills, and reduced IQ.

WORK A MUSCLE, IMPROVE A MIND

People who stay physically active maintain the highest level of cognitive function. When tested, their brain waves are remarkably youthful in patterning. The more years a person exercises, the greater the benefits in cognitive ability. Exercise increases blood flow, oxygen, and nutrients to the brain. It helps maintain low levels of stress hormones, while increasing levels of nerve chemicals such as norepinephrine. Exercise also increases the demand on the nervous system to maintain coordination and reaction times during exercise. Any of these responses could explain why physically active people have faster reaction times and retain more information than do sedentary people.

Vitally Thinking

"PREPARE YOURSELF FOR THE GREAT WORLD, AS THE ATHLETES USED TO DO FOR THEIR EXERCISES; OIL YOUR MIND AND YOUR MANNERS, TO GIVE THEM THE NECESSARY SUPPLENESS AND FLEXIBILITY; STRENGTH ALONE WILL NOT DO, AS YOUNG PEOPLE ARE TOO APT TO THINK."

Lord Chesterfield

Vitality often is the fuel that keeps a person thinking clearly. Those who read, travel, or expose themselves to new experiences at every age keep their minds active. They also live longer and are less likely to develop Alzheimer's disease. Our capacity to remember quantities of information declines somewhat as we age, which has more to do with disuse than with age. The average older person can remember only six items from a memory test compared to a younger person's eight items; the same older person after undergoing a memory training course can remember 30 items, while the younger person's recall jumps to 40. Age might make a difference, but not half as much as keeping the brain active and alert. The problem may not be that the mind fails as we age, but that we fail to keep our minds engaged.

USE EXPERIENCE TO MASTER AGING

Chapter 12

MIDDLE-AGE SPREAD

"Use, do not abuse; neither abstinence nor excess ever renders man happy."

Voltaire

The typical American gains 20 pounds between the ages of 25 and 55. Every extra pound of fat over 10 costs a person one month of life and affects the quality of life. More than 300,000 deaths each year in the United States are attributable to obesity, and that number is on the rise.

The percentage of obese people has jumped from one in four to one in three since the 1970s, or more than 60 million persons in the United States and 59 percent of the adult population, according to a 1995 report from the Institute for Medicine. The rates coincide with a similar increase in hours of television viewing and miles logged in automobiles and a drop in hours of physical activity. The obesity issue is one of lifestyle, not genetics. And the weight-loss goal is shedding fat and gaining muscle.

The Consequences of Trading Muscle for Fat

"LESS IS MORE. GOD IS IN THE DETAILS."
Ludwig Mies van der Rohe

People trade muscle for fat as they age. The fat increases disease risk, while the loss of muscle creates a spiral of increasing weight gain and leads a person to frailty and dependence. Excessive body fat significantly raises a person's risk of developing every major degenerative disease, from heart disease and cancer to diabetes and osteoarthritis. Obese people have up to a fourfold higher risk of developing cancer than their peers. In most cases, even a modest drop in weight of 15 to 20 pounds is all it takes to significantly reduce disease risk.

What's a Desirable Weight?

"SUCCESS RESTS IN HAVING THE COURAGE AND ENDURANCE AND, ABOVE ALL, THE WILL TO BECOME THE PERSON YOU ARE, HOWEVER PECULIAR THAT MAY BE. THEN YOU WILL BE ABLE TO SAY, 'I HAVE FOUND MY HERO AND HE IS ME.' "

George Sheehan, M.D.

The term *obesity* refers to a body weight that is 20 percent above the person's desirable weight. If someone's desirable weight is approximately 140 pounds, then that person is obese when the scale tips at 168 and the added 28 pounds are fat, not muscle.

Another measurement is the body mass index, or BMI, which calculates body fat by dividing body weight in kilograms by height squared. The American Health Foundation states that optimizing the cardiovascular risk profile corresponds to a BMI of 22.6 or less for men and 21.1 or less for women. A BMI greater than 27 is a warning for postmenopausal breast cancer, while the highest prevalence of diabetes occurs when the BMI is over 28. The lowest mortality and morbidity rates occur with BMIs between 19 and 25, which should be attained by 21 years old and maintained throughout life. As a reference point, for a 5'10" man to have a BMI of 19 to 25, his body weight must be 128 and 169 pounds, respectively. For a 5'5" women to reach a BMI of 19 to 25, her body must be 114 to 150 pounds.

WHAT'S A FEW EXTRA POUNDS?

While everyone is obsessing over how to lose weight, researchers at Cornell University report that a few extra pounds won't hurt you and might be healthier in the long run than being underweight. David Levitsky, Ph.D., the lead researcher of the Cornell study, says, "We found that people who were 20 to 30 pounds overweight were not more likely to die over a 30-year period than average-weight persons, . . . while the health risk of being moderately underweight is comparable to that of being quite overweight and looks more serious than most people realize."

Other studies, however, found a link between even moderate weight gain and disease risk. According to Walter Willett, M.D., Dr. P. H., and colleagues at Harvard Medical School, relying on only the Metropolitan Life Tables and other weight guidelines could give a false sense of security. In reviewing weights and disease rates in more than 115,000 women, the Harvard researchers found that modest weight gain (11 to 18 pounds) in the middle years, even though the women's weights were considered "normal," raised their risks for developing heart disease by 25 percent. An 18-pound gain raised disease risks even higher. The lowest disease rates were observed among women who weighed at least 15 percent less than the average for women of similar age and in women who maintained a stable weight throughout life.

The Cornell and Harvard findings may not be as contradictory as they appear. In a study conducted at the National Center for Chronic Disease Prevention and Health Promotion in Atlanta, researchers found that *intentional* weight loss that results from a well-planned diet results in reduced disease risks, while a study from the National Institute of Aging in Bethesda concluded that *involuntary* weight loss resulting from illness or cigarette smoking was a major contributor to disease and death.

Prevention is the best medicine when it comes to health and weight. The

American Health Foundation's Expert Panel on Healthy Weight states: "The healthiest weight is one that is attained by the age of 21 years old and maintained throughout life. . . ." If you are gaining a few pounds every year and those extra pounds are fat, not muscle, you should start and stick with a daily exercise routine and a low-fat diet. If you are already above your weight goal but are not yet at risk for weight-related diseases, the Expert Panel recommends losing between 10 and 16 pounds.

Are You an Apple or a Pear?

"MAKE THE BEST USE OF WHAT IS IN YOUR POWER, AND TAKE THE REST AS IT HAPPENS."

Epictetus

Recently researchers worldwide uncovered an important fact about fat: it's not only how much body fat you have, but where it's stored that influences how healthy you are and how long you live. The good news is that a few extra pounds in the hips and thighs might dent your vanity, but they won't hurt your health. On the other hand, a spare tire or beer belly, even in an otherwise slender person, could signal health problems.

Apple-shaped people carry most of their weight in the chest and abdomen (called an android pattern), while pear-shaped people store fat below the belt and remain relatively slender in their upper bodies (called a gynoid pattern). A man with a waist of 40 inches and a woman with a waist of 36 inches or greater are likely to be Apples.

Apples are more likely to be men or postmenopausal women. They also are more likely to develop heart disease, diabetes, high blood pressure, gallbladder disease, and possibly cancer; their diseases progress faster and more seriously; and they are more apt to die prematurely from disease than are Pears, even when the two have similar body weights and body fat percentages. In addition, blood cholesterol and triglyceride levels are high in Apples, while "good" cholesterol—HDL cholesterol—is low. The health risks apply to both slim and plump Apples.

The type of abdominal fat associated with health risks is called visceral fat, the firm fat that surrounds the internal organs. Subcutaneous fat that lies close to the skin is not the culprit. So, a firm, big belly is more indicative of health problems; one or two inches of pinchable fat around the middle might force you to loosen your belt, but it probably won't hurt your health.

Researchers can only speculate why upper-body fat is more harmful to health than lower-body fat. Fat above the waist is more likely to be stocked with saturated fats, so it's firmer than fat below the waist. This fat also is more metabolically active. Extra upper-body fat is associated with a condition called Syndrome X that includes increased blood levels of fats called free fatty acids, poor regulation of blood sugar and fat, and an increased risk for diabetes and heart disease. Upper-body fat increases both estrogen and testosterone levels, which elevate the risk for developing cancer.

THE ORIGIN OF FAT PATTERNS

Only 20 to 25 percent of the differences noted in fat distribution can be attributed to heredity, according to Claude Bouchard of Laval University in Quebec. Fat distribution is undoubtedly related to changes in the sex hormones secreted in puberty, since the male hormone testosterone is associated with an apple-shaped body and an increased risk for disease, while the female hormones produce more of a pear-shaped body and protect against disease. Once the adult fat-distribution pattern has been established, the amount of fat in the upper and lower body depends on diet, exercise, and other habits.

DIETING AND BODY SHAPE

Whether or not body shape changes when you lose weight depends on whether you're an Apple or a Pear. Dr. Thomas Wadden at Syracuse University monitored body measurements in overweight women who lost weight. Apple-shaped women lost more of their weight in the chest and abdomen; consequently, their body shapes noticeably changed as they lost weight. Women with big hips and thighs (Pears) lost as much if not more weight, but lost weight in both the upper and lower body, maintaining essentially the same shape as they slimmed down.

"They come into a weight-management program as large Pears and leave as small Pears," says Dr. Wadden.

Losing weight lowers what is called the "waist-to-hip ratio" (WHR), the proportion of fat above the waist compared to the fat at hip and thigh level (an Apple has a high WHR, while a Pear has a low WHR). Apples derive greater benefits from weight loss, because they lose more weight from the upper body; even a 10 percent reduction in weight significantly improves the Apple's health status. "In short, a person can get rid of the Apple shape, but a Pear will always be a Pear," states Dr. Wadden.

WHY CAN'T AN APPLE BE MORE LIKE A PEAR?

Pears tend to live healthful lives, while Apples are more likely to be smokers, to be stressed and sedentary, to drink alcohol, or to consume high-fat diets. The link with stress is particularly interesting.

Per Björntorp, M.D., Ph.D., at the University of Göteborg in Sweden, reports that monkeys exposed to stress accumulate abdominal fat and develop high blood sugar and cholesterol. Similarly, humans who are overly stressed, lose time from work, and struggle with anger or depression also tend to be Apples. Although the connections among stress, hormones, body fat, and health are poorly understood, what researchers do know is abdominal body fat and disease risk are reduced if a person stops the stressful behaviors. People who cut back on their fat intakes, stop watching television and start including exercise in their daily routines, stop smoking, and maintain weight loss lower their WHR and improve the length and quality of their lives.

Aerobic exercise significantly reduces the WHR (i.e., turns an Apple into more of a Pear) regardless of whether or not the person loses weight. Although the mechanism is poorly understood, reducing dietary fat might affect hormone levels in both men and women, which in turn changes fat distribution and lowers the risk for disease.

DIETING: SERIOUS BUSINESS

Dieting is likely to do more harm than good, unless a person maintains the weight loss. That doesn't mean you should give up on weight management. Weight loss is still recommended for Apples who are more than 20 percent above their desirable body weight. However, pear-shaped people who want to lose weight to improve their looks could have more to lose than just weight if they can't keep it off. If life is hectic, wait until you have the time and energy to commit to long-term weight management.

Obesity is still a health risk, regardless of body shape. Dr. Björntorp concludes that obesity and abdominal distribution of fat are two separate entities with different causes, different consequences, and possibly even different treatments. Apple-shaped people can greatly reduce their health risks and change their body shapes with diet, exercise, and stress management. "The only way a pear-shaped person can change body shape is to weight train and build the upper body so the lower body looks smaller," states Dr. Wadden. Learning to love your body the way it is might be a more healthful alternative to repeated dieting for Pears.

How to Lose Weight and Keep It Off

"EIGHTY PERCENT OF SUCCESS IS SHOWING UP."
Woody Allen

The only sound, time-proven skills for permanent weight management are:

1. burn more calories than you take in by exercising daily and cutting back on sugar and fat,
2. make changes gradually to allow for a one- to two-pound weight loss each week, and
3. establish an eating and exercise program that you can live with for life.

While you cut calories, you don't want to sacrifice your health by cutting vitamins and minerals. You must make every bite count! The Anti-Aging Diet can be tailored to your weight-management needs. But even this excellent eating plan can't guarantee optimal intake of all nutrients when calories drop too low. Consider taking a moderate-dose, well-balanced vitamin and mineral supplement if you're consuming fewer than 2,000 calories a day.

WEIGHT IN MOTION

Daily exercise is the number-one predictor of long-term weight-management success. Working out revs up your metabolism, builds muscle that burns calories, and keeps the weight off. Diet alone won't work and, in fact, might shrink muscles and slow metabolic rate. Diet without exercise means that up to half of the weight lost will be in lean muscle tissue, not fat weight. Metabolic rate slows, which means calories must be cut even more or you will gain back the weight. Combining cardiovascular exercise that burns fat, such as walking or jogging, with strength training that builds muscle and revs up the metabolic rate is the only way to maintain muscle and lose fat. Plan on exercising daily for the rest of your life!

JUST DO IT, THEN DO IT AGAIN

Permanent weight loss, like vitality, takes practice. You want an eating and exercise plan you can live with for life and that will allow a gradual weight loss of no more than two pounds a week. Make changes gradually, and do not consume fewer than 1,500 calories if you are a short or relatively inactive woman. Add 500 calories if you are a tall and/or active woman, and add up to 1,000 calories if you are an active man. You should increase exercise, not cut calories further, if you can't lose weight on this low-calorie plan.

IT ALL COMES BACK TO CALORIES AND FAT

Calories from fat, alcohol, and possibly sugar are more likely to end up as body fat than are similar amounts of carbs or protein. In addition to being twice as calorie-dense as other foods, dietary fat is more readily converted to body fat.

Starting Out

Before you begin a diet, review what really needs changing and where you should start. You want to lose the right kind of weight—fat weight—and you want to lose it for good without having to sacrifice your health. Here are the three pre-dieting steps to take before starting a weight-management plan:

Step One: Throw out the scale and check your body-fat percentage, that is how much of your total body weight is fat weight. Body-fat percentages can be calculated by trained professionals using a variety of techniques, including calipers and underwater weighing. Women should aim for a range somewhere between 20 to 30 percent. Men should aim for a range between 12 and 20 percent. Or, use the ball-park measure of "overfatness"— the waist-to-hip measurement, which requires nothing more than a tape measure and third-grade arithmetic skills. People can divide the waist measurement by the hip measurement; if the ratio is greater than .80 or, in women, if the total waist measurement is greater than 32 inches, you probably need to lose some fat weight.

Step Two: What are you eating? Any "no" answers to the following questions is a starting place for making dietary changes.

	Yes	No
1. Do you consume daily at least five servings of fresh fruits and vegetables?		
2. Of these five servings, is at least one a dark green vegetable and one a citrus fruit?		
3. Do you consume daily at least six servings of breads, pasta, cereals, and other grains?		
4. Do you consume more whole grains than refined grains?		
5. Do you consume daily at least three servings of nonfat or low-fat milk or other low-fat calcium-rich foods?		

Continued

	Yes	No
6. Do you consume daily at least three servings of iron-rich extra-lean meat, chicken, fish, or legumes?		
7. Do you almost always bake, steam, or broil rather than fry, sauté, or use sauces or gravies? When you use sauces, are they tomato-based rather than cream-based?		
8. Do you eat at fast-food restaurants less than once a week?		
9. Do you avoid or strictly limit butter, margarine, and other oils or fats?		
10. Do you read food labels and choose only foods that contain 3 grams of fat or less for every 100 calories?		
11. Do you strictly limit high-sugar or high-fat snack items?		
12. Do you limit (to less than one drink a day) or avoid alcohol?		

Step Three: The following questions might help you identify whether managing your emotions, thoughts, and stress should be at the forefront of your weight-loss plan. This time, any "yes" answer is a red flag.

	Yes	No
1. Do you eat with a frenzy when under stress?		
2. Do you constantly think about food and/or dieting?		
3. Do you eat when you're bored, tired, lonely, depressed, anxious, scared, or excited?		

	Yes	No
4. Do you eat to relax, as a reward or treat, or to calm down?		
5. Does extra body weight give you a sense of self-protection?		
6. Do you try to ignore hunger, but then feel deprived?		
7. Are you driven by a desire to be "fit" or "thin," and do you believe that thinness is synonymous with success, beauty, or personal power?		
8. Do you overeat in secret or when you are alone?		
9. Do you feel that physical hunger is more an enemy than a friend?		
10. Do you eat unconsciously, i.e., in front of the TV, while reading a book or magazine, or when preparing dinner?		

The combination of daily exercise plus a low-fat diet places the body in a fat deficit that promotes weight loss.

When you eat those calories also is important. Large, infrequent meals might set up a scenario in which the body stores more calories as fat as a safeguard against what it perceives as a famine. Dividing the same amount of calories into five or more little meals and snacks encourages the body to "burn" the food for immediate energy rather than store it in the hips and thighs. Space your meals similarly to those in the seven-day meal plan in Appendix A at the end of this book, starting with breakfast, so that no more than four hours go by between a light meal or snack.

Your ultimate goal is not just a certain figure or a number on the bathroom scale, it is a lifelong commitment to be the best and healthiest you.

*K*nowing Where You're Going

Goals are your roadmap to weight management. Without them you won't know where you are going or even if you got there. For a goal to be useful, it must be specific, realistic, and flexible. Instead of a vague goal to "exercise more" or "reduce fat intake," write specific goals that include what, when, where, and how, such as "I will jog for 30 minutes during my lunch hour, five days a week, for the next six months," or "To reduce my fat intake, I will spread apple butter instead of butter on my toast in the morning."

Realistic goals take into account where you are today and what you are likely to accomplish with reasonable effort. Unrealistic goals are a setup for failure, so avoid perfectionist goals that use words such as "always," "never," or "every day."

For a goal to be realistic, it should be broken down into mini-steps. For example, a long-term goal to lose 20 pounds can be broken down into short-term goals to lose one to two pounds a week for the next 10 to 20 weeks. Mini-steps also include walking an additional three miles a day to burn 250 calories, replacing negative thoughts with supportive ones, and substituting baby carrots for potato chips at the mid-afternoon snack.

Stay flexible. Modify your mini-steps if you find they are too easy or too difficult. Goals should be challenging, not overwhelming.

Little Meals

"DO WELL THE LITTLE THINGS NOW; SO SHALL GREAT THINGS COME
TO THEE BY AND BY ASKING TO BE DONE."

Persian proverb

The nibbler's diet has replaced the "three squares" diet as a better way for people in their second 50 years to manage their weight, cut their risk for heart disease, and curb cravings. Researchers at the University of Michigan School of Public Health report that women between the ages of 35 and 69 who divided their food intakes into several little meals and snacks throughout the day were leaner and had less body fat than were women who ate the same calories, but packed them

Sticking with It

"IF YOU ARE CHANGING ANY ASPECT OF YOUR LIFE, EXPECT SETBACKS AND BE PREPARED TO RECOVER. A SMART PERSON MINIMIZES MISTAKES. A SMARTER PERSON KNOWS HOW TO RECOVER."

Kelly D. Brownell, Ph.D., Professor of Psychology at Yale University

People who are most likely to successfully lose weight and maintain the weight loss (1) keep a daily food journal to monitor their eating habits, (2) learn from their slip-ups and return quickly to balanced eating and exercise patterns, (3) follow a low-fat, moderate-calorie eating plan, and (4) exercise regularly. Here are a few suggestions to help you steer your course to success.

MANAGING EATING AND THE ENVIRONMENT

- Sit at a designated place, such as the dining room table, to eat.
- Eat without reading, watching TV, driving, or doing other activities. Chew slowly and pay attention to flavors and textures.
- Make food less visible, convenient, and available. For example, store food out of sight, ask someone to clean up the leftovers, remove serving dishes from the table, or don't bring tempting foods into the house.
- Plan another activity, such as riding an exercycle, taking a bath, putting polish on your nails, writing a letter, or walking with a friend, during times of the day when you're prone to eat.
- Avoid or eliminate cues that signal you to eat inappropriately. If a doughnut shop on the way to work is too tempting, then take a different route to work.
- On returning home from work, go for a walk rather than opening the refrigerator.
- Bring nutritious foods to work or play, so you won't be tempted by the vending machine, fast-food restaurant, or cookie counter.

MANAGING THOUGHTS, EMOTIONS, ATTITUDES, AND BELIEFS

- Avoid using food as a reward, a treat, or a therapy.
- Listen to your body and eat only when you are physically hungry.
- List your beliefs about yourself and food. Replace negative beliefs (Everyone must like

me, I should be good at everything) that interfere with weight management with positive ones (Everyone doesn't have to like me, it's all right to make mistakes). Replace negative thoughts, such as "I can't do this" or "I deserve a treat," with positive ones, such as "I am in charge of my weight and health" or "I've worked hard and made progress in my weight management; I won't stop now!"

• Most people have one or more problem foods that are hard to refuse. Plan ahead when, where, and how much of a "trigger" food you will eat and how you will stop eating.

• Focus on what you can have, rather than what you can't have.

• Use thought stopping. Visualize a stop sign in your mind whenever you catch yourself thinking a negative thought about your weight-management efforts.

STAYING MOTIVATED

• Reward yourself frequently with nonfood rewards. Place tally marks on a calendar, tokens in a jar, or money in a piggy bank each time you accomplish a mini-step.

• Give yourself credit for daily successes.

• Visualize yourself ahead of time successfully handling food issues and social situations involving food.

• Recognize that changing habits will require an initial investment of time.

• Focus on gradual lifestyle changes rather than on dieting or weight loss.

into two or three big meals. The more little meals and snacks the women ate (up to six a day), the lower their body fat.

"It makes sense that the body is better adapted to small doses of fuel and nutrients all day long than trying to handle a glut of food every so often," says Sharon Edelstein, Sc.M., Research Scientist at George Washington University in Washington, D.C., and lead researcher on a study that linked snacking with a lower risk for disease. Our ancient ancestors evolved by grazing—not gorging—on nuts, berries, roots, and small game; feasts were rare. Our bodies were designed for nibbling on high-fiber, low-fat foods, not the "gorge 'n fast" eating style of modern society.

Common sense also is backed by scientific know-how. "Nibbling, compared to gorging on big meals, helps improve cholesterol metabolism and keep insulin levels low," says David Jenkins, M.D., Professor of Medicine and Nutritional Science and the Director of the Risk Factor Center at St. Michael's Hospital in Toronto.

Why nibbling benefits fat metabolism is poorly understood. One theory proposes that large, infrequent meals set up a feast-or-fast scenario in which the body stores more incoming calories as fat as a safeguard against what it perceives as a famine. Fat-building enzymes in adipose (fat) tissue might then be activated after a big meal, placing a person at greater risk for weight gain. Dividing the same amount of calories into five or more little meals and snacks encourages the body to "burn" the food for immediate energy rather than store it in the belly, hips, and thighs.

Body heat production after a meal, called diet-induced or postprandial thermogenesis, might be higher following multiple little meals than it is with a few big meals, so more calories are utilized as heat rather than stored as body fat. "The secret to triggering the thermogenic effect," says C. Wayne Callaway, M.D., Associate Clinical Professor of Medicine at George Washington University in Washington, D.C., "is to consume enough calories at each meal to get the burn off of calories." Dr. Callaway suggests that it is the mini-meals that contain about 25 percent of the day's total calories that increase thermogenesis by up to 20 to 25 percent.

SNACKS RULE

Unplanned nibbling can make or break your weight-management efforts and health. The secret is not to add more snacks to your usual diet, but to divide your current food intake into five or six little meals, while continuing to emphasize fiber and nutrients and to deemphasize fat, sugar, and salt. Have the oatmeal with raisins and orange juice for breakfast, but save the glass of milk and banana for a midmorning snack. Have a sandwich, raw vegetables, and tomato juice for lunch, but save the dessert of yogurt and fruit for a mid-afternoon snack. Dine on spaghetti, salad, and steamed vegetables in the evening, then have the slice of French bread and a cup of nonfat cocoa for a late-night snack. Looking good and feeling great might be as simple as leaving the house each day with your gym bag in one hand and a brown-bag snack and little meal in the other.

My Roadmap to Success

Complete the following worksheet each week. Use the checklist to monitor your success by summarizing your mini-steps in the left-hand column. Then give yourself credit by making a tally mark under the appropriate day each time you accomplish a mini-step. There can be more than one tally mark per day. (Use this sheet as a master copy.)

Date/Week: _____

Long-term Goal: _____

This week's short-term goal: _____

Each day's Mini-Steps (include details such as when, where, how often, with whom)

1. _____

2. _____

3. _____

	Mon.	Tues.	Wed.	Thurs.	Fri.	Sat.	Sun.
Mini-Step 1: _____							
Mini-Step 2: _____							
Mini-Step 3: _____							

25 OF THE BEST LITTLE MEALS AND SNACKS

Little meal or snack	*When?*	*Why?*
1. Bran muffin and ½ melon filled with 6 ounces vanilla low-fat yogurt or 2. English muffin topped with low-fat cheese, broiled, served with orange juice and fresh blueberries or 3. Crepe filled with low-fat ricotta cheese and two pieces of fresh fruit, chopped or 4. Equal parts wheat germ, peanut butter, and honey mixed and spread on whole-wheat toast, served with juice or a banana	Early to midmorning	Provides the right combination of protein and carbohydrate to sustain energy through early hours and curb hunger and cravings later in the day.
5. Low-fat yogurt and four Graham crackers or 6. One cup warmed almond-flavored milk and a banana or	Midmorning	A midmorning snack that includes carbohydrate and protein and little or no fat will sustain energy levels until lunch and will help avoid uncontrollable

Continued

Little meal or snack	When?	Why?
7. One soft cinnamon pretzel, an apple, and nonfat milk or 8. One ounce turkey slices, six fat-free crackers, and fresh strawberries		cravings and overeating later in the day, while not jeopardizing your calorie intake.
9. One-half tuna sandwich with salad (low-fat dressing), tomato slices, and nonfat milk or 10. Greek salad with feta cheese, cucumbers, tomatoes, and dressing (served on side), served with pita bread, fresh fruit, and nonfat milk or 11. One cup fat-free cottage cheese, served with fresh fruit, a whole-grain roll or bran muffin, and baby carrots or 12. Minestrone, served with bread, tossed salad, and nonfat milk	Lunchtime	To sustain energy and alertness during the afternoon, lunches should be low in fat and calories (500 calories or fewer) and high in flavor and nutrients.

Continued

Little meal or snack	When?	Why?

13. One whole-wheat raisin bagel topped with 1 tablespoon fat-free cream cheese and fruit slices
 	
    or
 	
14. One-half cup nonfat refried beans, served with 1 ounce oven-baked tortilla chips and salsa
 	
    or
 	
15. One cup kiwi-strawberry low-fat yogurt, mixed with two chopped kiwi fruits
 	
    or
 	
16. Two slices of whole-wheat toast, each topped with ¼ cup nonfat cottage cheese and ¼ cup crushed pineapple
	Midafternoon	Cravings for carbohydrates, salty, or crunchy foods are at an all-time high now. These snacks provide about 50 grams of complex carbs and help satisfy the need for something sweet, tasty, or crunchy. They also help avoid overeating at dinner.

17. Spaghetti with marinara sauce, served with French bread and salad or 18. Linguini with pesto sauce, served with tossed salad and a dinner roll	Evening	If your goal is a relaxing evening, these high-carb mini-meals will raise serotonin, a brain chemical that calms you down.

Continued

Little meal or snack	When?	Why?
19. Baked salmon, served with brown rice, steamed vegetables, and salad or 20. Split pea soup, served with cornbread, raw vegetables, and nonfat milk	Evening	If you have a late meeting or need to be alert in the evening, these mini-meals will provide the right mix of protein and carbohydrate to keep you energized.

21. A handful of Cheerios (no milk)
   or
22. Three fig bars with fruit juice
   or
23. One cinnamon-raisin English muffin with fruit
   or
24. One frozen whole-wheat waffle topped with 1 tablespoon maple syrup and berries
   or
25. One-half cup cooked maple and brown sugar instant oatmeal (no milk) and a banana.
	Nighttime	A small dose of carbohydrate, such as provided by these snacks, consumed an hour before bedtime will raise serotonin levels and help you sleep like a baby. By not overeating at night, you can reprogram your appetite clock and awake refreshed and comfortably hungry in the morning.

Chapter 13

MENOPAUSE: A CHANGE FOR THE BETTER

"We do not count a [wo]man's years, until [she] has nothing else to count."

Ralph Waldo Emerson

Forty million women will face menopause in the next 20 years; 60 million women will be in or through menopause by the year 2020. With that many women experiencing a major life transition, even the Change (as menopause is sometimes called) is undergoing a transformation.

As recently as the late 1800s, many women did not outlive their ovaries, so menopause was a moot point. Today, menopause, the cessation of ovulation, is only a halfway mark through life for many women. While our grandmothers weathered the experience in silence, women today have brought menopause into boardrooms and offices, onto magazine and book covers, and made it the topic of nationwide television talk shows. Many of the symptoms that women once suffered in silence are now preventable, or at least can be lessened, by a few simple changes in diet and activity.

Just Another Milestone

"KEEP CONSTANTLY IN MIND IN HOW MANY THINGS YOU YOURSELF
HAVE WITNESSED CHANGES ALREADY. THE UNIVERSE IS CHANGE, LIFE
IS UNDERSTANDING."

Marcus Aurelius

The term *menopause* literally means the cessation of menstruation. To be considered menopausal, a woman must be menstruation-free for 12 months. By the time she is officially diagnosed as menopausal, the experience is over. Of course, a woman knows long before this that something is different. Her memory or concentration might fail her at all the wrong times, causing her to doubt her competence or sanity. She might break out in drenching sweats during the day (called hot flashes or hot flushes) or at night (called night sweats). Her moods might fluctuate and intensify, while energy levels can fall to an all-time low.

To verify the causes of her symptoms, a woman can take a blood test that measures hormone levels, especially the female hormone called FSH (follicle stimulating hormone), which rises as estrogen levels fall. Menopausal symptoms can begin years before the actual cessation of menstruation, a period called the perimenopause.

The menopausal experience is as varied as the personalities of the women who pass this milestone. The average age at menopause is 52, but eight out of 100 women go through the Change before 40, while fertility has been documented in 57-year-old women. Often a women goes through menopause at about the same time as her mother, suggesting a strong genetic link.

Most of the symptoms can be traced to the hormonal roller coaster a woman rides during menopause. A woman's ovaries are the manufacturing center for the female hormone estrogen. As the ovaries begin to shut down, estrogen levels surge, fluctuate, and eventually decline. Anything that levels the surges in estrogen will help curb the symptoms of the menopause. While hormone replacement therapy (HRT) is by far the most effective method of balancing estrogen swells, diet and exercise also can play a role and might be a woman's first line of defense in handling menopausal discomforts.

The Soy Connection

"Change not the mass but change the fabric of your own soul and your own visions, and you change all."

Vachel Lindsay

The hot flash is the hallmark of menopause for many women. A hot flash is the sudden rise in body temperature accompanied sometimes by intense perspiration, a flushing of the skin, and waves of heat that can range from mild to tormenting. The hot flash is the external sign of internal swells in estrogen levels.

Recent evidence shows that estrogen-like compounds called phytoestrogens, found in soybeans, can help offset the drop in a woman's natural estrogen. While not exactly like estrogen, phytoestrogens act much like the female hormone, binding to the body's estrogen receptors and supplementing the effects of estrogen when levels are low.

This link between food and flush was first suspected when researchers noted the dramatic difference in the incidence of hot flashes across cultures. Only 14 to 18 percent of the women living in China and Japan ever experience a hot flash, while up to 80 percent of women in the United States and Europe can describe their last hot flash in detail. Women in Japan and China also add soy to their diets daily and excrete up to a thousand times more phytoestrogens in their urine. Studies report up to a 40 percent reduction in hot flashes when women add soy to their diets. An extra health bonus is that switching from hamburgers to soy burgers also reduces a woman's risk for heart disease and possibly breast cancer.

Preliminary evidence suggests that as little as 15 ounces of soy milk or two ounces of tofu daily might be all a woman needs to help dampen the hot flashes and curb the estrogen surges during menopause.

Food and Mood

"Time cools, time clarifies; no mood can be maintained quite unaltered through the course of hours."

Thomas Mann

Mood-Boosting and Energizing Snacks and Meals

- Six ounces grapefruit juice, two to three rice cakes, and one slice low-fat cheese
- Low-cholesterol egg salad made with one whole egg and two egg whites mixed with low-calorie mayonnaise, chopped celery, and seasoning on a whole-wheat roll
- Vegetable Medley Platter*
- Raisin bread toast topped with nonfat ricotta cheese, served with orange juice
- One bowl of Santa Fe Sweet Potato Soup* served with cheese and fat-free crackers
- One-half whole-wheat pita bread filled with Chicken and Grape Salad*
- Tuna sandwich made with whole-wheat bread, filled with water-packed tuna mixed with chives and celery, lemon, and a little olive oil, served with nonfat milk
- Chicken and Grape Salad*
- Greek salad made with nonfat feta cheese, tomatoes, cucumbers, a dash of olive oil, red wine vinegar, and seasonings, served with pita bread
- Jeanette's Spinach/Raspberry Salad*
- White bean soup served with cornbread and a mixed salad

*Recipes in Appendix B.

As hormones fluctuate, so does brain chemistry, including a powerful nerve chemical called serotonin. Peri- and postmenopausal women who struggle with mild depression might have lower serotonin levels than do other women. When serotonin levels are low, a woman is more likely to crave sweets and feel grumpy, while a rise in serotonin turns off the cravings and restores a more agreeable mood. Including a carbohydrate-rich snack, such as a cinnamon bagel with jam or a bowl of fat-free popcorn, could be all it takes to boost serotonin levels and mood.

Salt Cravings

"Your lordship, though not clean past your youth, hath yet some smack of age in you, some relish of the saltiness of time."
William Shakespeare, from The Merry Wives of Windsor

Women approaching and during menopause often report changes in taste and food preferences that reflect fluctuating estrogen levels. However, cravings for salty snack foods can interfere with a woman's attempts to maintain a desirable weight and can increase the risk for developing high blood pressure.

In some cases, the craving for salt is a biological drive to maintain health. Some pregnant women who restrict salt intake have more complications in the final months of their pregnancies than do those who satisfied their cravings for pickles and other salty foods. In menopause, fluctuating estrogen levels result in water retention, and the increased desire for salt might be the body's attempt to maintain the normal concentration of sodium in the expanded body fluids.

But cravings also can be a learned response, especially in the case of salt. The more you eat, the more you want, with the taste for salt gradually becoming more habit than need. Animals fed low-salt diets in infancy are less likely to overconsume salt later in life, while adult animals accustomed to salty diets crave the taste when salt is restricted. For most people who eat a highly salted diet, gradually weaning themselves off excessive salt is the best way to avoid cravings. Going "cold turkey" probably will upset taste buds, just as eliminating sugar too quickly from the diet can lead to sugar cravings.

Finally, salt cravings sometimes are a desire for tasty or crunchy foods. Try snacking on crunchy baby carrots dunked in flavored fat-free dips or oven-baked tortilla chips dipped in salsa. Try adding more spice to typical foods, such as adding an Ortega chili or gourmet mustard to your sandwich.

Boning Up on Calcium

"ONE IS NOT BORN A WOMAN, ONE BECOMES ONE."
Simone de Beauvoir

Women during and after menopause face an escalating risk for osteoporosis. Women who consumed ample calcium throughout life enter menopause with strong bones and are at low risk of developing osteoporosis. Unfortunately, however, most women don't get enough calcium. In fact, one of every two postmenopausal women consumes less than half the recommended calcium allotment of 1,200 to 1,500 milligrams needed to prevent age-related bone loss and osteoporosis. (See Chapter 10 for more about osteoporosis.)

Failing to consume enough calcium after menopause could have consequences beyond just bone loss. A study from the University of North Carolina at Chapel Hill found that lead, which accumulates gradually in the bones throughout life, is released as minerals dissolve out of the bones after menopause. This places a woman at increased risk for high lead levels in the blood, a condition associated with nerve damage, anemia, muscle wastage, and mental impairment. Consuming ample amounts of calcium during the early years inhibits lead absorption, and during and after menopause, optimal calcium and magnesium intake might help curb the release of lead from these tissues.

Protecting Your Heart

"IF I CAN STOP ONE HEART FROM BREAKING
I SHALL NOT LIVE IN VAIN.
IF I CAN EASE ONE LIFE THE ACHING
OR COOL ONE PAIN
OR HELP ONE FAINTING ROBIN
UNTO HIS NEST AGAIN
I SHALL NOT LIVE IN VAIN."

Emily Dickinson

The risk for heart disease escalates quickly as estrogen levels drop, catapulting heart disease to the number-one cause of death after menopause. Heart disease risk can be significantly reduced with hormone replacement therapy and/or diet and exercise. Adopting a low-fat, high-fiber diet based on a wide variety of fresh fruits and vegetables, whole-grain breads and cereals, legumes including soybeans, and nonfat dairy products can keep blood fat levels and heart disease risk low. Following the low-fat, high-fiber dietary guidelines outlined in the Anti-Aging Diet also will help maintain a trim, womanly figure, which is important for the prevention of heart disease.

Should Women Supplement During Menopause?

"Never try to impress a woman, because if you do she'll expect you to keep up the standard for the rest of your life."

W. C. Fields

Approximately one-half of middle-aged women do not consume even two-thirds of the recommended amounts for many vitamins, including the B vitamins, folic acid, vitamin C, vitamin D, and many minerals. Marginal dietary intake of these nutrients is linked to many mental, emotional, and physical problems, including memory loss, mood swings, depression, irritability, osteoporosis, and more. Taking a moderate-dose multiple vitamin and mineral supplement that contains extra vitamin E, plus a second supplement of calcium and magnesium, provides nutritional insurance on those days when a woman doesn't eat well enough.

The Dietary Nuts and Bolts for Menopause

*"WHEN SHE STOPPED CONFORMING TO THE CONVENTIONAL PICTURE
OF FEMININITY SHE FINALLY BEGAN TO ENJOY BEING A WOMAN."*

Betty Friedan

A woman who goes through "the Change" at 50 could theoretically have another 70 years of healthful living if she is aiming to reach her maximum life span of 120! The Anti-Aging Diet is the foundation for looking and feeling your best for that majority of life after menopause. Low in fat, salt, and sugar, it is high in fiber and the nutrients that help protect against mood swings, cancer, heart disease, and menopausal symptoms. The only adjustment menopausal women need to make is to add one to two servings of soy to the diet daily. Avoid or limit charcoal-cooked meats, processed meats, and smoked meats, all of which increase cancer risk.

THE HOT FLASH: THE DIETARY APPROACH

Except for including soy products in the daily diet, there is no way to eliminate hot flashes, but there are a few tricks that might ease the symptoms.

- First, avoid coffee, chocolate, alcohol, and spicy foods, all of which alter blood flow and can increase the symptoms of hot flashes.
- Second, eat small meals and snacks regularly throughout the day. Large meals increase body temperature and might aggravate a hot flash.
- Third, place a glass of ice water by the bed at night to drink at the first sign of an approaching night sweat. Try opening the bedroom window to keep the cool air flowing, use 100-percent cotton sheets, and try using a small fan by the bed.
- Fourth, be careful of what herbal teas you drink. Some herbs, such as black cohosh or dong quai, cause blood vessel dilation and could aggravate a hot flash.
- Some women report that vitamins E and C helped improve symptoms of hot flashes; however, this evidence is sketchy.
- Finally, dress in layers, so you can add or subtract clothes as your body's temperature fluctuates.

What's Exercise Got to Do with It?

"I HAD BEEN MY WHOLE LIFE A BELL, AND NEVER KNEW IT UNTIL AT
THAT MOMENT I WAS LIFTED AND STRUCK."

Annie Dillard, from Pilgrim at Tinker Creek

Women in their second 50 years not only can slow the aging process, they might even be able to reverse it with exercise. A weekly routine that combines some weight-bearing exercise, such as walking, with some strength-training exercise, such as lifting weights, helps prevent bone deterioration and even reverses bone loss in postmenopausal women. Exercise reduces the risk of developing heart disease, helps maintain a desirable weight, lowers the risk of losing your independence later in life due to frailty and weakness, and might even reduce cancer risk. In fact, an unfit woman at any age can reduce her risk of dying prematurely by up to 50 percent by becoming fit. Active women are two decades younger than sedentary couch potatoes.

Looking Forward to the Change

"ONE MUST NEVER LOSE TIME IN VAINLY REGRETTING THE PAST NOR
IN COMPLAINING ABOUT THE CHANGES WHICH CAUSE US DISCOM-
FORT, FOR CHANGE IS THE VERY ESSENCE OF LIFE."

Anatole France

The old myths about menopause causing hysteria and melancholy or signaling the end of life are quickly fading as healthy, active, and vital women approach the menopause and revel in the self-confidence and personal fulfillment that can come from maturity.

Many menopausal and postmenopausal women are actually more emotionally stable than women in their twenties and thirties. They are more at peace with and sure of themselves and happier with their lives than their younger counterparts, especially if they have nurtured their physical and emotional health. That's something to look forward to!

Menopause: Signs, Symptoms, and Solutions

MOOD SWINGS, DEPRESSION, IRRITABILITY, ANXIETY

Diet: Consume several small meals and snacks throughout the day. Include one or more servings of complex carbohydrate at each meal/snack. Avoid sugar, alcohol, and caffeine.

Supplements: Consider a multiple vitamin and mineral if daily intake is lower than 2,000 calories. Also, take a magnesium supplement if daily intake of dark green leafy vegetables, whole grains, legumes, wheat germ, and other magnesium-rich foods is low.

Exercise: Include regular aerobic exercise, such as walking, jogging, aerobic dance, or bicycling.

Habits: Reserve at least 20 minutes a day for relaxing, such as taking a hot bath, meditating, or doing deep breathing exercises. Avoid tobacco. Replace negative thoughts with more nurturing ones. Avoid taking on too many tasks and responsibilities.

FATIGUE

Diet: Eat breakfast and divide daily food intake into five to six small meals and snacks throughout the day. Avoid caffeine, sugar, and alcohol.

Supplements: A moderate-dose multiple vitamin and mineral might be useful.

Exercise: Daily exercise that includes either aerobic exercise, such as walking, or anaerobic exercise, such as weight lifting, can help boost energy levels.

Habits: Get at least seven to eight hours of sleep nightly. Take afternoon naps if possible. Set priorities, and avoid wasting emotional or physical energy on needless activities.

Other: Hormone replacement therapy (HRT) is sometimes helpful. Discuss this option with your physician.

SLEEP PROBLEMS

Diet: Avoid caffeine, alcohol, and sugar, especially after noon. Eat a light snack of carbohydrate-rich foods, such as fat-free popcorn or an English muffin with honey, an hour before bedtime. Avoid large evening meals or spicy foods at dinner.

Exercise: Daily exercise that includes some aerobic and some anaerobic activity, preferably in the morning or afternoon rather than at night, can help sleep.

Habits: Avoid tobacco. Take time to relax before bedtime. Develop a routine before bed that conditions the body for sleep.

Other: Herbs, such as catnip, chamomile, and valerian, might help improve sleep.

MENTAL FUNCTION, MEMORY, AND CONCENTRATION

Diet: Consume a low-fat, high-fiber diet that is rich in fruits, vegetables, whole grains, and nonfat dairy foods. Drink caffeinated beverages in moderation. Avoid sugar and alcohol.

Supplements: Take a moderate-dose multiple vitamin and mineral.

Exercise: Exercise should include some form of aerobic activity for at least 30 minutes daily.

Habits: Avoid tobacco. Sleep seven to eight hours nightly. Organize and use lists. Relax.

Other: HRT improves menopause-related memory loss and concentration problems.

DISEASE PREVENTION

Diet: Follow a low-fat, high-fiber diet. Limit sugar, cholesterol, saturated fat, and salt. Drink alcohol in moderation. Consume the calcium equivalent of three glasses of nonfat milk a day.

Supplement: Take a moderate-dose multiple vitamin and mineral. Consider taking extra amounts of calcium, magnesium, vitamin C, and vitamin E.

Exercise: Engage in weight-bearing aerobic activity for at least 30 minutes, four to five times a week.

Habits: Avoid tobacco. Relax and avoid excessive stress. Have an annual medical checkup.

Other: HRT is effective in reducing the risk of heart disease and osteoporosis, but might slightly increase a woman's risk for breast cancer.

Chapter 14

CAN DIET IMPROVE YOUR LOVE LIFE?

"So, lively brisk old fellow,
Don't let age get you down.
White hairs or not you can still be a lover."

Goethe

The greatest impediment to sexuality in the later years is illness, not ability. People who have an active sex life in their later years are the ones who are free from disease, are physically active, and enjoy life. These people report greater frequency of sexual activity and greater satisfaction compared to inactive people of the same age. If sexual ability wanes, is there anything you can do to stir the fires?

Looking for Mr. Good Potion

"WHEN I'M GOOD, I'M VERY GOOD, BUT WHEN I'M BAD I'M BETTER."

Mae West

For centuries, people have turned to food to enhance fertility and sexual prowess. Eating and loving are so closely entwined that we often speak of "eating our hearts out," "feasting our eyes," or having "lusty appetites." We call our lovers "spicy," "a dish," "a hot tomato," or "good enough to eat." The line separating sexual desire and physical hunger is a thin one.

"The age-old belief that a food or substance does what it looks like is called the Doctrine of Signatures," says Varro Tyler, Ph.D, Sc.D., Dean and Distinguished Professor Emeritus at Purdue University and author of *The Honest Herbal*. According to this belief, the universe reveals the use or virtues of a food by its shape and appearance.

Ginseng: Nice Buns!

[SEX] "THE MOST FUN I'VE EVER HAD WITHOUT LAUGHING."
Woody Allen, from the movie Annie Hall

Ginseng's notoriety comes from its shape: this root has leglike appendages and resembles the human body. "Occasionally a ginseng root will sprout an extra appendage that resembles the sexual organ," says Dr. Tyler. "That ginseng root is considered very precious and may sell for hundreds or even thousands of dollars in some countries.

"There is an enormous amount of research on the chemistry of ginseng and its effects on smaller animals," says Dr. Tyler. "But there is very little research on humans and without additional scientific studies we have no proof whether there is anything more to ginseng than just imagination." Even if ginseng is mildly effective, you can't be guaranteed that the ginseng you buy at the local health food store will work, since there is no quality control of herbs in the United States.

From Lusty Prunes to Rabbit Pie

"SEX AND BEAUTY ARE INSEPARABLE, LIKE LIFE AND CONSCIOUSNESS. AND THE INTELLIGENCE WHICH GOES WITH SEX AND BEAUTY, AND RISES OUT OF SEX AND BEAUTY, IS INTUITION."

D. H. Lawrence

A food doesn't necessarily have to look, taste, or even smell good to arouse lust. For example, people have dined on dried salamander and fat of camel's hump in preparation for a night of passion. During Elizabethan times, prunes were considered such a powerful aphrodisiac that they were served in brothels.

"If an animal is known for being fertile, such as rabbits, then their sexual organs and even their meat is believed to improve sexual potency," says George Armelagos, Ph.D., Professor of Anthropology at Emory University in Atlanta and author of *Consuming Passions: The Anthropology of Eating*. "Ancient mythology also has contributed to the aura of aphrodisiacs," he adds. Aphrodite, the goddess of beauty and love, whose name forms the root of the word *aphrodisiac*, was said to have risen from sea foam where Uranus's genitals had fallen in battle—hence the link between sexuality and oysters, clams, lobsters, fish eggs, eels, sea slugs, and almost anything else that comes from the ocean.

Modern Madness

"WOMEN COMPLAIN ABOUT SEX MORE OFTEN THAN MEN. THEIR GRIPES FALL INTO TWO MAJOR CATEGORIES: 1) NOT ENOUGH. 2) TOO MUCH."

Ann Landers, from Truth Is Stranger

Proponents of dietary aphrodisiacs may mix a little scientific jargon into the promotion of a food or food ingredient, but the same beliefs, myths, and magic are at play. For example, nutrient cocktails rich in vitamin C are billed as "quick-fix climax-enhancers." The active ingredients in many of these potions include caffeine or niacin, which appear to be potent only because they give you a temporary flushing of the skin.

There also is the belief that any food that contains hormone-like substances must trigger passions. For example, pheromones are hormone-like compounds naturally produced by many animals to attract members of the opposite sex. These chemicals also are found in minute amounts in some plants, such as parsley, celery, carrots, young parsnips, and anchovies. Truffles, a vegetable that looks like a homely version of the testes and has been promoted as a potent aphrodisiac for centuries, actually contains the male pig hormone androstenol. Unfortunately, these hormones have little or no effect on humans when eaten as food.

There is no scientific proof for any of these "remedies." The Food and Drug Administration reports that no product sold over the counter as an aphrodisiac (from ginseng and licorice to vitamins, chocolate, and choline) is effective. "It is very difficult to separate the effect of aphrodisiacs on the mind and their effect on the body," warns Dr. Tyler. "If people believe something is going to work, then it probably will." But was the passion caused by the food, your expectations, or just chance?

Candy Is Dandy, but Liquor Is Quicker

> "THOUGH I LOOK OLD, YET I AM STRONG AND LUSTY;
> FOR IN MY YOUTH I NEVER DID APPLY
> HOT AND REBELLIOUS LIQUORS IN MY BLOOD."
> *William Shakespeare, from* As You Like It

Liquor ranks among the most universal love potions of all time. Alcohol acts indirectly as a pseudo-aphrodisiac by its depressant effect on higher brain centers, thus suppressing any fear or guilt about improper behavior and allowing the imbiber to "loosen up." Ironically, more than a couple of drinks does not improve performance, since as a depressant drug, alcohol slows arousal, making for a clumsy and incompetent lover. As Shakespeare so succinctly wrote in *Macbeth:* "It [alcohol] provides the desire, but it takes away the performance."

Amorous Edibles: Foods That Really Work

THE HORN, THE HORN, THE LUSTY HORN
IS NOT A THING TO LAUGH OR SCORN."
William Shakespeare,
from As You Like It

When it comes to sexuality in the second 50 years, the real issue is not the aging process, but health. Nutritional deficiencies, from lack of vitamin A to insufficient zinc, can sap your mental and physical energy, while the nutrient-packed, low-fat eating plan outlined in the Anti-Aging Diet can put a spring in your step, a twinkle in your eye, and fuel your wildest desires. When it comes to wooing, even subtle nutritional problems can undermine desire, performance, and fertility. There is strong evidence that reversing the effects of poor nutrition will improve energy, mood, and even conception rates.

Researchers at the University of Utah School of Medicine report that blood testosterone levels plunged by 50 percent in a group of men after they drank milkshakes containing 57 percent fat calories. Testosterone levels remained constant in the same men when they downed low-fat shakes with only 1 percent fat calories. A. Wayne Meikle, M.D., Professor of Endocrinology and Metabolism and the head researcher for the study, concludes, "A high-fat diet over time might curb a man's interest in sex." Fatty diets also clog arteries, and arterial blockages are a common cause of impotence. In short, too little or too many calories, dietary fat, or body fat might interfere with a person's love life.

Oyster Ambrosia

"BE GOOD, SWEET MAID,
AND LET WHO WILL BE NAUGHTY.
IF YOU GROW BETTER EVERY DAY,
HOW GOOD YOU'LL BE AT FORTY."
William Hazlitt

The belief that oysters increase fertility might have some scientific basis. Oysters are the richest dietary source of zinc: one oyster supplies most people's daily requirement for the mineral. Several studies have shown that even short-term poor intake of this trace mineral reduces fertility, including reduced semen volume, blood testosterone (the male sex hormone) levels, and zinc concentrations in semen, and impaired ovulation and fertilization in women.

While consuming 15 to 25 milligrams of zinc each day will help sustain a person's normal sexual function, consuming larger doses will not produce superhuman fertility. It takes more than oysters, or any other food for that matter, to effectively treat serious sexual dysfunctions or infertility.

GALVANIZE YOUR REPRODUCTIVE SYSTEM

A person should consume approximately 15 milligrams of zinc each day. Here are a few ways to increase your zinc intake.

Food	Amount	Zinc (mg)
Oysters, raw	6 medium	76.70
Amaranth grain	1 cup	6.20
Wheat germ	½ cup	6.15
Ground beef, extra-lean	3 ounces	4.44
Baked beans, vegetarian	1 cup	3.55
Cashews	½ cup	3.09
Lentils, cooked	1 cup	2.50
Chicken, dark meat	3 ounces	2.38
Bean burrito	1	2.37
Rice, wild, cooked	1 cup	2.20
Clams, canned	½ cup	2.18
Yogurt, low-fat	1 cup	2.02
Tofu, firm	½ cup	1.98
Spinach, cooked	1 cup	1.37
Avocado, Florida	1	1.28
Oatmeal, cooked	1 cup	1.15
Chicken, light meat	3 ounces	1.05
Milk, nonfat	1 cup	.92
Cheese	1 ounce	.70–1.10

Candlelight, Soft Music, and a Smidgen of Nutrition

"AGE ONLY MATTERS WHEN ONE IS AGING. NOW THAT I HAVE ARRIVED AT A GREAT AGE, I MIGHT AS WELL BE TWENTY."

Pablo Picasso

Romance has a lot more to do with "chemistry," lingering glances, and subtle body language than it does with aphrodisiacs and zinc. The delicious complexities that attract you to someone are as much, if not more, likely to include qualities such as humor, intelligence, vulnerability, and integrity than sexual prowess alone. Good old common sense, combined with presentation when it comes to food, will go a lot farther than the most potent "love potion" in boosting energy and health. All you need is the nutrient-packed, low-fat Anti-Aging Diet, which supplies all the vitamins and minerals in optimal amounts; a moderate-dose multiple vitamin and mineral supplement; and to maintain a desirable weight.

Little Sexy Meals

Here are just a few ideas that are simple, elegant (or slightly risqué), and guaranteed to perk up your love life.

- Dim the lights and share a watermelon and dark chocolate salad on the floor in front of the TV.
- Have a backyard picnic of lemon pasta with steamed asparagus spears, sparkling apple cider, and caviar.
- Steam New Zealand Greenlip mussels in wine and herbs, serve with chunks of sourdough French bread, and let the juice dribble down your chin.
- Feed each other slices of Fruit Torte* blindfolded.
- Peel grapes and feed them to your lover one by one.
- Pack a picnic lunch that includes juicy fruits such as mangos, papaya, oranges, and honeydew melon. Eat the fruit with your fingers.
- Rent a copy of the movie *Tom Jones* and take notes during the "eating scene," then plan your own food orgy.

- Bring fresh strawberries and champagne to a drive-in movie.
- Serve your lover breakfast in bed, including fresh-squeezed orange juice and French toast topped with fresh raspberries.
- Eat plums, a bowl of custard, or a banana with your eyes closed, savoring the taste, texture, and smell.
- Eat mashed potatoes, pudding, spaghetti, or Glazed Fresh Fruit Parfait* with your fingers.

*Recipe in Appendix B.

LUSTY LIFESTYLES

People who are physically active engage in sexual activity more often and enjoy it more than couch potatoes. Additionally, daily relaxation (chronic stress interferes with sexual desire), avoidance of tobacco, limiting alcohol and caffeine, and limiting medications to only those prescribed by a physician will go much farther in boosting your desire, energy, and interest than rhino horn, ginseng, or fish eggs. According to Dr. Armelagos, "The most important sexual organ and the best aphrodisiac in the world is the imagination."

Lusty Tidbits

1. Have you used the term *horny* to describe an especially active sexual state? It is likely this term comes from Asian countries where there was a widespread belief that ground-up horns of various animals, such as rhinoceros and reindeer, could be powerful aphrodisiacs (probably because of their phallic shape). Some people went so far as to recommend unicorn horn; however, finding a supplier must have been difficult.

2. The ancient Greeks spread barley around the temple of Demeter to assure fertility. The custom was passed down to subsequent generations and today is perpetuated by the throwing of rice at the bride and groom during weddings. It's a nice custom, but a poor fertility pill.

3. Spicy foods raise the heart rate and cause a person to break out in a sweat, a physical condition similar to sexual excitement. You guessed it: Curry, chutney, pepper, chili, and cayenne pepper have at one time or another been linked to sexual prowess. Foods and spices linked to love usually are rare or exotic; that is, their very strangeness suggests the existence of secret powers. This is probably why the less-than-glamorous potato (and even white bread) were considered aphrodisiacs when they were introduced into England. Within a few decades, these foods usually sink to the level of delicious but prosaic edibles.

4. Researchers at the University of Wisconsin at Madison report that the combined effect of increasing vitamin D and calcium intake (i.e., to 400IU and 1,000mg, respectively) might improve fertility rates in men.

5. Both too much and too little selenium also might interfere with fertility, while consuming several selenium-rich foods, such as seafood, whole grains and extra-lean meats, enhances conception.

6. Men who smoke jeopardize their reproductive capability—that is, unless they also snack on vitamin C–rich foods, such as strawberries, orange juice, and broccoli. But, don't get carried away. Downing megadoses of vitamin C won't turn your couch potato into a Casanova. Since both smoking and exposure to other people's smoke can decrease fertilization rates, you're better off not smoking and avoiding passive smoke whenever possible.

BEYOND DIET AND EXERCISE

Chapter 15

MIND OVER AGING

"I don't know about you, but the way I figure, I can't change the world, but I can change the channel."

George Burns

The true light of vitality comes from within. There's a lot more to life, health, and longevity than just your reflection in the mirror. It is the shape of a person's inner life that shines through the body and keeps it fired with youth.

Attitude: The Science of Happiness

"OPTIMISM: AN INCLINATION TO PUT THE MOST FAVORABLE CONSTRUCTION UPON ACTIONS AND HAPPENINGS . . . TO ANTICIPATE THE BEST POSSIBLE OUTCOMES."

Webster's Third New International Dictionary

As discussed in Chapter 3, all of the qualities of vitality start with an optimistic and positive approach to life. Optimism is like a self-fulfilling prophecy. People who believe they have control over their health and lives take charge of their health, make changes in diet and exercise that will promote health, and experience fewer diseases and disabilities, take fewer medications, recover more quickly from illnesses, and have a lower incidence of depression. Pessimists who believe that their bodies automatically deteriorate with age are less likely to practice healthful behaviors, and their health suffers as a result. In one study, less than half of pessimists questioned were willing to make even simple changes in their diets even when they were told the changes would benefit their health.

Our thoughts literally help shape our bodies. The field of psychoneuroimmunology, which studies the connection between the brain and nervous system and the immune system, has found that the central nervous system communicates with the immune and endocrine systems through a network of neurotransmitters, hormones, and chemicals. The power of the mind to heal or hurt appears unlimited. Worry, depression, brooding or ruminating, feeling hopeless, or harboring pessimistic thoughts affect the heart rate, suppress the immune system, change skin temperature, and alter blood and brain chemistry. This toxic effect on the body leaves a person vulnerable to disease, abnormal cell growth, and organ damage.

On the other hand, positive attitudes, high hopes, humor, being carefree and light-hearted, and experiencing harmony, laughter, and peace of mind help healthy people stay that way. Vital people are more likely to educate and take care of themselves, and their attitudes also stimulate the immune system and allow the body to keep itself healthy.

BEYOND ATTITUDE

While agelessness springs from inner attitudes, there is something that underlies even this inner realm: the *will* to be vital. A person must first want to strive for vitality. From that determination blooms the drive to get there. As Leo Buscaglia says, "The only thing that stands between us and a happy life is the belief that we deserve it, that it is possible, and that the tools to achieve it exist."

Stress: Sorting Out the Good from the Bad

"IT IS MANY TIMES MORE IMPORTANT TO KNOW THE PATIENT WHO
HAS THE DISEASE, THAN WHAT KIND OF DISEASE THE PATIENT HAS."
Sir William Osler

Most people are born healthy. It is the stress, often self-imposed, of lifelong imbalances in perceptions, behaviors, and attitudes that tips the scale, allowing a person to slide gradually from health and vitality toward disease and despair. Many disorders once thought to be inevitable consequences of aging are now recognized as stress-inflicted and preventable. How you perceive and interpret stressful events, not the events themselves, determines the quality and longevity of your life.

WHAT IS STRESS?

To be alive is to be stressed. Stress is the body's response to any demand. The adaptive tools within the body were designed by nature millions of years ago as a protection against any danger, and this "fight-or-flight" response to any stressor rallies a wealth of physical, emotional, and mental resources to protect you from harm.

The fight-or-flight response is beneficial when it accompanies a real danger for which you need increased alertness, blood flow to the brain and muscles, improved vision and hearing, and other split-second responses that help ensure safety. The response also is beneficial when the stress is a positive one that incites us to stretch our limits, reach for our goals, and explore life. Positive stress actually encourages vitality. However, when stress results in worry, anger, and tension, then our fight-or-flight response might harm health, shorten life span, and undermine enjoyment of life even in someone who is otherwise vital.

STRESS AND YOUR HEALTH

High-level or chronic stress accelerates the body's natural aging process and contributes to the development of several disorders, including the major degenerative diseases. The early symptoms are as benign as:

- frequent colds and sore throats
- restless sleep or insomnia
- sudden emotional outbursts, hostility, or mood swings
- headaches or backaches
- heart palpitations
- fatigue
- skin problems
- stomach and digestive tract upset
- frequent use of alcohol or pills to help relax or sleep

Left unchecked, stress progresses and undermines vitality and long-term health.

Studies by Ancel Keys dating back to the early 1960s showed that stress raises blood cholesterol levels, increasing a person's risk for developing heart disease. Since then, hundreds of studies have confirmed the detrimental effects of stress on physical and emotional health, including a study from Duke University Medical Center in Durham, North Carolina, that found people who overreact to stress are much more likely to suffer heart attacks than those who let stress roll off their backs.

People who perceive a loss of control over their lives or are overcome by stress are more likely to suffer poor health, elevated blood cholesterol levels, hypertension, heart palpitations, sudden cardiac deaths, bleeding ulcers, colds and infections, asthma, kidney disorders, allergies, joint inflammation associated with arthritis, and possibly cancer. People who suppress their emotions in response to stress are more likely to die from heart disease. Stress also unleashes an army of free radicals, which further damage the body and contribute to disease.

"The effects of stress on aging may be greater than we think," warns Robert Russell, M.D., Professor of Medicine and Nutrition at Tufts University in Boston. For example, up until recently, women usually outlived their spouses. As women have entered the work force, the burden of juggling family and career has added heavy stress to their lives. Not surprisingly, life expectancy increases in women have begun to slow down as disease risk rates have begun to increase, not unlike the escalating rates of lung cancer that occurred after women began to smoke.

Future studies might find that many of the diet-related links with disease are more a matter of stress. Although many studies have linked red wine with a lowered risk of heart disease, researchers at the University Hospital in Leyden found that it has no direct link to heart disease; rather, the leisurely sipping of a glass of red wine is secondary to living a low-stress life that allows for such pleasantries.

IT'S UP TO YOU

Stress in itself doesn't cause disease; it is how we *react* to stress that determines illness or health. The secret to stress is to welcome it, work with it, and use it to reach your goals. As stress expert Dr. Robert Eliot recommends, "Don't sweat the small stuff, and remember everything is small stuff."

Change may be stressful, but it also is part of a vital life. The people who live their lives to the fullest are those who take the most calculated risks and thrive on positive stress, while minimizing harmful stress. Exercise may be the way to make peace with your body and prayer and meditation are ways to find peace with your soul, but reducing harmful stress is the way to make peace with your life.

How Not to Sweat the Small Stuff

Here is a partial list of ways to sidestep stress and enjoy life more.

1. Volunteer at a service that helps other people.
2. Get eight hours of restful sleep each night. Take a 20-minute cat nap mid-afternoon.
3. Have a pet. Pet owners live longer and are less prone to disease than people who live alone.
4. Develop a hobby.
5. Use time-management and organizational skills to more efficiently use time and energy.
6. Spend 20 minutes each day relaxing; for example, take a stroll outside, garden, throw a frisbee for the dog, practice a relaxation technique, read a novel, or play a game.
7. Meditate.
8. Cut back on caffeine, alcohol, and tobacco; they only aggravate the stress response.

Continued

9. Exercise more.

10. Let go of "all-or-nothing" thinking. No one is perfect, not even geniuses such as Mozart or Einstein.

11. Choose a physician with a positive attitude, one who will talk to you, answer your questions, and respond with sympathy.

12. If stress continues to be a problem, join a support group or get counseling.

13. Get married. People who are happily married are healthier and less stressed than single people.

Laugh or Lighten Up

"SO INSTEAD OF GETTING TO HEAVEN, AT LAST—I'M GOING, ALL ALONG."

Emily Dickinson

Anyone seeking to live long and vitally must embrace humor with a passion. Humor diffuses tension and conflicts, boosts morale, enhances relationships, relieves stress, and puts life in perspective. According to studies at Loma Linda University in California, laughter stimulates the immune system, boosting our resistance to infections and disease.

Laughter also is one of the best stress-management skills. It's almost impossible to be tense and laugh at the same time. Laughter is like internal jogging. It raises the heart rate, improves circulation and breathing, aids in the transport of oxygen to the brain and muscles, relaxes the muscles, and helps soothe headaches or back problems. Laughter also disrupts negative thoughts. Finally, a good laugh stimulates the release in the brain of endorphins, chemicals that produce a calming, euphoric feeling. Pain and inflammation are reduced and you feel relieved, more peaceful, and more alive. The more you laugh, the happier you are, the healthier you are, and the longer you're likely to live.

The Power of Prayer and Meditation

"THERE IS NOW SCIENTIFIC EVIDENCE THAT BELIEF IN PRAYER IS GOOD FOR YOU. FIRST THERE WAS EXERCISE AND EATING RIGHT, AND NOW BELIEF."

Herbert Benson, M.D.

Embracing strong spiritual beliefs, with or without belonging to an organized religion or going to church, is consistently associated with better health. People who regularly pray or meditate, who report they feel close to a Higher Power and feel connected or in harmony with the universe, and who define themselves as spiritual are happier and healthier than those with little or no spiritual component to their lives.

In a study from Dartmouth-Hitchcock Medical Center, survival of 232 patients undergoing open-heart surgery was most closely linked to the degree to which the patients said they derived comfort and strength from their spiritual beliefs. Those with strong beliefs had one-third the death rate of those with little faith. Coronary patients who pray and are prayed for often require less medication and are less prone to complications than other patients.

The link between prayer, meditation, and health goes beyond the operating table and mirrors the words of Dr. Albert Schweitzer, who said, "Each patient carries his own doctor inside him." People who develop an active spiritual life have lower blood pressures and half the risk of dying from heart disease, are less likely to suffer from depression or commit suicide, and tend to be in better physical health than those who infrequently pray or go to church. They are less likely to develop colorectal cancer and even if they do develop cancer, the quality of their lives is better during their illnesses than that of other people.

People with strong spiritual beliefs don't avoid tragedy or suffering, but they are generally better prepared to handle the pain of, and bounce back from, adversity than are others. Prayer and meditation are most effective when combined with, not used as a replacement for, traditional therapies.

A CLOSER LOOK AT MEDITATION

Meditation is the simple act of sitting still for 20 minutes each day with eyes closed, while focusing attention on either breathing or on a single word called a mantra (a mantra can be a sound such as "Om" or a gentle "Be still"), which the person repeats. When the mind wanders from this mantra, the meditator simply returns the attention to the mantra or breath. How can something so simple as doing nothing be so good for you?

Meditation aids healing because of its powerful calming effect on the body, which neutralizes the disabling effects of stress. It slows the heart rate, drops blood pressure, increases the flow of blood to the brain, and balances brain wave patterns. Meditation reduces a person's risk for developing arthritis, asthma, chronic pain, diabetes, digestive tract problems, hot flashes during menopause, infertility, and headaches. It also stimulates the immune system and improves memory and mental function.

By quieting the mind for 20 minutes or more each day, one becomes aware of internal thoughts, memories, attitudes, and beliefs that distort perceptions and undermine chances for vitality. Doubts, worries, regrets, desires, and other negative chatter that plague daily life are more easily replaced with positive thoughts when the mind is stilled each day. The result is that the emotional energy wasted on nonproductive thoughts is freed for more positive pursuits.

Forgiveness and Gratefulness

"TO OFFER FORGIVENESS IS THE ONLY WAY FOR ONE TO HAVE IT, FOR IN FORGIVENESS, GIVING AND RECEIVING ARE THE SAME."

James A. Knight, M.D.

Forgiveness and gratefulness are more than just good for the soul, they also are great for the body. People who hold onto anger, disapproval, grudges, thoughts of revenge, and disappointments pay a high price in their physical health, emotional energy, and loss of vitality. They are at much greater risk of developing chronic diseases, such as heart disease. Forgiving helps the forgiver more than the forgiven by diffusing harmful emotions and restoring the inner balance that encourages health.

*H*old *O*n *and* *L*et *G*o

How can you bring more gratefulness into your life?

1. Make a list of everything you have to be thankful for. Don't leave anything off, no matter how small. Value even the minor things.
2. Focus your thoughts throughout the day on the little things that make life wonderful. This is an example of how more comes from more; the more you emphasize all you have to be grateful for, the more you will find in life to appreciate.
3. Find a way to sympathize with the person who "did you wrong." Think of times you needed to be forgiven in your life. What do you have in common with your offender?
4. Write down how that person wronged you, but also list the unexpected good that came from the other person's actions.
5. Try the following visualization as a way to let go of anger:
   a. Close your eyes and visualize the person at whom you are angry.
   b. Fill yourself with love, then send that love and forgiveness to the other person.
   c. Ask that person to also forgive you for anything you might have said or done that may have caused pain.
   d. See yourself letting go of the person with love and forgiveness.
   e. Keep your eyes closed for a few moments to experience the feelings of love, lightness, and freedom.

A Suitcase Full of Vitality

"THE FARTHER ONE TRAVELS ALONG THE JOURNEY OF LIFE, THE MORE
JOY AND THE MORE PAIN ONE EXPERIENCES. HOWEVER, FOR ALL THAT
IS GIVEN UP EVEN MORE IS GAINED."

M. Scott Peck

The secret to a joyful journey in life is how you choose to pack your suitcase for the trip. The suitcase will hold only so much, so choose wisely the attitudes, beliefs, ideas, thoughts, and responses you want to bring. Keep in mind that how you choose to think about your life will determine how far down the road you get and, more importantly, to what extent you enjoy it.

Chapter 16

THE WORLD AROUND YOU

"When an old person dies, it is like a small library burning."
Alex Haley

I f there really is a River of Immortality in Eden, no one swims in it alone. A long and vital life always is intricately intertwined with the lives of others. The importance of developing and maintaining strong, supportive relationships with family, friends, co-workers, and community cannot be over-emphasized when it comes to longevity and vitality. We all need to give and receive love; that is what gives life meaning and purpose.

Unless people nurture these relationships when they are in their early and middle years, they are likely to spend the future alone, which can undermine any chances of living longer and healthier. As people age, they tend to loosen the connections they once had with their environments. They make and receive fewer phone calls, write and receive fewer letters, make and pursue fewer friendships, are involved less in other people's lives, participate in fewer meetings and social activities, and use their cars less. They touch and hug and are touched and hugged less, and they take fewer and fewer risks.

Sometimes the gradual isolation is caused by the insidious loss of hearing that can cause a person to slowly step back from social involvement. Physical infirmity, the loss of a loved one, disease, or some other crisis can start the gradual decline in social connections. Whatever the cause, isolation and the stress of lone-liness lead to mental and physical decline and an increased vulnerability to disease and premature death.

We humans are social animals, and much of our vitality comes from our connection to others. A person doesn't let go of life because he or she is old; rather, a person is old because he or she lets go of life. Make yourself useful to someone, something, or some cause; be necessary or even indispensable, and you'll always have a reason to live and will likely outlive your reclusive neighbors.

Home Life

"NEVER TAKE ANYTHING FOR GRANTED."
Benjamin Disraeli

Strong family ties and a satisfying and comforting homelife have been consistently linked to living a longer and healthier life. Happily married people live longer than do single people. Living in a loving home reduces a person's risk for developing heart disease and high blood pressure, aids in recovery and rehabilitation from illness, and speeds adaptation to life's changes, particularly in people after age 65 and especially in men.

The secret is to nurture a healthy household, one where open and supportive communication is welcomed. According to studies from the Ohio State University Medical School, couples who live with hostility and poor communication also have suppressed immune systems and are more susceptible to colds, infections, and diseases such as cancer. Developing ways to nurture support, love, and encouragement and to resolve disputes are critical not only to the life of the relationship, but to the health of the partners.

Developing a loving family life may be more important today than ever before. In past centuries, often several generations lived under one roof. People stayed, grew up, and grew old in the same neighborhoods. These built-in support groups have dwindled as our culture has become more mobile. It may be hard to imagine a need now to actively seek, develop, and nurture friendships for your health in later years, but cultivating those friendships could save your life and help in your quest for vitality.

Our ancestors never expected to live long enough to be grandparents. Today, most people should expect to become grandparents and, if they take care of themselves and/or are born with a good set of genes, they can look forward to being great- or even great-great-grandparents. Start planning how you want to live those later years as an integrated elder in a growing family.

Friends: How Well Have I Loved?

"YOU ARE NOT HERE TO MAKE A LIVING. YOU ARE HERE IN ORDER TO ENABLE THE WORLD TO LIVE MORE AMPLY, WITH GREATER VISION, WITH FINER SPIRIT OF HOPE, AND ACHIEVEMENT. YOU ARE HERE TO ENRICH THE WORLD, AND YOU IMPOVERISH YOURSELF IF YOU FORGET THE ERRAND."

Woodrow Wilson

More than money, possessions, job, status, or even sex, satisfaction with how well a person has loved and been loved determines the degree of meaning, purpose, and vitality he or she attributes to life.

Friends nourish and soothe the soul, providing a mirror from which to reflect on our path through life and a haven from daily problems. Women's ability to gather good friends might be one of the reasons they live longer than men.

People with strong, supportive relationships with family members and friends have one-quarter to one-half the risk of dying prematurely of lonely people. Women with strong, supportive friendships are less likely to develop fatal cancers; when cancer does strike, they are more likely to survive. In one study from Stanford University in Palo Alto, California, women with breast cancer who joined a support group lived twice as long as patients who received only medical care. Researchers at the University of Michigan have likened the effects of loneliness on health to the damaging effects of obesity, smoking, high blood pressure with elevated blood fats, and physical inactivity.

Maintaining good friends with open and honest communication also appears to shield us from other health problems. Menopausal symptoms are much more prevalent in women without strong social networks than in relatively symptom-free menopausal women with strong friendships. Even menstrual cramps, PMS

A healthy life is one that is balanced with inner joy,
outer health, and social connectedness.

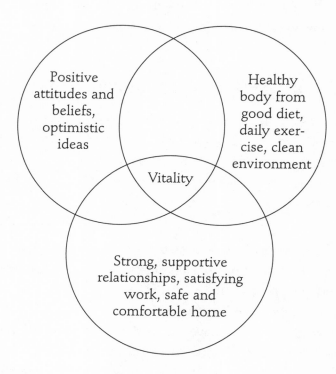

symptoms, and complications during pregnancy are more pronounced in women with poor social support. People need friends to stay healthy.

Developing a supportive community of friends helps encourage other healthful behaviors. A study from Cornell University found that women with strong social contacts were healthier and more likely to take charge of their health by reducing their dietary fat intake than were women who were more isolated. Even sharing life with a pet helps offset the aging process and can bring the humor, joy, meaning, and love necessary to keep us healthy and vital.

People who spend their leisure time in isolating pastimes, such as watching television, are most likely to develop high blood cholesterol levels, which doubles their risk for developing heart disease. Even moderate amounts of time in these sedentary, solo pursuits increase disease risk and could accelerate isolation and aging in later years, unless these habits are balanced with other, more social, activities.

How Does Your Environment Affect Your Health?

"IF LIFE IS A GAME, IT'S THE ONLY ONE I KNOW WHERE THE GOAL IS TO PROTECT THE PLAYING BOARD AND PRESERVE THE PLAYERS."

Kurt Vonnegut

If you're planning to live to be 100, you should plan to stay mentally and physically active so you can work at something you enjoy until you're 80 years old or older. People who report contentment and enjoyment in their work are more likely to live longer and healthier than people who are disgruntled with how they spend their time. Up to 250 hours or more each month are devoted to a job. You'd better like it, or the toll that the added stress takes on longevity could undermine the best of dietary and exercise practices.

The extra years you can expect to live when you adopt the healthful habits outlined in the book will mean you have more time to spend in fulfilling pastimes, including work. You'd better have a clear idea of what you want to do with that extra time, since there will be a lot of it. By conservative calculations, anyone planning to live vitally until at least the age of 100 will have an additional 35 years after the current retirement age of 65 to fill with meaningful pursuits.

Vital people keep working, change jobs, or attack retirement with the same passion with which they have lived their lives. Here are a few examples:

- Maggie Kuhn was 64 when she organized the Gray Panthers in 1970, a group dedicated to fighting age discrimination.
- At age 75, Golda Meir resigned as Israel's Prime Minister; two years later she accepted a position as head of the Labor Party.
- Victor Hugo, the French poet, novelist, and playwright, wrote his last great work at age 81.

- Maurice Chevalier, the French actor, starred in the movie *Gigi* at age 70.
- Arthur Rubenstein, the concert pianist, gave one of his finest performances at New York's Carnegie Hall at the age of 89.

How can your work support your longevity goals? Start today to aim for a type of work that you love. If your work could be anything you wanted, what would you like to do? Would you work outside or inside, with people or alone? Would you be self-employed or work for someone else? Would the job be a volunteer position? What talents and skills would you use? Once you have a clear idea of what you want to do, if it is something other than what you're doing now, start finding ways to bring that job vision into reality. As Kahlil Gibran said, "Work is love made visible."

When All Is Said and Done

"DON'T LEAD ME; I MAY NOT FOLLOW. DON'T WALK BEHIND ME; I MAY NOT LEAD. WALK BESIDE ME AND BE MY FRIEND."

Anonymous

As you venture on your journey toward a long and vital life, accumulate and bring with you the components that will give that life meaning and purpose, including special friends, family, satisfying work, and community involvement. Think of all the facets of a healthy life as threads in a tapestry. How you weave those threads will determine how beautiful and lasting a piece of work is created. For example, sharing meals with loved ones, or even starting a dinner club that meets weekly to share new healthful recipes, is a way to nurture relationships, express connections, and encourage well-being. It also satisfies one of the guidelines of the Anti-Aging Diet to "Enjoy food."

Nurture and build a social team of friends, family members, workmates, neighbors, and other loved ones. Look for healthy relationships everywhere. Select those friendships that make you feel good and that encourage you to stretch your wings and support your quest for health and vitality.

A FINAL WORD

"In the past few years, I have made a thrilling discovery . . .
that until one is over sixty, one can never really learn the
secret of living. One can then begin to live, not simply with
the intense part of oneself, but with one's entire being."

Ellen Glasgow

Most people want to hold on to a youthful appearance. How you live can affect how you look. But, at a more profound level, how you live, what you think, whom you choose to spend time with, and how you care for your body will be the deciding factors in how you feel, how much you enjoy your time here on earth, and to what extent others and the world are better off because you were here. Choosing healthful habits every day lets growing older become a greater opportunity for self-knowledge, balance, and joy than any other stage in life.

Never allow the tools for longevity to become your primary focus. When fitness and diet become a joyless quest for immortality, the deeper joy of passionate living gets lost in the process. You can never reduce the complexities, the wonder, and the magic of living to simple rules on how to eat or when to exercise. The guidelines in this book are a means to an end, not the end in itself.

Nothing can promise eternal life. Mortality is not an option. Embracing all of the guidelines in this book will push back the inevitable for a few years or even decades, but not forever. While we all must face life's exit at some point, by adopting healthful habits we can live life to its fullest and go out with a blaze of glory, with dignity intact, knowing we did well for ourselves and for others.

Albert Einstein once said, "When the solution is simple, God is answering." That truth applies to living a long and vital life and might be summed up in the following advice:

Dine well, stay fit, keep laughing, and enjoy life and the people you share it with. Another way of expressing it is to ask yourself, "How do I want to be remembered?" When you answer that question, you'll know how you want to live today.

My wish is that all of your highest dreams come true.

A WEEK'S WORTH OF ANTI-AGING MEALS

Items marked by an asterisk (*) are recipes found in Appendix B.

Day 1
BREAKFAST:

1 whole-wheat pita, cut in half, warmed, and filled with:

Eggbeaters (½ cup) scrambled with
> ½ cup chopped frozen spinach
> 1 ounce low-fat cheese
> Salt and pepper to taste

topped with 2 tablespoons salsa

Green tea with lemon

SNACK:

1 slice banana bread topped with:

1 tablespoon fat-free cream cheese

1 medium peach, skinned and sliced
1 glass water

LUNCH:
Tuna salad:

> 2 cups romaine lettuce
> ¼ cup thinly sliced carrots
> ¼ cup canned kidney beans, drained
> ¼ cup mung bean sprouts
> One 6-ounce can water-packed tuna, drained
> 2 tablespoons low-calorie Italian dressing

1 medium apple
8 ounces sparkling water with lime

SNACK:
Carrot-raisin salad with:

> ⅔ cup grated carrots
> 2 tablespoons raisins
> 2 tablespoons fat-free mayonnaise
> ½ teaspoon lemon juice
> Salt and pepper to taste

3 graham crackers
1 cup nonfat milk

DINNER:
1½ cups 3-Bean Market Soup*
1 piece (2½ × 2½ × 1½) cornbread
Tossed salad:

> 1 cup leaf lettuce, chopped
> ¼ cup canned mandarin orange slices, drained
> 2 tablespoons raspberry vinaigrette salad dressing

Sparkling water

Calories: 1,970
Protein: 25% of calories
Fat: 51 grams, 23% of calories
Carbohydrates: 52% of calories

Day 2

BREAKFAST:
⅔ cup low-fat granola
1 cup nonfat milk
½ cup cantaloupe, cubed
1 cup green tea

SNACK:
1 cup frozen blueberries
1 cup vanilla-flavored soy milk

LUNCH (NOTE: THIS LUNCH CAN BE PREPARED THE NIGHT BEFORE, PACKAGED IN LUNCH-SIZED CONTAINERS, AND REHEATED AT WORK THE NEXT DAY):
1 generous cup Linguini with Clams*
Grilled Eggplant:

⅔ eggplant, cut into ¾-inch strips and dusted with garlic powder and salt. Place in cast-iron skillet sprayed with vegetable oil spray. Grill for 4 minutes per side over medium heat.

1 cup tomato or V8 juice

SNACK:
3 cups fat-free microwave popcorn
1 glass water

DINNER:

2 cups Curried Broccoli Soup*

1 medium sweet potato, baked

1 slice French bread with:

    1 teaspoon butter

Cucumber salad:

    8 cucumber slices topped with:

        ¼ cup low-fat plain yogurt blended with 1 teaspoon dill and 1 teaspoon
            lemon juice

1 glass water

Calories: 2,010

Protein: 15% of calories

Fat: 64.6 grams, 28% of calories

Carbohydrates: 57% of calories

Day 3

BREAKFAST:

2 Breakfast Crepes*

1 cup orange juice

SNACK:

6 ounces strawberry-kiwi low-fat yogurt mixed with:

    1 kiwi, peeled and sliced

1 glass sparkling water

LUNCH:

Pita sandwich:

    1 whole-wheat pita cut in half and filled with:

        ½ cup garbanzo beans

        1 ounce cheddar cheese, grated

        3 cucumber slices

⅓ cup carrots, grated

3 sprigs fresh cilantro, chopped

2 medium tomatoes, sliced and topped with:

1 teaspoon basil

2 teaspoons olive oil

½ teaspoon red wine vinegar

1 cup nonfat milk

SNACK:

½ bagel topped with:

2 tablespoons fat-free cream cheese

1 cup vanilla-flavored soy milk

DINNER:

4 ounces grilled salmon topped with salsa made from:

1 green pepper, chopped

2 green onions, chopped

1 fresh jalapeño pepper, chopped

½ cup canned tomatoes

2 garlic cloves, chopped

3 tablespoons lime juice

1 tablespoon olive oil

Salt to taste

½ cup brown rice

1 cup steamed broccoli

1 cup coleslaw made with:

⅔ cup coleslaw mix

1 small apple, cut into ½-inch chunks

2 tablespoons low-fat or fat-free mayonnaise

½ teaspoon lemon juice

Salt to taste

1 cup nonfat milk

Calories: 1,990
Protein: 21% of calories
Fat: 54.5 grams, 25% of calories
Carbohydrates: 54% of calories

Day 4

BREAKFAST:
2 frozen whole-wheat waffles, toasted and topped with:

  1 banana, sliced
  2 teaspoons maple syrup

1 cup pink grapefruit sections
1 cup nonfat milk

SNACK:
½ whole-wheat bagel topped with:

  2 slices tomato
  1 thin slice red onion (optional)
  1 ounce low-fat cheese (broiled until cheese melts, if desired)

1 cup green tea or glass water

LUNCH:
Nachos:

  25 low-fat tortilla chips, topped and broiled with:
        ½ cup fat-free refried beans
        1 ounce low-fat cheese, grated
        Top this heated mixture with:
        ⅓ cup salsa
        2 tablespoons fat-free sour cream
1 cup orange juice

SNACK:

Fruit salad:

> 1 kiwi fruit, peeled and sliced
> 1 orange, peeled and sectioned
> ⅓ cup fruit cocktail, canned in juice

1 cup nonfat milk

DINNER:

Spaghetti with meatballs:

> 1 cup spaghetti noodles topped with:
> ½ cup spaghetti sauce with meatballs (2 ounces extra-lean meat)

Grilled Eggplant:

> ⅔ eggplant, sliced into ¾-inch slices, sprayed with vegetable spray and dusted with garlic powder and salt. Place in cast-iron skillet that is "greased" with 1 teaspoon olive oil. Heat 3 to 5 minutes per side or until browned.

1 cup fresh green beans, steamed
1 glass sparkling water flavored with lemon

Calories: 1,992
Protein: 17% of calories
Fat: 45.7 grams, 21% of calories
Carbohydrates: 62% of calories

Day 5

BREAKFAST:

Sunrise Smoothie (in a blender, blend the following):

> 1 cup low-fat coffee yogurt
> 1 cup fresh orange juice
> ½ banana
> 1 tablespoon marmalade
> 1 teaspoon freeze-dried coffee crystals (optional)

SNACK:
1 orange, sectioned
2 fig bars
1 glass sparkling water

LUNCH:
South-of-the-Border Sandwich (broil if desired):

    2 slices whole-wheat bread
    ½ chicken breast (roasted)
    2 ortega chilies
    1 slice Monterey Jack cheese

1½ cups Crunchy Chinese Salad*
1 glass sparkling water

SNACK:
½ whole-wheat pita with:
    ⅓ cup hummus dip

10 baby carrots

Iced green tea

DINNER:
1 beef fajita with:

    1 8-inch flour tortilla filled with grilled:
            2 ounces extra-lean roast beef
            ½ red bell pepper, sliced
            ½ green bell pepper, sliced
            ½ cup onion, sliced
            2 cloves garlic, minced
            ½ cup black beans, cooked
            ⅓ packet fajita sauce, prepared without oil
2 cups romaine lettuce, chopped and tossed with:

    1½ tablespoons olive oil and red wine vinegar

1 cup nonfat milk

Calories: 1,984
Protein: 20% of calories
Fat: 64 grams, 29% of calories
Carbohydrates: 51% of calories

Day 6

BREAKFAST:
⅔ cup oatmeal and ¼ cup wheat germ cooked in:

  1 cup nonfat milk

½ cup apricot halves
1 cup fresh orange juice

SNACK:
½ cup fat-free cottage cheese mixed with:

  1 apple, sliced
  1 teaspoon cinnamon
  1 ounce sliced almonds

6 ounces pineapple juice

LUNCH:
Sourdough Pizza Sandwich:

  1 sourdough roll, cut and spread in half, and topped with:
  2 tablespoons marinara sauce with garlic
  1 ounce low-fat mozzarella cheese, grated
  ½ cup zucchini, grated
  4 mushrooms, sliced

2 cups romaine lettuce salad with balsamic vinegar
Sparkling water

SNACK:

Three-Bean salad:

⅓ cup kidney beans
⅓ cup garbanzo beans
⅓ cup steamed green beans
2 tablespoons onion, chopped
Red wine vinegar
Salt and pepper to taste

3 celery stalks filled with:

2 tablespoons fat-free cream cheese

1 cup nonfat milk

DINNER:

1 large baked potato topped with:

½ cup steamed chopped spinach
1 ounce Parmesan cheese
1½ cups steamed baby vegetables seasoned with dill
2 medium tomatoes, sliced
1 cup soy milk

Calories: 1,985
Protein: 22% of calories
Fat: 45 grams, 20% of calories
Carbohydrates: 58% of calories

Day 7

BREAKFAST:

1 whole-wheat bran muffin
1 ounce cheese
1 cup fresh red raspberries
1 cup orange juice

SNACK:

1 slice Fruit Torte*

1 cup nonfat milk

LUNCH:

Oriental Chicken Salad:

   3 ounces roasted chicken breast, cubed and mixed with:

      ¼ cup celery, finely chopped

      2 tablespoon green onion, chopped

      2 tablespoons fat-free mayonnaise

      Salt and pepper to taste

   placed on top of tossed salad:

      2 cups romaine lettuce, chopped

      1 medium tomato, cut into wedges

   sprinkled with:

      1 tablespoon sesame seeds

½ papaya

1 caffè latte with ½ cup steamed nonfat milk

SNACK:

1 medium apple, sliced and sprinkled with:

   1½ teaspoons cinnamon sugar

1 ounce whole-wheat pretzels

1 glass sparkling water

DINNER:

Tofu Stir Fry:

In 1 tablespoon safflower oil, sauté until cooked, but crisp:

   4 ounces firm tofu, cubed

   ½ cup broccoli florets

   1 carrot, sliced diagonally into ½-inch slices

½ cup onion, chopped

3 garlic cloves, minced

¼ cup water chestnuts

¼ cup mung bean sprouts

2 tablespoons soy sauce

1 cup cooked brown rice

1 glass iced green tea

Calories: 1,993

Protein: 18% of calories

Fat: 55 grams, 24% of calories

Carbohydrates: 58% of calories

RECIPES

Snacks and Spreads

REFRESHING YOGURT SPREAD

1 quart nonfat plain yogurt
¼ cup walnuts, ground fine
1 small clove garlic, pressed through a garlic press
3 tablespoons fresh mint, finely chopped
1 tablespoon orange rind, grated
1 teaspoon honey
¼ teaspoon salt
⅛ teaspoon white pepper

Line a strainer with cheesecloth and place over a bowl. Place yogurt in cheese-cloth, pull up edges of cloth, and tie loosely to form a bag. Let yogurt drain until firm, approximately 4 hours. When yogurt is ready, mix the following in a bowl: yogurt, walnuts, garlic, 2½ tablespoons mint, 2 teaspoons orange rind, honey, salt, and pepper. Sprinkle remaining mint and orange rind over the top and refrigerate overnight. Use as a spread on crackers, celery sticks, fruit wedges, or toasted bread cubes.

Makes 16 servings (1 tablespoon each)

PER SERVING
Calories: 48
Protein: 3.8 grams (31% of calories)
Carbohydrate: 5.5 grams (46% of calories)
Fat: 1.2 grams (23% of calories)
Fiber: 0.136 grams

FRUIT-FILLED TORTILLA SNACKS

  4 flour tortillas, 8" round
  4 ounces fat-free cream cheese
  ⅓ cup fresh fruit, such as berries, peaches, or oranges
  1 medium banana, sliced

Grill tortillas on each side until they bubble. Fill each tortilla with ¼ of the cream cheese, fruit, and banana. Roll up tortillas and cut in half.

Makes 4 servings of 1 filled tortilla

PER SERVING
Calories: 170
Protein: 7.4 grams (18% of calories)
Carbohydrate: 29 grams (68% of calories)
Fat: 2.7 grams (14% of calories)
Fiber: 0.136 grams

Breakfast Items

BREAKFAST CREPES

Crepes

1¼ cups nonfat milk

1 cup all-purpose flour

1 egg (or use ¼ cup egg substitute)

1 teaspoon safflower oil

1½ teaspoons vanilla

1½ teaspoons sugar

¼ teaspoon baking powder

Filling

6 bananas, sliced

2 cups fresh or frozen strawberries, whole

2 cups fresh or frozen blueberries

1 packet NutraSweet (optional)

Cinnamon

In a blender, combine all ingredients for crepes. Cover and blend until smooth. Spray vegetable spray in an 8-inch nonstick skillet with flared sides and heat over medium heat. Remove from heat. Ladle 3 tablespoons of crepe batter into the center of the skillet; lift and tilt the skillet to evenly spread batter. Return to medium heat and cook for 1 minute on each side, or until the crepe is light brown. Place crepe on a paper towel. Repeat with remaining batter (with occasional re-spray of vegetable oil to prevent sticking). In a large bowl, mix filling ingredients. Fill crepes and sprinkle with cinnamon.

Makes about twelve 8-inch crepes; 1 serving = 2 crepes

Continued

PER SERVING
Calories: 231
Protein: 6.27 grams (10% of calories)
Carbohydrate: 45 grams (77% of calories)
Fat: 3.5 grams (13% of calories)
Fiber: 4.37 grams

BLUEBERRY PANCAKES À LA LEMON

Pancakes
1 cup all-purpose flour, sifted
2 teaspoons baking powder
¼ teaspoon salt
2 teaspoons sugar
3 tablespoons wheat germ
¼ cup egg substitute
1 cup nonfat buttermilk
1 tablespoon fresh lemon juice
1½ teaspoons lemon peel, grated
1 tablespoon canola oil
Nonstick vegetable spray

Topping
2 cups fresh or thawed frozen blueberries
1 cup nonfat plain yogurt
1 teaspoon lemon peel, grated
1 tablespoon lemon juice
2 teaspoons granulated sugar
Powdered sugar

For topping, thoroughly mix yogurt, lemon peel, lemon juice, and sugar together. Set aside.

Heat pancake griddle on medium-high.

For pancakes, sift flour, baking powder, salt, and sugar into a small bowl. Mix with wheat germ. In a medium bowl, combine egg substitute, buttermilk, lemon juice, lemon peel, and oil. Add flour mixture and mix only until flour is moistened. Batter will be lumpy. Spray griddle with vegetable spray. Pour approximately ¼ cup of batter for each pancake. Flip and brown other side after bubbles on top begin to break. Place two pancakes on plate and top with a dollop of yogurt topping and two heaping tablespoons of blueberries. Sprinkle lightly with powdered sugar, and serve.

Makes 6 servings (2 pancakes each)

PER SERVING
Calories: 200
Protein: 8 grams (16% of calories)
Carbohydrate: 33 grams (65% of calories)
Fat: 4 grams (19% of calories)
Fiber: 2.2 grams

Soups

THREE-BEAN MARKET SOUP

3 cups mixed beans (kidney, black, white, navy, soy, etc.)
Bouquet garni*
1 tablespoon salt
Ham hock (optional)
1 large can tomatoes
2 medium onions, chopped
6 stalks celery, chopped
4 cloves garlic, chopped
2 boneless chicken breasts, cut into ½" pieces
¾ cup fresh parsley, chopped

*Bouquet Garni: In a 5"×5" piece of cheesecloth, combine and tie into a bunch the following ingredients: 2 tablespoons dried parsley, 1 tablespoon thyme, 1 tablespoon marjoram, 2 bay leaves, and 2 tablespoons dried celery.

Continued

½ cup red wine
Salt and pepper

Wash and soak beans overnight. Drain. In a large covered saucepan, simmer beans, 3 quarts water, bouquet garni, and salt for approximately 3 hours. Add tomatoes, onions, celery, and garlic. Continue to simmer uncovered for another hour or until thick and creamy. Add chicken and simmer another 40 minutes. Add parsley and red wine. Remove from heat and let stand for 30 minutes before serving. Season with salt and pepper. (The flavor of this soup enhances with age. It is best made the day before and reheated.)

Makes 6 servings (approximately 1½ cups each)

PER SERVING
Calories: 337
Protein: 24.5 grams (29% of calories)
Carbohydrate: 50.5 grams (60% of calories)
Fat: 4.32 grams (11% of calories)
Fiber: 17 grams

CURRIED BROCCOLI SOUP

1 green pepper, chopped
½ cup onion, chopped
2 clove garlic, minced
1 tablespoon olive oil
3½ cups broccoli, chopped
¾ cup water
1 cup low-fat milk
1½ teaspoons curry powder
Salt and pepper to taste
1 tablespoon parsley, chopped

In a large saucepan, sauté pepper, onion, and garlic in olive oil until onion is transparent. Add broccoli and water. Cover and simmer until broccoli is tender, but still bright green. Blend mixture until smooth. Return to saucepan and add milk, curry, salt, and pepper. Reheat and garnish with parsley.

Makes 2 servings (1½ cups each)

PER SERVING
Calories: 187
Protein: 9 grams (19% of calories)
Carbohydrate: 18 grams (38% of calories)
Fat: 8.93 grams (43% of calories)
Fiber: 5.57 grams

SANTA FE SWEET POTATO SOUP

3 tablespoons olive oil
1 cup onion, chopped
3 sweet potatoes, peeled and chopped (about 8 cups)
7 cups chicken broth
1 can Ortega chilies, chopped, or 1 jalapeño pepper, seeded and thinly sliced
1 10-ounce package frozen corn kernels
½ cup low-fat milk
Salt and pepper to taste
3 tablespoons fresh cilantro, finely chopped (optional)
¼ cup fat-free sour cream (optional)

Heat olive oil in a large saucepan over medium heat. Add onions and sauté until transparent. Add sweet potatoes and chicken broth. Bring to a boil, lower heat, and simmer until potatoes are tender, about 25 minutes. Place potato mixture in a blender with broth (in small batches) and blend until smooth. Return to saucepan and add chilies and corn. Simmer 10 minutes. Stir in milk, salt, and pepper. Serve immediately. If desired, top with cilantro and sour cream. Makes 8 servings

PER SERVING
Calories: 322
Protein: 12.5 grams (15% of calories)
Carbohydrate: 53 grams (65% of calories)
Fat: 7.3 grams (20% of calories)
Fiber: 6.4 grams

Salads

CRUNCHY CHINESE SALAD

1 cup Chinese pea pods, washed and de-stemmed
1 cup fresh spinach, washed
1 medium tomato, cut into wedges
1 tablespoon olive oil
2 teaspoons red wine vinegar
1 teaspoon soy sauce
½ teaspoon honey

Steam pea pods for 1 minute. Cover and refrigerate. Fill bowl with spinach and top with pea pods and tomato wedges. Mix oil, vinegar, soy sauce, and honey, and drizzle dressing over the top and serve.

Makes one 1½ cup serving

PER SERVING
Calories: 234
Protein: 7 grams (11% of calories)
Carbohydrate: 22 grams (37% of calories)
Fat: 13.5 grams (52% of calories)
Fiber: 7 grams

SUNRISE SALAD

1½ cups orange juice (fresh or from concentrate)

8 large carrots, peeled and cut into 1" diagonal slices (if in a hurry, use
   1 pound of baby carrots, uncut)

2 teaspoons butter

1½ teaspoons grated fresh ginger

¼ teaspoon red pepper flakes (optional)

⅔ cup pea pods, cut in half diagonally

½ teaspoon salt

1 11-ounce can of mandarin oranges, drained

½ cup fresh parsley, finely chopped

Place orange juice, carrots, butter, ginger, and pepper flakes in a deep-dish frying pan. Bring to slow boil and cook for 20 minutes. Add pea pods and cook for another 10 minutes, or until carrots and pea pods are still slightly crisp and juice has evaporated. Remove from heat and cool to room temperature. Add orange slices and parsley, and toss. Salt to taste. Serve at room temperature or chill before serving. Makes 4 servings

PER SERVING
Calories: 163
Protein: 3.55 grams (8% of protein calories)
Carbohydrate: 32.5 grams (79% of carb calories)
Fat: 2.5 grams (13% of fat calories)
Fiber: 6.3 grams

JEANETTE'S SPINACH/RASPBERRY SALAD

4 cups fresh spinach, washed and dried

6 large mushrooms, washed, dried, and sliced thin

3 slices red onion

¼ cup fresh or frozen raspberries

2 tablespoons fat-free raspberry vinaigrette salad dressing

Continued

Arrange spinach leaves on a large serving platter. Place sliced mushrooms around the edges. Add red onion rings. Place raspberries in a decorative fashion in and around spinach leaves. Drizzle dressing over top, and serve. (For variety, replace raspberries with fresh peaches or winter pears.)

Makes 4 servings

PER SERVING
Calories: 34
Protein: 2 grams (23% of calories)
Carbohydrate: 5.78 grams (68% of calories)
Fat: 0.34 grams (9% of calories)
Fiber: 2.34 grams

CHICKEN AND GRAPE SALAD

2 chicken breasts (about 3 cups), cooked and cubed
1½ cups red grapes, halved
1½ cups celery, chopped fine
⅓ cup golden raisins
1½ cups apple, chopped
2½ teaspoons curry powder
4 tablespoons nonfat mayonnaise
Salt to taste
5 cups mixed greens, washed and torn into bite-size pieces

In a large bowl, combine all ingredients except greens and mix well. Serve chilled on a bed of greens.

Makes 5 servings

PER SERVING
Calories: 187
Protein: 13 grams (28% of calories)
Carbohydrate: 26 grams (55% of calories)
Fat: 3.7 grams (17% of calories)
Fiber: 3.5 grams

Entrées

LINGUINI WITH CLAMS

8 ounces linguini

4 cloves garlic, minced

2 tablespoons olive oil

3 tablespoons dry white wine

3 tablespoons fresh parsley, chopped

Pinch basil or thyme

One 8-ounce can minced clams

Salt and pepper to taste

1 tablespoon fresh parsley, chopped

Parmesan cheese, grated (optional)

Boil water in a large saucepan, and cook linguini until tender. While water is rising to a boil, gently cook garlic in the oil over low heat. When garlic is tender, add wine, parsley, and herbs. Simmer for 4 minutes. Add clams with their juice and heat through. Season with salt and pepper. Spoon sauce over pasta, sprinkle with fresh parsley, and serve with Parmesan, if desired.

Makes 3 servings (1 generous cup each)

PER SERVING

Calories: 370

Protein: 18 grams (20% of calories)

Carbohydrate: 49 grams (53% of calories)

Fat: 10.9 grams (27% of calories)

Fiber: 3 grams

SPINACH LASAGNA ROLL-UPS

2 teaspoons canola oil

¼ cup all-purpose flour

1 cup chicken broth, divided

Continued

1¼ cups nonfat milk

1 teaspoon dried basil or 2 teaspoons fresh basil, chopped fine

10 lasagna noodles

1 cup onions, chopped

5 cloves garlic, chopped

1½ cups zucchini, grated

1 cup carrots, grated

1 package frozen spinach, thawed and drained well

1 cup fat-free ricotta cheese

¾ cup fat-free mozzarella cheese, grated

2 egg whites

3 tablespoons fresh parsley, chopped fine

Heat oven to 375°F.

For sauce, heat oil in a medium saucepan over medium heat. Stir in flour, using a wire whisk. Gradually stir in ¾ cup chicken broth, milk, and basil. Cook over medium heat, stirring constantly until mixture is slightly thick. Bring to a gentle boil and stir for another 2 minutes. Set aside.

Cook lasagna noodles according to directions on package, drain and rinse briefly with cool water.

For vegetable mixture, pour the remaining chicken broth into a large skillet and heat over medium heat until hot. Add onions and garlic and cook until tender. Remove from heat and add zucchini, carrots, spinach, ricotta, ½ cup mozzarella, and egg whites. Mix thoroughly.

Pour half of the sauce into the bottom of an ungreased 11" × 7" × 1½" baking dish. Spread approximately ¼ cup of vegetable mixture along each lasagna noodle to within 1 inch of one short end. Roll the noodle/vegetable mixture beginning at end with vegetable mixture and place each roll seam-side down in baking dish. Pour remaining sauce over the rolls. Cover with aluminum foil and bake for 30 minutes. Uncover and bake another 15 minutes, or until hot and bubbly. Sprinkle remaining mozzarella and parsley over top and serve.

Makes 5 servings of 2 lasagna rolls each

PER SERVING
Calories: 394
Protein: 36.4 grams (37% of calories)
Carbohydrate: 51.8 grams (52% of calories)
Fat: 4.68 grams (11% of calories)
Fiber: 4.88 grams

VEGETABLE PIZZA

1 Boboli pizza crust
5 small packets Boboli Traditional Pizza Sauce
6 ounces fat-free mozzarella cheese, grated
1 green pepper, seeded and chopped
4 slices red onion, chopped
1 zucchini, sliced thin
6 mushrooms, sliced
1 cup tomatoes, chopped

Spread the packets of sauce evenly over pizza crust. Top with grated cheese, then top with pepper, onion, zucchini, and mushrooms. Bake at 450°F for 15 to 20 minutes, or until cheese is melted and vegetables are crisp. Top with tomatoes and cut into 8 slices.

Makes 8 servings

PER SERVING
Calories: 211
Protein: 15.5 grams (29% of calories)
Carbohydrate: 31 grams (58% of calories)
Fat: 3 grams (13% of calories)
Fiber: 2.54 grams

SALMON STEAKS WITH PARSLEY SAUCE

2 salmon steaks (approximately 1 pound total)
Vegetable spray

Continued

½ onion, sliced thin

2 carrots, peeled and sliced in thin diagonals

2 cloves garlic, minced

½ cup dry white wine

⅓ cup water

2 tablespoons fresh parsley, chopped fine

2 tablespoons fresh cilantro, chopped fine

Salt and pepper to taste

Place salmon steaks in a deep, nonstick frying pan sprayed with vegetable spray. On medium-high heat, sear on one side until brown, flip, and sear on other side. Remove salmon steaks from pan, drain any oil, and place onion, carrots, and garlic in pan. Cook on medium heat until soft and slightly brown (approximately 5 minutes). Add wine, water, and salmon. Heat for another 10 minutes or until salmon is cooked through. Remove steaks from pan. Continue to cook sauce until reduced to ⅓ cup. Add parsley, cilantro, salt, and pepper. Let sit for 2 minutes. Pour over salmon and serve with rice and steamed vegetables.

Makes 2 servings

PER SERVING
Calories: 491
Protein: 56 grams (46% of calories)
Carbohydrate: 15 grams (12% of calories)
Fat: 23 grams (42% of calories)
Fiber: 3 grams

Vegetables

VEGETABLE MEDLEY PLATTER

Topping:

1½ teaspoons olive oil

½ medium onion, chopped

½ tablespoon flour

3 tablespoons low-sodium tamari soy sauce
½ cup tomato juice
3 tablespoons water

Vegetables:
2 celery stalks, cut into 1" slices
2 large carrots, cut into ¾" diagonal slices
½ cup cauliflower florets
1 cup broccoli florets
½ cup crookneck squash, cut into ¾" slices
¾ cup spinach leaves, washed and stemmed
1 medium tomato, cut into wedges
2 tablespoons cheddar cheese, grated
1 cup steamed brown rice

Topping: Heat olive oil in a nonstick skillet over medium heat. Add onions and cook until tender. Reduce heat and slowly add flour, stirring to thoroughly coat onions. Continue to stir while slowly adding soy sauce, tomato juice, and water. Simmer for 20 minutes, stirring frequently.

Vegetables: Heat water in a large steamer. Add celery and carrots, and steam 5 minutes before adding cauliflower and broccoli. Continue to steam for another 5 minutes, then add squash. Steam another 5 minutes, then add spinach. Steam 5 more minutes. Add tomatoes and steam for 3 minutes. (All vegetables should be cooked, but crunchy, and spinach and tomato should be heated through.) Remove from heat, transfer to a heated bowl, and toss lightly to mix colors. Pour topping evenly over vegetables and sprinkle with grated cheese. Serve immediately over rice.

Makes 4 (¾ cup) servings, including rice

PER SERVING
Calories: 163
Protein: 6 grams (15% protein calories)

*These vegetables are merely suggestions. Be creative and experiment by adding your favorite choices, including mushrooms, asparagus, or cabbage.

Continued

Carbohydrate: 25 grams (61% carb calories)
Fat: 4.4 grams (24% fat calories)
Fiber: 5 grams

SQUASH ON THE ROCKS

    1 acorn squash, cut in half and seeded
    1 teaspoon butter
    2 teaspoons brandy
    ½ teaspoon salt

Lightly rub inside of both halves of squash with butter. Pour in brandy and sprinkle with salt. Cover and bake for 45 minutes at 350°F.

Makes 2 servings

PER SERVING
Calories: 130
Protein: 2 grams (6% of calories)
Carbohydrate: 26 grams (79% of calories)
Fat: 2.17 grams (15% of calories)
Fiber: 16 grams

GARLIC SPINACH

    ¾ cup chicken broth
    4 bunches fresh spinach, washed, stemmed, and dried
    3 cloves garlic, minced
    1 teaspoon olive oil
    ¼ teaspoon dried red pepper flakes
    ½ teaspoon salt

In a small saucepan, bring chicken broth to a boil. Set aside. Place spinach in a large, deep nonstick frying pan and heat, turning frequently, until soft but still dark green. Set aside.

In a saucepan over medium heat, sauté garlic in olive oil until golden. Add chicken broth, pepper flakes, and salt and stir. Pour garlic mixture over spinach, stir gently, let stand for 3 minutes, and serve.

Makes 8 servings, each serving slightly more than ½ cup

PER SERVING
Calories: 40
Protein: 3.8 grams (38% of calories)
Carbohydrate: 3.8 grams (38% of calories)
Fat: 1.1 grams (24% of calories)
Fiber: 3 grams

MASHED POTATOES WITH ROASTED GARLIC

4 large potatoes
5 unpeeled garlic cloves
¾ cup nonfat sour cream
1 tablespoon horseradish
⅔ cup nonfat milk
Salt and pepper to taste

Heat oven to 375°F. Scrub potatoes. Wrap garlic cloves in tin foil. Place potatoes and garlic in oven. Bake potatoes for one hour, or until soft. Bake garlic for 45 minutes. Cut potatoes in half and scoop out insides. Discard skins. Scoop softened garlic cloves from skins and add to potatoes. Add sour cream, horseradish, milk, salt, and pepper and blend until fluffy. Add more milk if needed for desired consistency.

Makes 4 servings

PER SERVING
Calories: 199
Protein: 7.7 grams (15% protein calories)
Carbohydrate: 40.5 grams (81% carb calories)
Fat: 0.9 grams (4% fat calories)
Fiber: 2.5 grams

Desserts

FRUIT TORTE

1 package pizza dough mix for 10-inch to 12-inch pizza, sweetened
   with 2 teaspoons granulated sugar
Two 6-ounce containers lemon-flavored nonfat yogurt
3 cups sliced fresh fruit, including kiwi, strawberries, bananas, halved
   grapes, mandarin oranges, and cantaloupe balls
3 tablespoons orange juice concentrate
1 tablespoon powdered sugar
1 sprig mint

Prepare pizza dough mix according to package directions, with addition of sugar. Shape dough into a large circle on a round pizza pan or stone, forming a ½-inch-high edge. Bake according to package directions. Cool. Spread crust evenly with a layer of yogurt to within ½-inch of raised edge. Beginning with kiwi, arrange each grouping of sliced fruit in concentric circles on top of crust. Mix orange juice concentrate with powdered sugar until smooth. Drizzle over top of fruited torte. Finish with mint sprig in center. Chill.

Makes 4 servings of ¼ torte

PER SERVING
Calories: 309
Protein: 10.8 grams (14% protein calories)
Carbohydrate: 59 grams (77% carb calories)
Fat: 3.02 grams (9% fat calories)
Fiber: 3 grams

GLAZED FRESH FRUIT PARFAIT

1 tablespoon orange marmalade
1 kiwi, peeled and sliced
2 apricots (fresh or canned in light syrup), halved
½ banana, sliced

4 fresh strawberries
½ medium orange, peeled and sectioned
1 tablespoon light whipping cream

Melt marmalade in the microwave on high for about 3 minutes. Cool, then pour over fruit, tossing gently to coat. Fill a parfait or stemmed water glass with the fruit and top with whipping cream.

Makes 1 serving

PER SERVING
Calories: 274
Protein: 3 grams (4% of calories)
Carbohydrate: 58 grams (85% of calories)
Fat: 3.5 grams (11% of calories)
Fiber: 9.4 grams

Appendix C

ANTI-AGING SUPERFOODS

Tired of only hearing about the foods you can't have, should cut back on, or should avoid like the plague? Well, here's a list of foods scientists report we should be eating much *more* of. From chin-dribbling strawberries to sweet, chewy figs, these selections are Mother Nature's superfoods, supplying lots of anti-aging nutritional punch for very few calories and little fat.

Broccoli: A one-cup serving of steamed broccoli supplies 20 percent of a person's folic acid needs, 193 percent of vitamin C needs, and 15 percent of the requirements for vitamins B_2 and B_6, all for only 43 calories! Broccoli also contains sulforaphane and indoles, phytochemicals that block the growth of cancerous tumors.

Tomatoes: Tomatoes top the list as a source of a carotene-like substance called lycopene, which is one of the most potent antioxidants in preventing damage to cells and tissues. One tomato supplies only 25 calories and no fat, but packs more than 10 percent of a person's daily need for vitamin A, folic acid, vitamin C, and potassium.

Greens: It is almost impossible to meet all your nutritional needs without at least one to two servings daily of dark green leafies. Spinach and other greens (such as collards, chard, mustard, and turnip) are the best dietary sources of lutein, another carotene-like compound that has antioxidant capabilities. Green leafies also boost your intake of folic acid, vitamin A, vitamin C, calcium, iron, magnesium, potassium, and fiber. Layer them into lasagna; steam, chop, and whip them into mashed potatoes; blend them with tofu for a vegetarian quiche; add them to a stir fry; or sauté them in a little olive oil and garlic.

Nonfat plain yogurt: A one-cup serving supplies 488 milligrams of calcium (50 percent of a person's daily need), plus ample amounts of vitamins B_2, B_{12}, and B_6; magnesium, potassium, selenium, and zinc; and protein, all for under 150 calories. If cultured with lactobacillus acidophilus, yogurt also might reduce the risk for cancer, heart disease, and yeast infections. Go easy on the fruited brands, since their high sugar content might increase urinary loss of magnesium. Instead, mix commercial or homemade nonfat yogurt with all-fruit jam, fresh fruit, or flavoring extracts such as almond or vanilla for a nutritional punch without the fat or sugar.

Wheat germ: The heart of the wheat kernel is a goldmine of nutrition. Adding one-quarter cup of wheat germ to hot cereal, meatloaf, or pancake batter supplies a whopping dose of all the B vitamins, most of the trace minerals (such as zinc, selenium, chromium, manganese, and iron), magnesium, and fiber, and 90 percent of the daily requirement for vitamin E. Sprinkle wheat germ on cold cereal, cook it into hot cereal, and mix into pancake, cookie, or biscuit batters. Blend it into meatloaf, meatballs, or hamburger patties before cooking.

Onions and garlic: It's not just folklore—a wealth of research shows that garlic and onions are packed with sulfur-containing compounds, including alliin and allicin, that help prevent numerous diseases, including infections, heart disease, and cancer. Garlic also may stimulate the immune system, thus strengthening the body's natural defense against a host of other ills.

Whole-grain bread: They both tally 70 calories, but compared to white bread, 100-percent whole-wheat bread contains three times as much fiber, magnesium, vitamin B_6, vitamin E, and chromium, and lots more zinc, copper, manganese, folic acid, and pantothenic acid (a B vitamin).

Tofu: Ounce for ounce, tofu has over three times more iron, magnesium, manganese, and folic acid than does red meat, yet remains an excellent source of the

B vitamins, magnesium, zinc, and protein typically supplied by meat, and for about half the fat and calories. An added benefit of tofu is that, like other soybean-made products, it contains an arsenal of anti-breast-cancer compounds called phytoestrogens. Blend it with fat-free sour cream for dips, crumble it into cottage or ricotta cheese in recipes, mix it with eggs before scrambling, toss it into salads, add chunks of it to casseroles and stir fry, or toss cubes into soup and stews.

Pacific salmon: In addition to being delicious, a 4-ounce salmon steak provides up to 2.2 grams of a eicosapentaenoic acid (EPA), a type of fish oil known to lower blood cholesterol and triglyceride and possibly raise HDL (the "good" cholesterol) levels. Eaten canned with the bones, salmon is also an excellent source of calcium (3 ounces contain more than 200 milligrams).

Oatmeal: Oatmeal is an excellent source of oat fiber (one cup supplies 24 percent of a person's daily fiber need), which helps lower blood cholesterol and the risk for heart disease. Cooked in low-fat milk and topped with wheat germ, this hot cereal is an excellent way to fuel the morning and help fend off carb cravings later in the day.

Strawberries: This juicy, delicious fruit is also an excellent source of folic acid, B vitamins, and iron. Surprisingly, cup for cup, strawberries have more vitamin C and fiber than do oranges. They also contain the phytochemical ellagic acid, which scavenges cancer-causing substances. Add to fruit salads, use as a topping for fat-free cheesecakes, layer with other fruits to make a parfait, or just eat with your fingers!

Cinnamon-raisin bagel: This sweet-tasting bagel can curb sugar cravings midday and fuel your workouts by supplying up to 30 grams of carbohydrates. Top with a drizzle of honey, all-fruit jam, or a smear of peanut butter. Or, dunk in cinnamon-apple yogurt.

Orange juice: The classic source of vitamin C has an added nutritional punch: one cup also supplies 109mcg of folic acid, a B vitamin often sorely lacking in people's diets. Orange juice also is a source of limonene and bioflavonoids, phytochemicals that activate detoxifying enzymes in the body and possibly lower the risk for cancer.

Lentils: These legumes are a fat- and cholesterol-free alternative to red meat. One cup of cooked lentils supplies 2.5 milligrams of zinc, as well as ample amounts of calcium, iron, magnesium, folic acid and other B vitamins, fiber, protein, and complex carbohydrates, all for under 225 calories. Besides the proverbial lentil soup, cook a pot of lentils and store in the refrigerator to add to rice dishes, stews, salads, burritos, Indian dals, and chili.

Chocolate: Maybe it's the phenylethylamine (PEA) that produces love-like emotions, or the endorphin release that produces feelings of euphoria, or maybe it's just the melt-in-your-mouth taste and aroma. Whatever it is, chocolate is the number-one most craved food, and nothing else satisfies the craving. So work with, rather than against, chocolate cravings. Dip two cups of fresh fruit in ¼ cup low-fat chocolate syrup, eat chocolate with a meal (you're likely to eat less), or have a cup of low-fat, sugar-free hot chocolate.

Figs: If you're looking for something sweet and chewy, four dried figs is a healthy choice. For just under 200 calories, this snack provides 7 grams of fiber and more than 10 percent of your daily requirements for vitamin B_6, calcium, iron, magnesium, and potassium.

Kidney beans: One cup, sprinkled onto a salad, added to vegetable soup, mixed with couscous to make a meal, or rolled into a tortilla with cheese and salsa, supplies almost one-third of a premenopausal woman's daily need for iron, but only 219 calories and no fat! Beans also contain a wealth of other health-enhancing chemicals called phytochemicals, including saponins that lower blood cholesterol and phytosterols that reduce your risk for cancer.

Quinoa ("keen-wa"): This birdseed-shaped, mild-flavored grain far surpasses other grains in nutritional content. Ounce for ounce, quinoa contains 700 percent more iron than enriched white rice. It also is an excellent source of protein, calcium, and other minerals. Use as a substitute for rice in all casseroles, stuffed bell peppers, side dishes, or soups and stews, or as a hot breakfast cereal.

Brewer's yeast: Though not a typical inclusion in many people's daily fare, a quarter-cup of this nutritional yeast mixed into orange juice contains more zinc than two cups of green peas, five slices of white bread, or 21 cups of cabbage. It also contains more vitamin B_1 than 27 pounds of hamburger or 45 slices of vitamin B_1–enriched bread. Brewer's yeast is equally high in the other B vitamins, as well as being an excellent source of iron, calcium, and selenium. For that kind of nutritional punch, it might be worth getting used to the taste!

Bananas: This fruit is one of the few plants that is high in vitamin B$_6$, a nutrient essential for red blood cell formation, nerve function, energy metabolism, and the regulation of mood and sleep. A banana with a whole-wheat bagel and juice is an excellent after-workout way to restock glycogen stores and fuel your energy level.

Resources:
Organizations, Books, and Related Materials

AGING

Administration on Aging, 330 Independence Avenue, SW, Washington, D.C., 20201. (202) 619-0724.

Aging Network Services, 4400 East-West Highway, Bethesda, MD 20814. (301) 657-4329.

American Association of Retired Persons (AARP), 601 E Street, NW, Washington, D.C., 20049. (202) 434-2277.

National Alliance for Senior Citizens, 1744 Riggs Place, NW, 3rd Floor, Washington, D.C. 20009. (202) 986-0117.

National Association of Area Agencies on Aging, 11112 16th Street, NW, Washington, D.C. 20036. (202) 296-8130.

National Council of Senior Citizens, 8430 Colesville Road, Suite 1200, Silver Springs, MD 20910. (310) 578-8800.

National Council on Aging, 409 Third Street, SW, Suite 200, Washington, D.C. 20024. (800) 424-9046 or (202) 479-1200.

National Institutes of Health, National Institute on Aging, Information Center, P.O. Box 8057, Gaithersburg, MD 20898-8057. (800) 222-2225 (for information on publications) or (301) 496-1752 (for the Center).

Older Women's League (OWL), 666 11th Street, NW, Suite 700, Washington, D.C. 20001. (202) 783-6686.

ARTHRITIS

The Arthritis Foundation, 1314 Spring Street, Atlanta, GA 30309, or P.O. Box 19000, Atlanta, GA 30326. (800) 283-7800 or (404) 872-7100.

CANCER

American Cancer Society, Inc., National Headquarters, 1599 Clifton Road, NE, Atlanta, GA 30329-4251. (404) 320-3333. For local Cancer Society, call (800) 227-2345.

American Institute for Cancer Research, 1759 R Street, NW, Washington, D.C. 20009. (800) 843-8114.

National Cancer Institute, Cancer Information Service, Bldg. 31, Room 10A24, 9000 Rockville Pike, Bethesda, MD 20892. (800) 422-6237.

The Wellness Community, 2716 Ocean Park Boulevard, Suite 1040, Santa Monica, CA 90405. (310) 314-2555.

DIABETES

American Diabetes Association, 1660 Duke Street, Alexandria, VA 22314. (800) DIA-BETES.

EXERCISE

American College of Sports Medicine, P.O. Box 1440, Indianapolis, IN 46206. (317) 637-9200.

Evans, W., and Rosenberg, I.: *Biomarkers: The 10 Keys to Prolonging Vitality*. New York: Fireside Books, 1991.

President's Council on Physical Fitness and Sports, 701 Pennsylvania Avenue, NW, Room 250, Washington, D.C. 20004. (202) 272-3421.

Rippe, J.: *Fit over Forty*. New York: William Morrow, 1996.

HEALTH AND MEDICINE

American Holistic Medical Association, 4101 Lake Boone Trail, Suite 201, Raleigh, NC 27607. (919) 787-5181.

Center for Mind/Body Medicine, 5225 Connecticut Avenue, NW, Suite 414, Washington, D.C. 20015. (202) 966-7338.

National Institutes of Health, Office of Alternative Medicine (OAM) Clearinghouse, P.O. Box 8218, Silver Springs, MD 20907-8218. (800) 531-1794.

National Women's Health Network, 514 10th Street, NW, Suite 400, Washington, D.C. 20004. (202) 347-1140.

National Women's Health Resource Center, 2425 L Street, NW, 3rd Floor, Washington, D.C. 20037. (202) 293-6045.

HEARING

Better Hearing Institute, P.O. Box 1840, Washington, D.C. 20013. (800) EARWELL.

International Hearing Society, 20361 Middlebelt Road, Livonia, MI 48152. (810) 478-2610.

HEART DISEASE AND HYPERTENSION

American Association of Cardiovascular and Pulmonary Rehabilitation, 7611 Elmwood Avenue, Suite 201, Middleton, WI 53562. (608) 831-6989.

American Heart Association, 7272 Greenville Avenue, Dallas, TX 75231-4596. (214) 373-6300. For local Heart Association, call (800) AHA-USA1. Also provides a free booklet on "How To Choose a Nutrition Counselor."

National Heart, Lung, and Blood Institute Information Center, P.O. Box 30105, Bethesda, MD 20824-0105. (301) 251-1222.

National Hypertension Association, 324 East 30th Street, New York, NY 10016. (212) 889-3557.

MENOPAUSE

North American Menopause Society, P.O. Box 94527, Cleveland, Ohio 44101-4527. (216) 844-8748.

MENTAL HEALTH

Alzheimer's Association, 919 North Michigan, Chicago, IL 60611. (800) 272-3900.

American Psychological Association, 750 First Street, NE, Washington, D.C. 20002. (202) 336-5500.

National Depressive and Manic-Depressive Association, 730 North Franklin, Chicago, IL 60610. (800) 826-3632.

National Foundation for Depressive Illness, Inc., P.O. Box 2257, New York, NY 10116. (800) 248-4344.

National Institute on Aging's Alzheimer's Disease Education and Referral Center, P.O. Box 8250, Silver Springs, MD 20907-8250. (800) 438-4380.

National Institute of Neurological Disorders and Stroke, 31 Center Drive, MSC 2540, Bethesda, MD 20892-2540. (800) 352-9424.

NUTRITION AND DIET

The American Dietetic Association, 216 West Jackson Boulevard, Suite 800, Chicago, IL 60606. (301) 899-0040. Nutrition hotline (800) 366-1655, 10 A.M. to 5 P.M. EST, Monday through Friday.

Dietary Guidelines for Americans, Consumer Information Center, Pueblo, CO 81009. (Free with SASE.)

The Food Guide Pyramid, Superintendent of Documents, Consumer Information Center, Department 150-Y, Pueblo, CO 81009. (Price: $1.00 check or money order.)

The Food Guide Pyramid: Beyond the Basic 4. Food Marketing Institute, 800 Connecticut Avenue, NW, Washington, D.C. 20006. (Price: $0.50 with SASE.)

OSTEOPOROSIS

National Osteoporosis Foundation, 1150 17th Street, NW, Suite 500, Washington, D.C. 20036-4603. (202) 223-2226. For listings of your nearest bone density testing sites, call (800) 464-6700.

Osteoporosis and Related Bone Diseases National Resource Center, 1150 17th Street, NW, Suite 500, Washington, D.C. 20036-4603. (800) 624-BONE or (202) 223-0344.

OTHER DISORDERS AND PROBLEMS

National Kidney and Urologic Diseases Information Clearinghouse, 3 Information Way, Bethesda, MD 20892-3560. (301) 654-4415.

National Organization for Rare Disorders, 100 Route 37, P.O. Box 8923, New Fairfield, CT 06812-8923. (800) 999-NORD.

SKIN

American Academy of Dermatology, 930 N. Meacham Road, P.O. Box 4014, Schaumberg, IL 60168-4014. (847) 330-0230.

The Skin Cancer Foundation, 245 Fifth Avenue, Suite 1403, New York, NY 10016. (800) SKIN-490 or (212) 725-5176.

SLEEP DISORDERS

American Sleep Disorders Association, 1610 14th Street, NW, Rochester, MN 55901. (507) 287-6006.

STRESS

American Institute of Stress, 124 Park Avenue, Yonkers, NY 10703. (800) 24-RELAX.

Anxiety Disorders Association of America, Dept. B, P.O. Box 96505, Washington, D.C. 20077-7140. (301) 231-9350.

VISION

American Academy of Ophthalmology, P.O. Box 7424, San Francisco, CA 94120-7424. (800) 684-9788 or (415) 561-8500.

National Eye Institute, Information Office, Building 31, Room 6A32, 31 Center Drive MSC 2510, Bethesda, MD 20892-2510. (301) 496-5248.

VITALITY

Benson, H.: *Timeless Healing: The Power and Biology of Belief.* New York: Scribner, 1996.

Burns, D.: *Feeling Good: The New Mood Therapy.* New York: William Morrow, 1990.

Jeffers, S.: *Feel the Fear and Do it Anyway.* New York: Fawcett Columbine, 1987.

Maslow, A.: *Toward a Psychology of Being,* 2nd edition. New York: D. Van Nostrand, 1962.

Moore, T.: *The Re-Enchantment of Everyday Life.* New York: HarperCollins, 1996.

Omega Institute, 260 Lake Drive, Rhinebeck, NY 12572. (914) 266-4444.

Seligman, M.: *Learned Optimism.* New York: Pocket Books, 1992.

Spiritual Eldering Institute, 7318 Germantown Avenue, Philadelphia, PA 19919. (215) 248-9308.

Selected References

CHAPTER 1

Akisaka M, Asato L, Chan Y, et al.: Energy and nutrient intakes of Okinawan centenarians. *J Nutr Sc V* 1996;42:241–248.

Burchfield S, Holmes T, Harrington R: Personality differences between sick and rarely sick individuals. *Social Sci M* 1981;15E:145–148.

Butler R: Quality of life: Can it be an endpoint? How can it be measured? *Am J Clin N* 1992;55:1267S–1270S.

Casper R: Nutrition and its relationship to aging. *Exp Geront* 1995;30:299–314.

Glaser J, Brind J, Vogelman J, et al.: Elevated serum DHEA levels in practitioners of the Transcendental Meditation (TM) and TM-Sidhi programs. *J Behav Med* 1992;15:327.

Harman D: Aging and disease: Extending functional lifespan. *Ann NY Acad* 1996;786: 321–336.

Harman D: Role of antioxidant nutrients in aging: Overview. *Age* 1995;18:51–62.

Johnson M, Brown M, Poon L, et al.: Nutritional patterns of centenarians. *Int J Aging* 1992;34:57–76.

Katz S, Branch L, Brannon M, et al.: Active life expectancy. *N Eng J Med* 1983;309: 1218–1224.

Manadhar M: Functional ability and nutritional status of free-living elderly people. *P Nutr Soc* 1995;54:677–691.

Murray M, Murray A: Diet and cardiovascular disease in centenarians of Hunza. *Arterioscle* 1984;4:546a.

CHAPTER 2

Barnett Y, King C: An investigation of antioxidant status, DNA repair capacity and mutation as a function of age in humans. *Mut R-DNAGI* 1995;338:115–128.

Bernardis L, Davis P: Aging and the hypothalamus: Research perspectives. *Physl Behav* 1996;59:523–536.

Cals M, Bories P, Devanlay M, et al.: Extensive laboratory assessment of nutritional status in fit, health-conscious, elderly people living in the Paris area. *J Am Col N* 1994;13:646–657.

Campbell W: Dietary protein requirements of older people: Is the RDA adequate? *Nutr Today* 1996;31:192–196.

Ebeling P, Sandgren M, DiMagno E, et al.: Evidence of an age-related decrease in intestinal responsiveness to vitamin D: Relationship between serum 1,25-dihydroxyvitamin D3 and intestinal vitamin D receptor concentrations in normal women. *J Clin End* 1992;75:176–182.

Fishman P: Detecting malnutrition's warning signs with simple screening tools. *Geriatrics* 1994;49:39–45.

Greenstein R, Ybanez M, Zhang R, et al. Is aging preprogrammed? Observations from the brain/gut axis. *Mech Age D* 1991;61:113–121.

Hanger H, Sainsbury R, Gilchrist N, et al.: A community study of vitamin B_{12} and folate levels in the elderly. *J Am Ger So* 1991;39:1155–1159.

Lipofuscin, the age pigment. *Nutr Rev* 1993;51:205–212.

Lopez-Torres L, Perez-Campo R, Rojas C, et al.: Maximum life span in vertebrates. *Mech Age D* 1993;70:177–199.

Monti D, Troiano L, Tropea F, et al.: Apoptosis—programmed cell death: A role in the aging process? *Am J Clin N* 1992;55:1208S–1214S.

Need A, Morris H, Horowitz M, et al.: Effects of skin thickness, age, body fat, and sunlight on serum 25-hydroxyvitamin D. *Am J Clin N* 1993;58:882–885.

Olivieri O, Stanzial A, Girelli D, et al.: Selenium status, fatty acids, vitamins A and E, and aging: The Nove Study. *Am J Clin N* 1994;60:510–517.

Oreopoulos D, Lindeman R, VanderJagt D, et al.: Renal excretion of ascorbic acid: Effect of age and sex. *J Am Col N* 1993;12:537–542.

Reid D, Conrad S, Hendricks S: Tracking nutrition trends, 1989–1994: An update on Canadians' attitudes, knowledge and reported actions. *Can J Publ* 1996;87:113–118.

Rosenberg I: Sarcopenia: Origins and clinical relevance. *J Nutr* 1997;127:S990–S991.

Russell R, Suter P: Vitamin requirements of elderly people. An update. *Am J Clin N* 1993;58:4–14.

Szweda L: Age-related increase in liver retinyl palmitate. *J Biochem* 1994;269:8712–8715.

Tucker D, Penland J, Sandstead H, et al.: Nutrition status and brain function in aging. *Am J Clin N* 1990;52:93–102.

Varela-Moreiras G, Perez-Olleros L, Garcia-Cuervas M, et al.: Effects of aging on folate metabolism in rats fed a long-term folate deficient diet. *Int J Vit N* 1994;64:294–299.

Vellas B, Balas D, Albarede J: Effects of aging process on digestive functions. *Compreh Ther* 1991;17:46–52.

Wood R, Suter P, Russell R: Mineral requirements of elderly people. *Am J Clin N* 1995; 62:493–505.

CHAPTER 3

Butler R: Quality of life: Can it be an endpoint? How can it be measured? *Am J Clin N* 1992;55:1267S–1270S.

Dahlof C, Dimenas E: Migraine patients experience poorer subjective well-being/quality of life even between attacks. *Cephalalgia* 1995;15:31–36.

Donaldson S, Blanchard A: The seven health practices, well-being, and performance at work: Evidence for the value of reaching small and underserved worksites. *Prev Med* 1995;24:270–277.

Fisher B: Successful aging, life satisfaction, and generativity in later years. *Int J Aging* 1995;41:239–250.

Lee K, Lentz M, Taylor D, et al.: Fatigue as a response to environmental demands in women's lives. *Image J Nurs Sch* 1994;26:149–154.

Ravaja N, Keltikangas-Jarvinen L: Temperament and metabolic syndrome precursors in children: A three-year follow-up. *Prev Med* 1995;24:518–527.

Rose G, Sivik T, Delimar N: Gender, psychological well-being and somatic cardiovascular risk factors. *Integ Ph Be* 1994;29:423–430.

Sarkisian C, Lachs M: Failure to thrive in older adults. *Ann Int Med* 1996;124:1072–1078.

Tsana K, Garraway W: Impact of benign prostatic hyperplasia on general well-being in men. *Prostate* 1993;23:1–7.

Vallerand R, O'Connor B, Hamel M: Motivation in later life: Theory and assessment. *Int J Aging* 1995;41:221–238.

van Tulder M, Aaronson N, Bruning P: The quality of life of long-term survivors of Hodgkin's disease. *Ann Oncol* 1994;5:152–158.

CHAPTER 4

Ames B, Shigenaga M, Hagen T: Oxidants, antioxidants, and the degenerative diseases of aging. *P NAS US* 1993;90:7915–7922.

Azhar S, Cao L, Reaven E: Alteration of the adrenal antioxidant defense system during aging in rats. *J Clin Inv* 1995;96:1414–1424.

Barnett Y, King C: An investigation of antioxidant status, DNA repair capacity and mutation as a function of age in humans. *Mut R-DNAGI* 1995;338:115–128.

Battisti C, Dotti M, Manneschi L, et al.: Increase of serum levels of vitamin E during human aging: Is it a protective factor against death? *Arch Ger G* 1994; Suppl 4:13–18.

Bergamini E, Gori Z: Towards an understanding of the anti-aging mechanism of dietary restriction: A signal transduction theory of aging. *Aging* 1995;7:473–475.

Campbell D, Bunker V, Thomas A, et al.: Selenium and vitamin E status of healthy and institutionalized elderly subjects: Analysis of plasma, erythrocytes and platelets. *Br J Nutr* 1989;62:221–227.

D'Costa A, Ingram R, Lenham J, et al.: The regulation and mechanisms of action of growth hormone and insulin-like growth factor 1 during normal ageing. *J Repr Fert* 1993;46:87–98.

Frei B: Reactive oxygen species and antioxidant vitamins: Mechanisms of action. *Am J Med* 1994;97;suppl 3A:5S–13S.

Gadkari J, Joshi V: Effect of ingestion of raw garlic on serum cholesterol level, clotting time and fibrinolytic activity in normal subjects. *J Postgrad Med* 1991;37:128–131.

Greenberg E, Baron J, Karagas M, et al.: Mortality associated with low plasma concentration of beta carotene and the effect of oral supplementation. *J Am Med A* 1996; 275:699–703.

Hallfrisch J, Muller D, Singh V: Vitamin A and E intakes and plasma concentrations of retinol, beta carotene, and alpha tocopherol in men and women of the Baltimore Longitudinal Study of Aging. *Am J Clin N* 1994;60:176–182.

Harman D: Aging: Prospects for further increases in the functional lifespan. *Age* 1994; 17:119–146.

Harman D: Role of antioxidant nutrients in aging: Overview. *Age* 1995;18:51–62.

Hass B, Lewis S, Duffy P, et al.: Dietary restriction in humans: Report on the Little Rock Conference on the value, feasibility, and parameters of a proposed study. *Mech Age D* 1996;91:79–94.

Hertog M: Epidemiological evidence on potential health properties of flavonoids. *P Nutr Soc* 1996;55:385–397.

Ishikawa T, Suzukamo M, Ito T, et al.: Effect of tea flavonoid supplementation on the susceptibility of low-density lipoprotein to oxidative modification. *Am J Clin N* 1997; 66:261–266.

Jacques P, Halpner A, Blumberg J: Influence of combined antioxidant nutrient intakes on their plasma concentrations in an elderly population. *Am J Clin N* 1995;62:1228–1233.

Junyao L, Bing L, Blot W, et al.: Preliminary report on the results of nutrition prevention trials of cancer and other common diseases among residents in Linxian, China. *Chin Med J* 1995;108:780.

Kakkar R, Bains J, Sharma S: Effect of vitamin E on life span, malondialdehyde content and antioxidant enzymes in aging Zaprionus paravittiger. *Gerontology* 1996;42:312–321.

Kirkwood T: Comparative life spans of species: Why do species have the life spans they do? *Am J Clin N* 1992;55:1191S–1195S.

Knekt P, Jarvinen R, Reunanen A, et al.: Flavonoid intake and coronary mortality in Finland: A cohort study. *Br Med J* 1996;312:478.

Knekt P, Jarvinen R, Seppanen R. et al.: Dietary flavonoids and the risk of lung cancer and other malignant neoplasms. *Am J Epidem* 1997;146:223–230.

Lau B, Tadi P, Tosk J: Allium sativum (garlic) and cancer prevention. *Nutr Res* 1990;10:937–948.

Lawson L, Ransom D, Hughes B: Inhibition of whole blood platelet-aggregation by compounds in garlic clove extracts and commercial garlic products. *Thromb Res* 1992; 65:141–156.

Liu J, Lin R, Milnr J: Inhibition of 7,12-dimethylbenzaanthracene-induced mammary tumors and DNA adducts by garlic powder. *Carcinogene* 1992;13:1847–1851.

Losonczy K, Harris T, Havlik R: Vitamin E and vitamin C supplement use and risk of all-cause and coronary heart disease mortality in older persons: The Established Populations for Epidemiologic Studies of the Elderly. *Am J Clin N* 1996;64:190–196.

Lynn W, Wallwork J: Does food restriction retard aging by reducing metabolic rate? *J Nutr* 1992;122:1917–1918.

Masoro E: Dietary restriction and aging. *J Am Ger So* 1993;41:994–999.

Masoro E: McCay's hypothesis: Undernutrition and longevity. *P Nutr Soc* 1995;54:657–664.

Mezzetti A, Lapenna D, Romano F, et al.: Systemic oxidative stress and its relationship with age and illness. *J Am Ger So* 1996;44:823–827.

Mobarhan S, Hupert J, Friedman H: Effects of aging on beta carotene and vitamin A status. *Age* 1991;14:13–16.

Nakagami T, Nanaumi-Tamura N, Toyomura K, et al.: Dietary flavonoids as potential natural biological response modifiers affecting the autoimmune system. *J Food Sci* 1995;60:653–656.

Olivieri O, Stanzial A, Girelli D, et al.: Selenium status, fatty acids, vitamins A and E, and aging: The Nove Study. *Am J Clin N* 1994;60:510–517.

Pandey D, Shekelle R, Selwyn B, et al.: Dietary vitamin C and beta carotene and risk of death in middle-aged men: The Western Electric Study. *Am J Epidem* 1995;142: 1269–1278.

Peretz A, Neve J, Desmedt J, et al.: Lymphocyte response is enhanced by supplementation of elderly subjects with selenium-enriched yeast. *Am J Clin N* 1991;53:1323–1328.

Peters E, Seidell J, Menotti A, et al.: Changes in body weight in relation to mortality in 6441 European middle-aged men: The Seven Countries Study. *Int J Obes* 1995; 19:862–868.

Pinto J, Qiao C, Xing J, et al.: Effects of garlic thioallyl derivatives on growth, glutathione concentration, and polyamine formation of human prostate carcinoma cells in culture. *Am J Clin N* 1997;66:398–405.

Poulin J, Cover C, Gustafson M, et al.: Vitamin E prevents oxidative modification of brain and lymphocyte band 3 proteins during aging. *P NAS US* 1996;93:5600–5603.

Pryor W: Measurement of oxidative stress status in humans. *Cancer Epidem: Biomarkers Prevention* 1993;2:289–292.

Rao K, Ayyagari S, Raji N, et al.: Undernutrition and aging: Effects on DNA repair in human peripheral lymphocytes. *Current Sci* 1996;71:464–469.

Schmuck A, Fuller C, Devaraj S, et al.: Effect of aging on susceptibility of low density lipoproteins to oxidation. *Clin Chem* 1995;41:1628–1632.

Snowdon D, Gross M, Butler S: Antioxidants and reduced functional capacity in the elderly: Findings from the Nun Study. *J Geront S* 1996;51:M10–M16.

Sonntag W, Xu X, Ingram R, et al.: Moderate caloric restriction alters the subcellular distribution of somatostatin mRNA and increases growth hormone pulse amplitude in aged animals. *Neuroendocr* 1995;61:601–608.

Starkere-Reed P: Aging. *J Nutr* 1996;126:2593–2594.

Svendsen L, Rattan S, Clark B: Testing garlic for possible anti-aging effects on long-term growth characteristics, morphology, and macromolecular synthesis of human fibroblasts in culture. *J Ethnophar* 1994;43:125–133.

Wachsman J: The beneficial effects of dietary restriction: Reduced oxidative damage and enhanced apoptosis. *Mut R-DNAGI* 1996;350:25–34.

Weber N, Andersen D, North J, et al.: In vitro virucidal effects of allium sativum (garlic) extract and compounds. *Planta Med* 1992;58:417–423.

Weindruch R: Immunogerontologic outcomes of dietary restriction started in adulthood. *Nutr Rev* 1995;53:S66–S71.

Weisburger J, Hara Y, Dolan L, et al.: Tea polyphenols as inhibitors of mutagenicity of major classes of carcinogens. *Mut Res-G T* 1997;371:57–63.

Yu B: Aging and oxidative stress: Modulation by dietary restriction. *Free Rad B* 1996; 21:651–668.

CHAPTER 5

Araneo B, Dowell T, Woods M, et al.: DHEAS as an effective vaccine adjuvant in elderly humans: Proof of principal studies. *Ann NY Acad* 1995;774:232–248.

Arvat E, Gianotti L, Grottoli S, et al.: Arginine and growth hormone-releasing hormone restored the blunted growth hormone-releasing activity of hexarelin in elderly subjects. *J Clin End* 1994;79:1440–1443.

Barrett-Connor E, Khaw K, Yen S: A prospective study of dehydroepiandrosterone sulfate, mortality, and cardiovascular disease. *N Eng J Med* 1986;315:1519–1524.

Baulieu E: Studies on dehydroepiandrosterone (DHEA) and its sulphate during aging. *CR Ac S III* 1995;318:7–11.

Beneking M, Oellerich M, Binder L, et al.: Inhibition of mitochondrial carnitine acyl-carnitine translocase by hypoglycaemia-inducing substances. *J Clin Chem* 1990;28: 323–327.

Bonello R, Marcus R, Bloch D, et al.: Effects of growth hormone and estrogen on T lymphocytes in older women. *J Am Ger So* 1996;44:1038–1042.

Boonen S, Aerssens J, Dequeker J: Age-related endocrine deficiencies and fractures of the proximal femur: Implications of growth hormone deficiency in the elderly. *J Endocr* 1996;149:7–12.

Borst S, Millard W, Lowenthal D: Growth hormone, exercise, and aging: The future of therapy for the frail elderly. *J Am Ger So* 1994;42:528–535.

Braun B, Clarkson P, Freedson P, et al.: Effects of coenzyme Q10 supplementation on exercise performance, VO_2max, and lipid peroxidation in trained cyclists. *Int J Sp Nu* 1991;1:353–365.

Caroleo M, Doria G, Nistico G: Melatonin restores immunodepression in aged and cyclophosphamide-treated mice. *Ann NY Acad* 1994;719:343–352.

Cartee G, Bohn E, Gibson B, et al.: Growth hormone supplementation increases skeletal muscle mass of old male Fischer 344/brown Norway rats. *J Gerontol* 1996;51:B214–B219.

Casson P, Faquin L, Stentz F, et al.: Replacement of dehydroepiandrosterone enhances T-lymphocyte insulin binding in postmenopausal women. *Fert Steril* 1995;63:1027–1031.

Corpas E, Harman S, Blackman M: Human growth hormone and human aging. *Endocr Rev* 1993;14:20–239.

Costell M, Grisolia S: Effect of carnitine feeding on the levels of heart and skeletal muscle carnitine of elderly mice. *FEBS Letter* 1993;315:43–46.

DeAngelis C, Scarfo C, Falcinelli M, et al.: Acetyl-L-carnitine prevents age-dependent structural alterations in rat peripheral nerves and promotes regeneration following sciatic nerve injury in young and senescent rats. *Exp Neurol* 1994;128:103–114.

Djakoure C, Guibourdenche J, Porquet D, et al.: Vitamin A and retinoic acid stimulate within minutes camp release and growth hormone secretion in human pituitary cells. *J Clin End* 1996;81:3123–3126.

Ebeling P, Kolvisto V: Physiological importance of dehydroepiandrosterone. *Lancet* 1994;343:1479–1481.

Esposti D, Mariani M, Dermartini G, et al.: Modulation of melatonin secretion by acetyl-L-carnitine in adult and old rats. *J Pineal R* 1994;17:132–136.

Fischer M, Adkins W, Scaman P, et al.: Improved selenium, carnitine and taurine status in an enterally fed population. *J Parent En* 1990;14:270–274.

Garcia-Patterson A, Puig-Domingo M, Webb S: Thirty years of human pineal research: Do we know its clinical relevance? *J Pineal R* 1996;20:1–6.

Gelato M: Aging and immune function: A possible role for growth hormone. *Hormone Res* 1996;45:46–49.

Glaser J, Brind J, Vogelman J, et al.: Elevated serum dehydroepiandrosterone sulfate levels in practitioners of the Transcendental Meditation (TM) and TM-Sidhi programs. *J Behav Med* 1992;15:327.

Hartman M, Pezzoli S, Hellmann P, et al.: Pulsatile growth hormone secretion in older persons is enhanced by fasting without relationship to sleep stages. *J Clin End* 1996; 81:2694–2701.

Heinonen O: Carnitine and physical exercise. *Sport Med* 1996;22:109–132.

Ho K, Hoffman D: Aging and growth hormone. *Hormone Res* 1993;40:80–86.

Holmes S, Shalet S: Factors influencing the desire for long-term growth hormone replacement in adults. *Clin Endocr* 1995;43:151–157.

Hornsby P: Biosynthesis of DHEAS by the human adrenal cortex and its age-related decline. *Ann NY Acad* 1995;774:29–46.

Imagawa M, Naruse S, Tsuji S, et al.: Coenzyme Q10, iron, and vitamin B_6 in genetically-confirmed Alzheimer's disease. *Lancet* 1992;340:671.

Ishihara F, Komatsu M, Yamada T, et al.: Role of dehydroepiandrosterone and dehydroepiandrosterone sulfate for the maintenance of axillary hair in women. *Hormone Met* 1993;25:34.

Jorgensen J, Christiansen J: Growth hormone therapy: Brave new senescence, GH in adults. *Lancet* 1993;341:1247–1248.

Majewska M: Neuronal actions of dehydroepiandrosterone. Possible roles in brain development, aging, memory, and affect. *Ann NY Acad* 1995;774:111–120.

McMillin J, Taffet G, Taegtmeyer H, et al.: Mitochondrial metabolism and substrate competition in the aging Fischer rat heart. *Cardio Res* 1993;27:2222–2228.

Miklos S: Dehydroepiandrosterone sulphate in the diagnosis of osteoporosis. *Acta Biomed At* 1995;66:139–146.

Molina A, Munoz A, Uberos J, et al.: Pineal functioning (melatonin levels) in healthy children of different ages: An update and the value of pineal gland study in pediatrics. *An Esp Pediatr* 1996;45:33–44.

Morales A, Nolan J, Nelson J, et al.: Effects of replacement dose of dehydroepiandrosterone in men and women of advancing age. *J Clin End* 1994;78:1360–1367.

Oaknin-Bendahan S, Anis Y, Nir I, et al.: Effects of long-term administration of melatonin and a putative antagonist on the aging rat. *Neuroreport* 1995;6:785–788.

Odiet J, Boerrigter M, Wei J: Carnitine palmitoyl transferase-I activity in the aging mouse heart. *Mech Age D* 1995;79:127–136.

Orentreich N, Matias J, DeFelice A, et al.: Low methionine ingestion by rats extends life span. *J Nutr* 1993;123:269–274.

Papadakis M, Grady D, Black D, et al.: Growth hormone replacement in healthy older men improves body composition but not functional ability. *Ann Int Med* 1996;124:708–716.

Paradies G, Ruggiero F, Petrosillo G, et al.: Effect of aging and acetyl-L-carnitine on the activity of cytochrome oxidase and adenine nucleotide translocase in rat heart mitochondria. *FEBS Letter* 1994;350:213–215.

Pierpaoli W, Regelson W: Pineal control of aging: Effect of melatonin and pineal grafting on aging mice. *P NAS US* 1994;91:787–791.

Ravaglia G, Forti P, Maioli F, et al.: The relationship of dehydroepiandrosterone sulfate (DHEAS) to endocrine-metabolic parameters and functional status in the oldest-old. Results from an Italian study on healthy free-living over-ninety-year-olds. *J Clin End* 1996;81:1173–1178.

Rebouche C: Carnitine function and requirements during the life cycle. *FASEB J* 1992;6:3379–3386.

Reiter R: The pineal gland and melatonin in relation to aging: A summary of the theories and of the data. *Exp Geront* 1995;30:199–212.

Reiter R, Melchiorri D, Sewerynek E, et al.: A review of the evidence supporting melatonin's role as an antioxidant. *J Pineal R* 1995;18:1–11.

Reiter R, Pablos M, Agapito T, et al.: Melatonin in the context of the free radical theory of aging. *Ann NY Acad* 1996;786:362–378.

Riedel M, Brabant G, Rieger K, et al.: Growth hormone therapy in adults: Rationales, results, and perspectives. *Exp Clin En* 1994;102:273–283.

Rosen T, Eden S, Larson G, et al.: Cardiovascular risk factors in adult patients with growth hormone deficiency. *Acta Endocr* 1993;129:195–200.

Rosen T, Hansson T, Granhed H, et al.: Reduced bone mineral content in adult patients with growth hormone deficiency. *Acta Endocr* 1993;129:201–206.

Rudman D, Feller A, Nagraj H, et al.: Effects of human growth hormone in men over 60 years old. *N Eng J Med* 1990;323:1–6.

Salvini S, Stampfer M, Barbieri R, et al.: Effects of age, smoking, and vitamins on plasma DHEAS levels: A cross-sectional study in men. *J Clin End* 1992;74:139–143.

Schneider-Rivas S, Rivas-Arancibia S, Vazquez-Pereyra F, et al.: Modulation of long-term memory and extinction responses induced by growth hormone (GH) and growth hormone releasing hormone (GHRH) in rats. *Life Sci* 1995;56:PL433–PL441.

Spagnoli L, Orlandi A, Marino B, et al.: Propionyl-L-carnitine prevents the progression of atherosclerotic lesions in aged hyperlipemic rabbits. *Atheroscler* 1995;114:29–44.

Swenson C, Gottesman S, Belsito D, et al.: Relationship between humoral immunoaugmenting properties of DHEAS and IgD-receptor expression in young and aged mice. *Ann NY Acad* 1995;774:249–258.

Taaffe D, Pruitt L, Reim J, et al.: Effect of recombinant human growth hormone on the muscle strength response to resistance exercise in elderly men. *J Clin End* 1994;79:1361–1366.

Toogood A, Adams J, O'Neill P, et al.: Body composition in growth hormone deficient adults over the age of 60 years. *Clin Endocr* 1996;45:399–405.

Toogood A, O'Neill P, Shalet S: Beyond the somatopause: Growth hormone deficiency in adults over the age of 60 years. *J Clin End* 1996;81:460–465.

Vermeulen A: Dehydroepiandrosterone sulfate and aging. *Ann NY Acad* 1995;774:121–127.

Walker R, Ness G, Zhao Z, et al.: Effects of stimulated growth hormone secretion on age-related changes in plasma cholesterol and hepatic low density lipoprotein messenger RNA concentrations. *Mech Age D* 1994;75:215–226.

Wawrzenczyk A, Nalecz K, Nalecz M: Effect of externally added carnitine on the synthesis of acetylcholine in rat cerebral cortex cells. *Neurochem I* 1995;26:635–641.

Weber C, Jakobsen T, Mortensen S, et al.: Antioxidative effect of dietary coenzyme Q10 in human blood plasma. *Int J Vit N* 1994;64:311–315.

Weksler M: Immune senescence and adrenal steroids: Immune dysregulation and the action of dehydroepiandrosterone (DHEA) in old animals. *Eur J Cl Ph* 1993;45(suppl 1):S21–S23.

Welle S, Thornton C, Statt M, et al.: Growth hormone increases muscle mass and strength but does not rejuvenate myofibrillar protein synthesis in healthy subjects over 60 years old. *J Clin End* 1996;81:3239–3243.

Yarasheski K, Zachwieja J: Growth hormone therapy for the elderly: The fountain of youth proves toxic. *J Am Med A* 1993;270:1694.

Yarasheski K, Zachwieja J, Campbell J, et al.: Effect of growth hormone and resistance exercise on muscle growth and strength in older men. *Am J Physl* 1995;268:E268–E276.

Yen S, Morales A, Khorram O: Replacement of DHEA in aging men and women: Potential remedial effects. *Ann NY Acad* 1995;774:128–142.

CHAPTER 6

Ascherio A, Hennekens C, Buring J, et al.: Trans-fatty acids intake and risk of myocardial infarction. *Circulation* 1994;89:94–101.

Enig M, Atal S, Keeney M, et al.: Isomeric trans fatty acids in the U.S. diet. *J Am Col N* 1990;9:471–486.

Grover S, Gray-Donald K, Joseph L, et al.: Life expectancy following dietary modification or smoking cessation. *Arch In Med* 1994;154:1697–1704.

Hunter J, Applewhite T: Reassessment of trans fatty acid availability in the US diet. *Am J Clin N* 1991;54:363–369.

Judd J, Clevidence B, Muesing R, et al.: Dietary trans fatty acids: Effects on plasma lipids and lipoproteins of healthy men and women. *Am J Clin N* 1994;59:861–868.

Kromhout D, Menotti A, Bloemberg B, et al.: Dietary saturated and trans fatty acids and cholesterol and 25-year mortality from coronary heart disease: The 7 countries study. *Prev Med* 1995;24:308–315.

Lizard G, Deckert V, Dubrez L, et al.: Induction of apoptosis in endothelial cells treated with cholesterol oxides. *Am J Path* 1996;148:1625–1638.

Margetts B, Beilin L, Vandongen R, et al.: Vegetarian diet in mild hypertension: A randomized controlled trial. *Br Med J* 1986;293:1468–1471.

Pronczuk A, Kipervarg Y, Hayes C: Vegetarians have higher plasma alpha-tocopherol relative to cholesterol than do nonvegetarians. *J Am Col N* 1992;11:50–55.

Snowdon D, Phillips R, Fraser G: Meat consumption and fatal ischemic heart disease. *Prev Med* 1984;13:490–500.

Stender S, Dyerberg J, Holmer G, et al.: The influence of trans fatty acids on health: A report from the Danish Nutrition Council. *Clin Sci* 1995;88:375–392.

Summary of the second report of the National Cholesterol Education Program (NCEP) expert panel on detection, evaluation, and treatment of high blood cholesterol in adults (adult treatment panel ii). *J Am Med A* 1993;269:3015–3023.

Thorogood M, Mann J, Appleby P, et al.: Risk of death from cancer and ischemic heart disease in meat and non-meat eaters. *Br Med J* 1994;308:1667–1671.

Walter P: Effects of vegetarian diets on aging and longevity. *Nutr Rev* 1997;55:67S–68S.

Willett W, Ascherio A: Trans fatty acids: Are the effects only marginal? *Am J Pub He* 1994;84:722–724.

Willett W, Stampfer M, Manson J, et al.: Intake of trans fatty acids and risk of coronary heart disease among women. *Lancet* 1993;341:581–585.

CHAPTER 7

Ackroff K, Sclafani A: Sucrose-induced hyperphagia and obesity in rats fed a macro-nutrient self-selection diet. *Physl Behav* 1988;44:181–187.

Anderson R, Kozlovsky A, Moser P: Effects of diets high in simple sugars on urinary chromium excretion of humans. *Fed Proc* 1985;44:751.

Baghurst K, Baghurst P, Record S: Demographic and nutritional profiles of people consuming varying levels of added sugars. *Nutr Res* 1992;12:1455–1465.

Benton D, Haller J, Fordy J: Vitamin supplementation for 1 year improves mood. *Neuropsychob* 1995;32:98–105.

Birlouez-Aragon I, Girard F, Ravelontseheno L, et al.: Comparison of two levels of vitamin C supplementation on antioxidant vitamin status in elderly institutionalized subjects. *Int J Vit N* 1995;65:261–266.

Block G, Abrams B: Vitamin and mineral status of women of childbearing potential. *Ann NY Acad* 1993;678:244–254.

Dawson-Hughes B: Calcium and vitamin D nutritional needs of elderly women. *J Nutr* 1996;126:1165–1167.

Dekker J, Eggink L, Dewaart F, et al.: Use of vitamin and mineral supplements and mortality in Dutch elderly. *Am J Epidem* 1996;143;182 (Meeting abstract).

Dittus K, Hillers V, Beerman K: Benefits and barriers to fruit and vegetable intake: Relationship between attitudes and consumption. *J Nutr Educ* 1995;27:120–126.

Dragstead L, Strube M, Larsen J: Cancer protective factors in fruits and vegetables. *Am J Card* 1992;70:869–874.

Edelstein S, Barrett-Connor E, Wingard D, et al.: Increased meal frequency associated with decreased cholesterol concentrations; Rancho Bernardo, CA, 1984–1987. *Am J Clin N* 1992;55:664–669.

Frankel E, Kanner J, German J, et al.: Inhibition of oxidation of human low-density lipoprotein by phenolic substances in red wine. *Lancet* 1993;341:454–456.

Jenkins D, Wolever T, Vuksan V, et al.: Nibbling versus gorging: Metabolic advantages of increased meal frequency. *N Eng J Med* 1989;321:929–934.

Kant A, Block G, Schatzkin A, et al.: Association of fruit and vegetable intake with dietary fat intake. *Nutr Res* 1992;12:1441–1454.

Kant A, Schatzkin A, Harris T, et al.: Dietary diversity and subsequent mortality in the First National Health and Nutrition Examination Survey Epidemiologic Follow-Up Study. *Am J Clin N* 1993;57:434–440.

Katschinski B, Logan R, Edmond M, et al.: Duodenal ulcer and refined carbohydrate intake: A case-control study assessing dietary fibre and refined sugar intake. *Gut* 1990;31:993–996.

Kruis W, Forstmaier G, Scheurlen C, et al.: Effect of diets low and high in refined sugars on gut transit, bile acid metabolism, and bacterial fermentation. *Gut* 1991;32:367–371.

LaForge R, Greene G, Prochaska J: Psychosocial factors influencing low fruit and vegetable consumption. *J Behav Med* 1994;17:361–374.

Mangels A, Holden J, Beecher G, et al.: Carotenoid content of fruits and vegetables: An evaluation of analytic data. *J Am Diet A* 1993;93:284–296.

Massie H: Effect of dietary boron on the aging process. *Envir H Per* 1994;102:45–48.

McDonald R: Influence of dietary sucrose on biological aging? *Am J Clin N* 1995;62:284S–293S.

Meydani S, Meydani M, Rall L, et al.: Assessment of the safety of high-dose, short-term supplementation with vitamin E in healthy older adults. *Am J Clin N* 1994;60:704–709.

Mobarhan S: Micronutrient supplementation trials and the reduction of cancer and cerebrovascular incidence and mortality. *Nutr Rev* 1994;52:102–105.

Patterson B, Block G, Rosenberger W, et al.: Fruit and vegetables in the American diet: Data from the NHANES II survey. *Am J Pub He* 1990;80:1443–1449.

Pennington J, Young B, Wilson D, et al.: Mineral content of foods and total diets: The Selected Minerals in Foods Survey, 1982–1984. *J Am Diet A* 1986;86:876–891.

Serdula M, Coates R, Byers T, et al.: Fruit and vegetable intake among adults in 16 states: Results of a brief telephone survey. *Am J Pub He* 1995;85:236–239.

Shibata A, Paganini-Hill A, Ross R, et al.: Intake of vegetables, fruits, beta-carotene, vitamin C and vitamin supplements and cancer incidence among the elderly: A prospective study. *Br J Canc* 1992;66:673–679.

Singh R, Niaz M, Ghosh S, et al.: Effect of central obesity and associated disturbances of low-energy, fruit- and vegetable-enriched prudent diet in North Indians. *Postgr Med J* 1994;70:895–900.

Sparks J, Sparks C, Kritchevsky D: Hypercholesterolemia and aortic glysosaminoglycans of rabbits fed semi-purified diets containing sucrose and lactose. *Atheroscler* 1986;60:183–196.

Survival beyond age 70 in relation to diet. *Nutr Rev* 1996;54:211–212.

Woodward M, Tunstall-Pedoe H: Alcohol consumption, diet, coronary risk factors, and prevalence of coronary heart disease in men and women in the Scottish Heart Health study. *J Epidem C* 1995;49:354–362.

Yudkin J, Eisa O, Kang S, et al.: Dietary sucrose affects plasma HDL cholesterol concentration in young men. *Ann Nutr M* 1986;30:261–266.

CHAPTER 8

Aoyagi U, Shephard R: Aging and muscle function. *Sport Med* 1992;14:376–396.

Calles-Escandon J, Arciero P, Gardner A, et al.: Basal fat oxidation decreases with aging in women. *J App Physl* 1995;78:266–271.

Christensen H, Mackinnon A: The association between mental, social and physical activity and cognitive performance in young and old subjects. *Age Ageing* 1993;22: 175–182.

Evans W: Functional and metabolic consequences of sarcopenia. *J Nutr* 1997;127:S998–S1003.

Fielding R: The role of progressive resistance training and nutrition in the preservation of lean body mass in the elderly. *J Am Col N* 1995;14:587–594.

Giada F, Vigna G, Vitale E, et al.: Effect of age on the response of blood lipids, body composition, and aerobic power to physical conditioning and deconditioning. *Metabolism* 1995;44:161–165.

Horber F, Kohler S, Lippuner K, et al.: Effect of regular physical training on age-associated alteration of body composition in men. *Eur J Cl In* 1996;26:279–285.

Heitkamp H, Schmid K, Scheib K: Beta endorphin and adrenocorticotropic hormone production during marathon and incremental exercise. *Eur J A Phy* 1993;66:269–274.

Ilmarinen J, Pohjonen T, Punakallio A, et al.: Habitual physical activity, psychomotor performance, and older workers. *Nutr Rev* 1996;54:32S–36S.

King A, Taylor C, Haskell W: Effects of differing intensities and formats of 12 months of exercise training on psychological outcomes in older adults. *Health Psyc* 1993;12: 292–300.

Lee I, Hsieh C, Paffenbarger R: Exercise intensity and longevity in men: The Harvard Alumni Health Study. *J Am Med A* 1995;273:1179–1184.

Meydani M, Evans W, Handelman G, et al.: Protective effect of vitamin E on exercise-induced oxidative damage in young and older adults. *Am J Physl* 1993;264:R992–R998.

Owens J, Matthews K, Wing R, et al.: Can physical activity mitigate the effects of aging in middle-aged women? *Circulation* 1992;85:1265–1270.

Paffenbarger R, Kampert J, Lee I, et al.: Changes in physical activity and other lifestyle patterns influencing longevity. *Med Sci Spt* 1994;7:857–865.

Paolisso G, Gambardella A, Balbi V, et al.: Body composition, body fat distribution, and resting metabolic rate in healthy centenarians. *Am J Clin N* 1995;62:746–750.

Pate R, Pratt M, Blair S, et al.: Physical activity and public health: A recommendation from the Centers for Disease Control and Prevention and the American College of Sports Medicine. *J Am Med A* 1995;273:402–407.

Poehlman E, Goran M, Gardner A, et al.: Determinants of decline in resting metabolic rate in aging females. *Am J Physl* 1993;264:E450–E455.

Shephard R, Shek P: Exercise, aging, and immune function. *Int J Sp M* 1995;16:1–6.

Silverman H, Mazzeo R: Hormonal responses to maximal and submaximal exercise in trained and untrained men of various ages. *J Gerontol* 1996;51A:B30–B37.

Stillman R, Lohman T, Slaughter M, et al.: Physical activity and bone mineral content in women aged 30 to 85 years. *Med Sci Spt* 1986;18:576–580.

Venkatraman J, Fernandes G: Exercise, immunity and aging. *Aging-Clin* 1997;9:42–56.

Wallace J, Raglin J, Jastremski C: Twelve month adherence of adults who joined a fitness program with a spouse versus without a spouse. *J Sport Med* 1995;35:206–213.

CHAPTER 9

Beisel W: Nutrition and immune function: An overview. *J Nutr* 1996;126:2611S–2615S.

Bogden J: Studies on micronutrient supplements and immunity in older people. *Nutr Rev* 1995;53:S59–S65.

Chandra R, Excessive intake of zinc impairs immune responses. *J Am Med A* 1984;252:1443–1446.

Fata F, Herzlich B, Schiffman G, et al.: Impaired antibody responses to pneumococcal polysaccharide in elderly patients with low serum vitamin B_{12} levels. *Ann Int Med* 1996;124:299–304.

Fernandes G: Effects of calorie restriction and omega-3 fatty acids on autoimmunity and aging. *Nutr Rev* 1995;53:S72–S79.

Goodwin J: Decreased immunity and increased morbidity in the elderly. *Nutr Rev* 1995;53:S41–S46.

Herskind A, McGue M, Iachine I, et al.: Untangling genetic influences on smoking, body mass index and longevity: A multivariate study of 2464 Danish twins followed for 28 years. *Hum Genet* 1996;98:467–475.

Kelley D, Bendich A: Essential nutrients and immunological functions. *Am J Clin N* 1996;63:994S–996S.

Lesourd B: Nutrition and immunity in the elderly: Modification of immune responses with nutritional treatments. *Am J Clin N* 1997;66:4785–4845.

Licastro F, Chiricolo M, Morini M, et al.: Influence of age and health on immune functions and trace elements. *Gerontology* 1995;41:235–241.

Meydani S: Vitamin E enhancement of T cell-mediated function in healthy elderly. Mechanisms of action. *Nutr Rev* 1995;53:S52–S58.

Meydani S: Vitamin/mineral supplementation, the aging immune response, and risk of infection. *Nutr Rev* 1993;51:106–109.

Meydani S, Wu D, Santos M, et al. Antioxidants and immune response in aged persons: Overview of present evidence. *Am J Clin N* 1995;62:1462S–1476S.

Pike J, Chandra R: Effect of vitamin and trace element supplementation on immune indices in healthy elderly. *Int J Vit N* 1995;65:117–121.

Santos M, Meydani S, Leka L, et al.: Natural killer cell activity in elderly men is enhanced by beta carotene supplementation. *Am J Clin N* 1996;64:772–777.

Thomas J: Drug-nutrient interactions. *Nutr Rev* 1995;53:271–282.

Tucker K: Micronutrient status and aging. *Nutr Rev* 1995;53:S9–S15.

CHAPTER 10

The Big 4 (Heart Disease, Hypertension, Diabetes, and Cancer)

Baird D, Umbach D, Lansdell L, et al.: Dietary intervention study to assess estrogenicity of dietary soy among postmenopausal women. *J Clin End* 1995;80:1685–1690.

Chajes V, Lhuillery C, Sattler W, et al.: Alpha tocopherol and hydroperoxide content in breast adipose tissue from patients with breast tumors. *Int J Canc* 1996;67:170–175.

Clarkson T, Anthony M, Hughes C: Estrogenic soybean isoflavones and chronic disease: Risk and benefits. *Trends Endo* 1995;6:11–16.

Davis D, Dinse G, Hoel D: Decreasing cardiovascular disease and increasing cancer among whites in the United States from 1973 through 1987. *J Am Med A* 1994;271:431–437.

Flavonoids and cancer risk in the Zutphen Elderly Study. *Nutr Cancer* 1996;22:175–184.

Freudenheim J, Marshall J, Graham S, et al.: Lifetime alcohol consumption and risk of breast cancer. *Nutr Cancer* 1995;23:1–11.

Grover S, Coupal L, Hu X: Identifying adults at increased risk of coronary disease. *J Am Med A* 1995;274:801–806.

Hall J, Brands M, Zape D, et al.: Insulin resistance, hyperinsulinemia, and hypertension. *P Soc Exp M* 1995;208:317–329.

Hennig B, Toborek M, McClain C, et al.: Nutritional implications in vascular endothelial cell metabolism. *J Am Col N* 1996;15:345–358.

Herman C, Adlercreutz T, Goldin B, et al.: Soybean phytoestrogen intake and cancer risk. *J Nutr* 1995;125:757S–770S.

Hertog M, Kromhout D, Aravanis C, et al.: Flavonoid intake and long-term risk of coronary heart disease and cancer in the Seven Countries Study. *Arch In Med* 1995;155:381–386.

Herzlich B, Lichstein E, Schulhoff N, et al.: Relationship among homocyste(e)ine, vitamin B_{12}, and cardiac disease in the elderly: Association between vitamin B_{12}

deficiency and decreased left ventricular ejection fraction. *J Nutr* 1996;126:1249S–1253S.

Kuller L, Meilahn E, Bunker C, et al.: Development of risk factors for cardiovascular disease among women from adolescence to older ages. *Am J Med Sc* 1995;310:S91–S100.

Letiexhe M, Scheen A, Gerard P, et al.: Postgastroplasty recovery of ideal body weight normalizes glucose and insulin metabolism in obese women. *J Clin End* 1995;80:364–369.

Morrison H, Schaubel D, Desmeules M, et al.: Serum folate and risk of fatal coronary heart disease. *J Am Med A* 1996;275:1893–1896.

Paolisso G, Gambardella A, Giugliano D, et al.: Chronic intake of pharmacological doses of vitamin E might be useful in the therapy of elderly patients with coronary heart disease. *Am J Cin N* 1995;61:848–852.

Rose D, Goldman M, Connolly J, et al.: High-fiber diet reduces serum estrogen concentrations in premenopausal women. *Am J Clin N* 1991;43:520–525.

Stephens F: Phytoestrogens and prostate cancer: Possible preventive role. *Med J Aust* 1997;167:138–140.

Willett W, Hunter D: Prospective studies of diet and breast cancer. *Cancer* 1994;74:1085–1089.

Wing R, Blair E, Bononi P, et al.: Caloric restriction per se is a significant factor in improvements in glycemic control and insulin sensitivity during weight loss in obese NIDDM patients. *Diabet Care* 1994;17:30–36.

Zheng W, Doyle T, Kushi L, et al.: Tea consumption and cancer incidence in a prospective cohort study of postmenopausal women. *Am J Epidem* 1996;144:175–182.

Arthritis

Flynn M, Irvin W, Krause G: The effect of folate and cobalamine on osteoarthritic hands. *J Am Col N* 1994;13:351–356.

Heliovaara M, Knekt P, Aho K, et al.: Serum antioxidants and risk of rheumatoid arthritis. *Ann Rheum Dis* 1994;53:51–53.

Kjeldsen-Kragh J, Haugen M, Borchgrevink C, et al.: Vegetarian diet for patients with rheumatoid arthritis status: Two years after introduction of the diet. *Clin Rheuma* 1994;13:475–482.

Kjeldsen-Kragh J, Mellbye O, Haugen M, et al.: Changes in laboratory variables in rheumatoid arthritis patients during a trial of fasting and one-year vegetarian diet. *Sc J Rheum* 1995;24:85–93.

Kroger H, Penttila I, Alhava E: Low serum vitamin D metabolites in women with rheumatoid arthritis. *Sc J Rheum* 1993;22:172–177.

McAlindon T, Jacques P, Zhang Y, et al.: Do antioxidant micronutrients protect against the development and progression of knee osteoarthritis? *Arth Rheum* 1996;39: 648–656.

Mulherin D, Thurnham D, Situnayake R: Glutathione reductase activity, riboflavin status, and disease activity in rheumatoid arthritis. *Ann Rheum D* 1996;55:837–840.

Nielsen C, Faarvang K, Thomsen B, et al.: The effects of dietary supplementation with n-3 polyunsaturated fatty acids in patients with rheumatoid arthritis: A randomized, double-blind trial. *Eur J Cl In* 1992;22:687–691.

Roubenoff R, Roubenoff R, Selhub J, et al.: Abnormal vitamin B_6 status in rheumatoid cachexia. *Arth Rheum* 1995;38:105–109.

Cataracts and Macular Degeneration

Friedrichson T, Kalbach H, Buck P, et al.: Vitamin E in macular and peripheral tissues of the human eye. *Curr Eye R* 1995;14:693–701.

Maitra I, Serbinova E, Trischler H, et al.: Alpha-lipoic acid prevents buthionine sulfoximine-induced cataracts formation in newborn rats. *Free Rad B* 1995;18:823–829.

Mares-Perlman J, Brady W, Klein R, et al.: Dietary fat and age-related maculopathy. *Arch Ophth* 1995;113:743–748.

Mares-Perlman J, Brady W, Klein R, et al.: Serum antioxidants and age-related macular degeneration in a population-based case-control study. *Arch Ophth* 1995;113:1518–1523.

Mares-Perlman J, Klein R, Klein B, et al.: Association of zinc and antioxidant nutrients with age-related maculopathy. *Arch Ophth* 1996;114:991–997.

Seddon J, Ajani U, Sperduto R, et al.: Dietary carotenoids, vitamins A, C, and E, and advanced age-related macular degeneration. *J Am Med A* 1994;272:1413–1420.

Seddon J, Christen W, Manson J, et al.: The use of vitamin supplements and the risk of cataract among US male physicians. *Am J Pub He* 1994;84:788–792.

Snodderly D: Evidence for protection against age-related macular degeneration by carotenoids and antioxidant vitamins. *Am J Clin N* 1995;62:1448S–1461S.

Taylor A, Jacques P, Epstein E: Relations among aging, antioxidant status, and cataract. *Am J Clin N* 1995;62:1439S–1447S.

Dental Health

Barone J, Taioli E, Herbert J, et al.: Vitamin supplement use and risk for oral and esophageal cancer. *Nutr Cancer* 1992;18:31–41.

Garewal H: Antioxidants in oral cancer prevention. *Am J Clin N* 1995;62:1410S–1416S.

Gridley G, McLaughlin J, Block G, et al. Vitamin supplement use and reduced risk of oral and pharyngeal cancer. *Am J Epidem* 1992;135:1083–1092.

Kaugars G, Silverman S, Lovas J, et al.: Use of antioxidant supplements in the treatment of human oral leukoplakia. *Oral Surg O* 1996;81:5–14.

Konig K, Navia J: Nutritional role of sugars in oral health. *Am J Clin N* 1995;62:275S–282S.

Kune G, Kune S, Field B, et al.: Oral and pharyngeal cancer, diet, smoking, alcohol, and serum vitamin A and beta carotene levels: A case control study in men. *Nutr Cancer* 1993;20:61–70.

Leggott P, Robertson P, Jacob R, et al.: Effects of ascorbic acid depletion and supplementation on periodontal health and subgingival microflora in humans. *J Dent Res* 1991;70:1531–1536.

MacEntee M, Clark D, Glick N: Predictors of caries in old age. *Gerodontology* 1993;10:90–97.

Takezaki T, Hirose K, Inque M, et al.: Tobacco, alcohol, and dietary factors associated with the risk of oral cancer among Japanese. *Jpn J Canc* 1996;87:555–562.

Depression

Bell I, Edman J, Morrow F, et al.: Brief communication: Vitamin B_1, B_2, and B_6 augmentation of tricyclic antidepressant treatment in geriatric depression with cognitive dysfunction. *J Am Col N* 1992;11:159–163.

Christensen L, Somers S: Adequacy of the dietary intake of depressed individuals. *J Am Col N* 1994;13:597–600.

Delgado P, Price L, Miller H, et al.: Serotonin and the neurobiology of depression: Effects of tryptophan depletion in drug-free depressed patients. *Arch G Psyc* 1994;51:865–874.

Heseker H, Kubler W, Pudel V, et al.: Psychological disorders as early symptoms of a mild to moderate vitamin deficiency. *Ann NY Acad* 1992;669:352–357.

Lewis C, Park Y, Dexter P, et al.: Nutrient intakes and body weights of persons consuming high and moderate levels of added sugars. *J Am Diet A* 1992;92:708–713.

Pivonka E, Grunewald K: Aspartame- or sugar-sweetened beverages: Effects on mood in young women. *J Am Diet A* 1990;90:250–254.

Wurtman J: Depression and weight gain: The serotonin connection. *J Affect D* 1993;29:183–192.

Fatigue

Barclay C, Loisell D: Dependence of muscle fatigue on stimulation protocol: Effect of hypocaloric diet. *J App Physl* 1992;72:2278–2284.

Golub M, Takeuchi P, Keen C, et al.: Activity and attention in zinc-deprived adolescent monkeys. *Am J Clin N* 1996;64:908–915.

Hallberg L, Rossander-Hulten L: Iron requirements in menstruating women. *Am J Clin N* 1991;54:1047–1058.

Manore M, Besenfelder P, Wells C, et al.: Nutrient intakes and iron status in female long-distance runners during training. *J Am Diet A* 1989;89:257–259.

Morley J: Nutrition and the older woman: A review. *J Am Col N* 1993;12:337–343.

Newhouse J, Clement D, Lai C: Effects of iron supplementation and discontinuation on serum copper, zinc, calcium, and magnesium levels in women. *Med Sci Spt* 1993; 25:562–571.

Hearing

Brookes G.: Vitamin D deficiency: A new cause of cochlear deafness. *J Laryng Ot* 1983; 97:405–420.

Joachims Z, Netzer A, Ising H, et al.: Oral magnesium supplementation as prophylaxis for noise-induced hearing loss: Results of a double blind field study. *Schriftenr Ver Wasser Boden Lufthyg* 1993;88:503–516.

Lautermann J, McLaren J, Schacht J: Glutathione protection against gentamicin ototoxicity depends on nutritional status. *Hearing Res* 1995;86:15–24.

Shambaugh G: Zinc, an essential nutrient for hearing and balance. *Int J Bios M* 1991; 13:192–199.

Shemesh Z, Attias J, Ornan M, et al.: Vitamin B_{12} deficiency in patients with chronic tinnitus and noise-induced hearing loss. *Am J Otolar* 1993;14:94–99.

Insomnia

Bhanot J, Chhina G, Singh B, et al.: REM sleep deprivation and food intake. *Ind J Physl Ph* 1989;33:139–145.

Driver H, Taylor S: Sleep disturbances and exercise. *Sport Med* 1996;21:1–6.

Garfield D, Laudon M, Nof D, et al.: Improvement of sleep quality in elderly people by controlled-release melatonin. *Lancet* 1995;346:541–544.

Haimov I, Lavie P: Potential of melatonin replacement therapy in older patients with sleep disorders. *Drug Aging* 1995;7:75–78.

Karklin A, Driver H, Buffenstein R: Restricted energy intake affects nocturnal body temperature and sleep patterns. *Am J Clin N* 1994;59:346–349.

Ohta T, Ando K, Iwata T, et al.: Treatment of persistent sleep-wake schedule disorders in adolescents with methylcobalamin (vitamin B_{12}). *Sleep* 1991;14:414–418.

Penland J: Effects of trace element nutrition on sleep patterns in adult women. *FASEB J* 1988;2:A434.

Wetter D, Young T: The relation between cigarette smoking and sleep disturbance. *Prev Med* 1994;23:328–334.

Kidney Stones

Curhan G, Willett W, Rimm E, et al.: A prospective study of the intake of vitamins C and B_6, and the risk of kidney stones in men. *J Urol* 1996;155:1847–1851.

Curhan G, Willett W, Rimm E, et al.: Prospective study of beverage use and the risk of kidney stones. *Am J Epidem* 1996;143:240–247.

Curhan G, Willett W, Speitzer F, et al.: A prospective study of dietary and supplemental calcium and the risk of kidney stones in women. *Am J Epidem* 1996;143:57.

Lemann J, Pleuss J, Worcester E, et al.: Urinary oxalate excretion increases with body size and decreases with increasing dietary calcium intake among healthy adults. *Kidney Int* 1996;49:200–208.

Shah G, Ross E, Sabo A, et al. Effects of ascorbic acid and pyridoxine supplementation on oxalate metabolism in peritoneal dialysis patients. *Am J Kidney* 1992;20:42–49.

Osteoporosis

Boonen S, Lesaffre E, Aerssens J, et al.: Deficiency of the growth hormone-insulin-like growth factor-I axis potentially involved in age-related alterations in body composition. *Gerontology* 1996;42:330–338.

Bourgoin B, Evans D, Cornett J, et al.: Lead content of 70 brands of dietary calcium supplements. *Am J Pub He* 1993;83:1155–1160.

Dawson-Hughes B: Calcium and vitamin D nutritional needs of elderly women. *J Nutr* 1996;126:1165S–1167S.

Devine A, Criddle R, Dick I, et al.: A longitudinal study of the effect of sodium and calcium intakes on regional bone density in postmenopausal women. *Am J Clin N* 1995;62:740–745.

Gooth F, Tobin J: Vitamin D deficiency in older people. *J Am Ger So* 1995;43:822–828.

Heaney R: Age considerations in nutrient needs for bone health: Older adults. *J Am Col N* 1996;15:575–578.

Liu B, Gordon M, Labranche J, et al.: Seasonal prevalence of vitamin D deficiency in institutionalized elderly. *J Am Ger So* 1997;45:598–603.

Meunier P: Prevention of hip fractures by correcting calcium and vitamin D insufficiencies in elderly people. *Sc J Rheum* 1996;25(suppl 103):75–78.

Newnham R: Essentiality of boron for healthy bones and joints. *Envir H Per* 1994;102(suppl):83–85.

Strause L, Saltman P, Smith K, et al.: Spinal bone loss in postmenopausal women supplemented with calcium and trace minerals. *J Nutr* 1994;124:1060–1064.

Skin and Hair

Clement-Lacroix P, Michel L, Moysan A, et al.: UVA-induced immune suppression in human skin: Protective effect of vitamin E in human epidermal cells in vitro. *Br J Derm* 1996;134:77–84.

Colven R, Pinnell S: Topical vitamin C in aging. *Clin Dermat* 1996;14:227–234.

Darr D, Dunston S, Faust H, et al.: Effectiveness of antioxidants (vitamin C and vitamin E) with and without sunscreens as topical photoprotectants. *Act Der-Ven* 1996;76: 264–268.

Gensler H, Gerrish K, Williams T, et al.: Prevention of photocarcinogenesis and UV-induced immunosuppression in mice by topical tannic acid. *Nutr Cancer* 1994;22: 121–130.

Kadunce D, Burr R, Gress R, et al.: Cigarette smoking: Risk factor for premature facial wrinkling. *Ann Int Med* 1991;14:840–844.

Marks R, Foley P, Jolley D, et al.: The effect of regular sunscreen use on vitamin D levels in an Australian population. *Arch Dermat* 1995;131:415–421.

Noonan F, Webber L, DeFabo E, et al.: Dietary beta carotene and ultraviolet-induced immunosuppression. *Clin Exp Im* 1996;35:54–60.

Pence B, Delver E, Dunn D: Effects of dietary selenium on UVA-induced skin carcinogenesis and epidermal antioxidant status. *J Inves Der* 1994;102:759–761.

Strickland F, Pelley R, Kripke M: Prevention of ultraviolet radiation-induced suppression of contact and delayed hypersensitivity by aloe barbadensis gel extract. *J Inves Der* 1994;102:197–204.

Werninghaus K, Meydani M, Bhawan J, et al.: Evaluation of the photoprotective effect of oral vitamin E supplementation. *Arch Dermat* 1994;130:1257–1261.

Wright S: Essential fatty acids and the skin. *Br J Derm* 1991;124:503–515.

CHAPTER 11

Carmetl R, Gott P, Waters C, et al.:The frequently low cobalamin levels in dementia usually signify treatable metabolic, neurologic, and electrophysiologic abnormalities. *Eur J Haem* 1995;54:245–253.

Eipper B, Mains R: The role of ascorbate in the biosynthesis of neuroendocrine peptides. *Am J Clin N* 1991;54:1153S–1156S.

Etnier J, Landers D: Brain function and exercise: Current perspectives. *Sport Med* 1995; 19:81–85.

Forbes W, Agwani N: A suggested mechanism for aluminum biotoxicity. *J Theor Bio* 1994;171:207–214.

Froscher W, Maier V, Laage M, et al.: Folate deficiency, anticonvulsant drugs, and psychiatric morbidity. *Clin Neur* 1995;18:165–182.

Gold M, Chen M, Johnson K: Plasma and red blood cell thiamine deficiency in patients with dementia of the Alzheimer's type. *Arch Neurol* 1995;52:1081–1086.

Green M, Rogers P: Impaired cognitive functioning during spontaneous dieting. *Psychol Med* 1995;25:1003–1010.

Jama J, Launer L, Witteman J, et al.: Dietary antioxidants and cognitive function in a population-based sample of older persons. *Am J Epidem* 1996;144:275–280.

Kalmijn S, Feskens E, Launer L, et al.: Polyunsatured fatty acids, antioxidants, and cognitive function in very old men. *Am J Epidem* 1997;145:33–41.

Kleijnen J, Knipschild P: Ginkgo biloba for cerebral insufficiency. *Br J Clin Pharmacol* 1992;34:352–358.

LaRue A, Koehler K, Wayne S, et al.: Nutritional status and cognitive functioning in a normally aging sample: A 6-y reassessment. *Am J Clin N* 1997;65:20–29.

Li L, Johnson D: The effect of caffeine, choline, and caffeine with choline on short term memory in humans. *FASEB J* 1996;10:4139.

Means L, Higgins J, Fernandez T: Mid-life onset of dietary restriction extends life and prolongs cognitive functioning. *Physl Behav* 1993;54:503–508.

Penland J: Dietary boron, brain function, and cognitive performance. *Envir H Per* 1994; 102(Suppl):83–85, 65–72.

Perrig W, Perrig P, Stahelin H: The relation between antioxidants and memory performance in the old and very old. *J Am Ger So* 1997;45:718–724.

Pollitt E: Iron deficiency and cognitive function. *Ann R Nutr* 1993;13:521–537.

Poulin J, Cover C, Gustafson M, et al.: Vitamin E prevents oxidative modification of brain and lymphocyte band 3 proteins during aging. *P NAS US* 1996;93:5600–5603.

Riggs K, Spiro A, Tucker K, et al.: Relations of vitamin B_{12}, vitamin B_6, folate, and homocysteine to cognitive performance in the Normative Aging Study. *Am J Clin N* 1996;63:306–314.

Snowdon D, Kemper S, Mortimer J, et al.: Linguistic ability in early life and cognitive function and Alzheimer's disease in late life. *J Am Med A* 1996;275:528–532.

Wahlin A, Winblad B, Hill R, et al.: Effects of serum vitamin B_{12} and folate status on episodic memory performance in very old age: A population based study. *Psychol Ag* 1996;11:487–496.

Wing R, Vazquez J, Ryan C: Cognitive effects of ketogenic weight-reducing diets. *Int J Obes* 1995;19:811–816.

Zeisel S: Choline: An important nutrient in brain development, liver function and carcinogenesis. *J Am Col N* 1992;11:473–481.

CHAPTER 12

Abernathy R, Black D: Healthy body weights: An alternative perspective. *Am J Clin N* 1996;63:S448–S451.

Aloia J, Vaswani A, Ma R, et al.: Aging in women: The four compartment model of body composition. *Metabolism* 1996;45:43–48.

Astrup A, Beuemann B, Western P, et al.: Obesity as an adaptation to a high-fat diet: Evidence from a cross-sectional study. *Am J Clin N* 1994;59:350–355.

Carey D, Jenkins A, Campbell L, et al.: Abdominal fat and insulin resistance in normal and overweight women: Direct measurements reveal a strong relationship in subjects at both low and high risk of NIDDM. *Diabetes* 1996;45:633–638.

Drent M, Zelissen P, Koppeschaar H, et al.: The effect of dexfenfluramine on eating habits in a Dutch ambulatory android overweight population with an overconsumption of snacks. *Int J Obes* 1995;19:299–304.

Edelstein S, Barrett-Connor E, Wingard D, et al.: Increased meal frequency associated with decreased cholesterol concentrations; Rancho Bernardo, CA, 1984–1987. *Am J Clin N* 1992;55:664–669.

Ford E, Williamson D, Liu S: Weight change and diabetes incidence: Findings from a national cohort of US adults. *Am J Epidem* 1997;146:214–222.

Horton T, Drougas H, Brachey A, et al.: Fat and carbohydrate overfeeding in humans: Different effects on energy storage. *Am J Clin N* 1995;62:19–29.

Iribbarren C, Sharp D, Burchfiel C, et al.: Association of weight loss and weight fluctuation with mortality among Japanese-American men. *N Eng J Med* 1995;333:686–692.

Jenkins D, Khan A, Jenkins A, et al.: Effect of nibbling versus gorging on cardiovascular risk factors: Serum uric acid and blood lipids. *Metabolism* 1995;44:549–555.

Losonczy K, Harris T, Cornoni-Huntley J, et al.: Does weight loss from middle age to old age explain the inverse weight mortality relation in old age? *Am J Epidem* 1995;141:312–321.

Manson J, Willett W, Stampfer M, et al.: Body weight and mortality among women. *N Eng J Med* 1995;333:677–685.

Meisler J, St Jeor S: Summary and recommendations from the American Health Foundations' Expert Panel on Healthy Weight. *Am J Clin N* 1996;63:474S–477S.

Saris W: Physical inactivity and metabolic factors as predictors of weight gain. *Nutr Rev* 1996;54:S110–S115.

Schlundt D, Hill J, Sbrocco T, et al.: The role of breakfast in the treatment of obesity: A randomized clinical trial. *Am J Clin N* 1992;55:645–651.

Willett W, Manson J, Stampfer M, et al.: Weight, weight change, and coronary heart disease in women. *J Am Med A* 1995;273:461–465.

Williamson D, Pamuk E, Thun M, et al.: Prospective study of intentional weight loss and mortality in never-smoking overweight US white women aged 40–64 years. *Am J Epidem* 1995;141:1128–1141.

CHAPTER 13

Frye C, Demolar G: Menstrual cycle and sex differences influence salt preferences. *Physl Behav* 1994;55:193–197.

Fukutake M, Takashahi M, Ishida K, et al.: Quantification of genistein and genistein in soybeans and soybean products. *Food Chem T* 1996;34:457–461.

Gavaler J: Alcohol and nutrition in postmenopausal women. *J Am Col N* 1993;12: 349–356.

Knight D, Eden J: Phytoestrogens: A short review. *Maturitas* 1995;22:167–175.

Morley J: Nutrition and the older female: A review. *J Am Col N* 1993;12:337–343.

Murkies A, Lombard C, Strauss B, et al.: Dietary flour supplementation decreases post-menopausal hot flushes: Effect of soy and wheat. *Maturitas* 1995;21:189–195.

Svendsen O, Hassager C, Christiansen C: Age associated and menopause associated variations in body composition and fat distribution in healthy women as measured by dual energy X ray absorptiometry. *Metabolism* 1995;44:369–373.

Woods M, Barnett J, Spiegelman D, et al.: Hormone levels during dietary changes in premenopausal African-American women. *J Nat Canc* 1996;88:1369–1374.

CHAPTER 14

Apgar J: Zinc and reproduction: An update. *J Nutr Bioc* 1992;3:266–278.

Brown J: Preconceptual nutrition and reproductive outcomes. *Ann NY Acad* 1993;678: 286–292.

Cumming D, Wheeler G, Harber V: Physical activity, nutrition, and reproduction. *Ann NY Acad* 1994;709:55–76.

Dawson E, Harris W, Teter M, et al.: Effects of ascorbic acid supplementation on the sperm quality of smokers. *Fert Steril* 1992;58:1034–1039.

Hatch E, Bracken M: Association of delayed conception with caffeine consumption. *Am J Epidem* 1993;138:1082–1092.

Hunt C, Johnson P, Herbel J, et al.: Effects of dietary zinc depletion on seminal volume and zinc loss, serum testosterone concentrations, and sperm morphology in young men. *Am J Clin N* 1992;56:148–157.

Meikle A: Effects of a fat-containing meal on sex hormones in men. *Metabolism* 1990; 39:943–946.

Rosevear S, Holt D, Lee T, et al.: Smoking and decreased fertilization rates in vitro. *Lancet* 1992;340:1195–1196.

Zaadstra B, Seidell J, Van Noord P, et al.: Fat and female fecundity: Prospective study of effect of body fat distribution on conception rates. *Br Med J* 1993;306:484–487.

CHAPTER 15

Campbell A, Busby W, Robertson M, et al.: Control over future health in old age: Characteristics of believers and skeptics. *Age Ageing* 1995;24:204–209.

Davison G, Williams M, Nezami E, et al.: Relaxation, reduction in angry articulated thoughts and improvements in borderline hypertension and heart rate. *J Behav Med* 1991;14:453–466.

Denollet J, Sys S, Stroobant N, et al.: Personality as independent predictor of long-term mortality in patients with coronary heart disease. *Lancet* 1996;347:417–421.

Jella S, Shannahoff-Khalsa D: The effects of unilateral forced nostril breathing on cognitive performance. *Int J Neuros* 1993;73:61–68.

Johnson T, Lithgow G, Murakami S: Interventions that increase the response to stress offer the potential for effective life prolongation and increased health. *J Gerontol* 1996;51A:B392–B395.

Krause N, Tran T: Stress and religious involvement among older blacks. *J Geront S* 1989;44:S4–S13.

Mabry T, Gold P, McCarty R: Age-related changes in plasma catecholamine responses to chronic intermittent stress. *Physl Behav* 1995;58:49–56.

Morris J, Cook D, Shaper A: Loss of employment and mortality. *Br Med J* 1994;308: 1135–1139.

Morris T, Greer S, Pettingale K, et al.: Patterns of expression of anger and other psychological correlates in women with breast cancer. *J Psychosom* 1981;25:111–117.

Muldoon M, Bachen E, Manuck S, et al.: Acute cholesterol responses to mental stress and change in posture. *Arch In Med* 1992;152:775–780.

Patterson S, Zakowski S, Hall M, et al.: Psychological stress and platelet activation: Differences in platelet reactivity in healthy men during active and passive stressors. *Health Psyc* 1994;13:34–38.

Rosengren A, Orth-Gomer K, Wedel H, et al.: Stressful life events, social support, and mortality in men born in 1933. *Br Med J* 1993;307:1102–1105.

Siegman A: Cardiovascular consequences of expressing, experiencing, and repressing anger. *J Behav Med* 1993;16:539–545.

Yeung A, Vekshtein V, Krantz D, et al.: The effect of atherosclerosis on the vasomotor response of coronary arteries to mental stress. *N Eng J Med* 1991;325:1551–1556.

CHAPTER 16

Berkman L, et al.: Emotional support and survival after myocardial infarction. *Ann Int Med* 1992;117:1003–1009.

Berkman L, Syme S: Social networks, host resistance and mortality: A nine-year follow-up study of Alameda County residents. *Am J Epidem* 1979;109:186–204.

Blazer D: Social support and mortality in an elderly community population. *Am J Epidem* 1982;115:684–694.

Brown P, Smith T: Social influence, marriage, and the heart: Cardiovascular consequences of interpersonal control in husbands and wives. *Heal Psych* 1992;11:88–96.

Kiecolt-Glaser J: Negative behavior during marital conflict is associated with immunological down-regulation. *Psychos Med* 1993;55:395–409.

Maunsell E: Social support and survival among women with breast cancer. *Cancer* 1995; 76:631–637.

Spiegel D, Bloom J, Kraemer H, et al.: Effect of psychosocial treatment on survival of patients with metastic breast cancer. *Lancet* 1989;2:888–891.

Tucker L, Bagwell M: Relationship between serum cholesterol levels and television viewing in 11,947 employed adults. *Am J He Pro* 1992;6:437–442.

Venters M: Family life and cardiovascular risk: Implications for the prevention of chronic disease. *Social Sc M* 1986;22:1067–1074.

Index